Vascular Surgery: Current Concepts and Treatments for Venous Disease

Editor

MARC A. PASSMAN

SURGICAL CLINICS
OF NORTH AMERICA

www.surgical.theclinics.com

Consulting Editor
RONALD F. MARTIN

April 2018 • Volume 98 • Number 2

ELSEVIER

1600 John F. Kennedy Boulevard ● Suite 1800 ● Philadelphia, Pennsylvania, 19103-2899

http://www.surgical.theclinics.com

SURGICAL CLINICS OF NORTH AMERICA Volume 98, Number 2
April 2018 ISSN 0039–6109, ISBN-13: 978-0-323-58328-2

Editor: John Vassallo, j.vassallo@elsevier.com
Developmental Editor: Meredith Madeira

Surgical Clinics of North America (ISSN 0039–6109) is published bimonthly by Elsevier Inc., 360 Park Avenue South, New York, NY 10010-1710. Months of publication are February, April, June, August, October, and December. Business and Editorial Offices: 1600 John F. Kennedy Blvd., Suite 1800, Philadelphia, PA 19103-2899. Periodicals postage paid at New York, NY and additional mailing offices. Subscription prices are $350.00 per year for US individuals, $802.00 per year for US institutions, $100.00 per year for US students and residents, $420.00 per year for Canadian individuals, $1015.00 per year for Canadian institutions, $475.00 for international individuals, $1015.00 per year for international institutions and $225.00 per year for Canadian and foreign students/residents. To receive student/resident rate, orders must be accompanied by name of affiliated institution, date of term, and the *signature* of program/residency coordinator on institution letterhead. Orders will be billed at individual rate until proof of status is received. Foreign air speed delivery is included in all *Clinics* subscription prices. All prices are subject to change without notice. POSTMASTER: Send address changes to *Surgical Clinics*, Elsevier Health Sciences Division, Subscription Customer Service, 3251 Riverport Lane, Maryland Heights, MO 63043. **Customer Service (orders, claims, online, change of address): Telephone: 1-800-654-2452 (U.S. and Canada); 314-447-8871 (outside U.S. and Canada). Fax: 314-447-8029. E-mail: journalscustomerservice-usa@elsevier.com (for print support); journalsonline support-usa@elsevier.com (for online support).**

Reprints. For copies of 100 or more, of articles in this publication, please contact the Commercial Reprints Department, Elsevier Inc., 360 Park Avenue South, New York, New York 10010-1710. Tel. 212-633-3874, Fax: 212-633-3820, E-mail: reprints@elsevier.com.

The Surgical Clinics of North America is also published in Spanish by McGraw-Hill Interamericana Editores S.A., P.O. Box 5-237 06500 Mexico D.F. Mexico; and in Portuguese by Interlivros Edicoes Ltda., Rua Comandante Coelho 1085, CEP 21250, Rio de Janeiro, Brazil; and in Greek by Paschalidis Medical Publications, Athens Greece.

The Surgical Clinics of North America is covered in *MEDLINE/PubMed (Index Medicus)*, *EMBASE/Excerpta Medica*, *Current Contents/Clinical Medicine*, *Current Contents/Life Sciences*, *Science Citation Index*, and *ISI/BIOMED*.

Contributors

CONSULTING EDITOR

RONALD F. MARTIN, MD, FACS
Colonel (ret.), United States Army Reserve, Department of Surgery, York Hospital, York, Maine

EDITOR

MARC A. PASSMAN, MD
Professor of Surgery, Division of Vascular Surgery and Endovascular Therapy, The University of Alabama at Birmingham, Birmingham, Alabama

AUTHORS

ADHAM N. ABOU ALI, MD
Resident Physician, Division of Vascular Surgery, University of Pittsburgh Medical Center, Pittsburgh, Pennsylvania

EFTHYMIOS D. AVGERINOS, MD
Associate Professor of Surgery, Division of Vascular Surgery, University of Pittsburgh Medical Center, Pittsburgh, Pennsylvania

SAMIR BITTAR, MD
ProMedica Jobst Vascular Institute, Toledo, Ohio

RABIH A. CHAER, MD
Professor of Surgery, Division of Vascular Surgery, University of Pittsburgh Medical Center, Pittsburgh, Pennsylvania

MICHAEL C. DALSING, MD
Professor Emeritus, Division of Vascular Surgery, Department of Surgery, Indiana University School of Medicine, Indianapolis, Indiana

ELLEN D. DILLAVOU, MD
Associate Professor of Surgery, Division of Vascular Surgery, Duke University Hospital, Durham, North Carolina

RAUDEL GARCIA, MD, RPVI
Phlebology Fellow, Division of Vascular and Endovascular Surgery, Department of Surgery, Stony Brook University Hospital, Stony Brook, New York

DANIEL F. GEERSEN, MPAP, PA-C
Associate Program Director, PA-Surgical Residency, Co-Administrator, APP Services, Department of Surgery, Division of Vascular and Endovascular Surgery, Duke University Medical Center, Durham, North Carolina

KATHLEEN GIBSON, MD, FACS
Lake Washington Vascular Surgeons, Bellevue, Washington

PETER GLOVICZKI, MD
Joe M. and Ruth Roberts Emeritus Professor of Surgery, Mayo Clinic College of Medicine & Science, Rochester, Minnesota

KRISSA GUNDERSON, BS
Lake Washington Vascular Surgeons, Bellevue, Washington

CINDY P. HA, MD
Vascular Surgery Fellow, Division of Vascular and Endovascular Surgery, The University of Texas Southwestern Medical Center, Dallas, Texas

PETER K. HENKE, MD
Professor, Department of Surgery, Section of Vascular Surgery, University of Michigan, Ann Arbor, Michigan

BEN JACOBS, MD
Department of Surgery, Section of Vascular Surgery, University of Michigan, Ann Arbor, Michigan

MICHAEL JOLLY, MD, FACC
OhioHealth Heart and Vascular Physicians, Riverside Methodist Hospital, Columbus, Ohio

MANJU KALRA, MBBS
Professor, Vascular and Endovascular Surgery, Mayo Clinic, Rochester, Minnesota

GREGORY KASPER, MD
ProMedica Jobst Vascular Institute, Toledo, Ohio

MISAKI M. KIGUCHI, MD
Assistant Professor of Surgery, Department of Vascular Surgery, MedStar Washington Hospital Center, Washington, DC

MATTHEW C. KOOPMANN, MD
Vascular Surgeon, VA Portland Health Care System, Assistant Professor of Surgery, Oregon Health & Science University, Portland, Oregon

NICOS LABROPOULOS, PhD, DIC, RVT
Director, Vascular Laboratory, Division of Vascular and Endovascular Surgery, Professor of Surgery and Radiology, Department of Surgery, Stony Brook University Hospital, Stony Brook, New York

KATHERIN E. LECKIE, MD
Vascular Surgery Resident, Division of Vascular Surgery, Department of Surgery, Indiana University School of Medicine, Indianapolis, Indiana

FEDOR LURIE, PhD, MD
ProMedica Jobst Vascular Institute, Toledo, Ohio; University of Michigan, Ann Arbor, Michigan

ROBERT B. McLAFFERTY, MD
Chief of Surgery, VA Portland Health Care System, Professor of Surgery, Oregon Health & Science University, Portland, Oregon

ANDREA OBI, MD
Assistant Professor, Department of Surgery, Section of Vascular Surgery, University of Michigan, Ann Arbor, Michigan

JOHN PHILLIPS, MD, FSCAI
OhioHealth Heart and Vascular Physicians, Riverside Methodist Hospital, Columbus, Ohio

JOSEPH D. RAFFETTO, MD
Associate Professor of Surgery, Harvard Medical School, VA Boston Healthcare System, Brigham and Women's Hospital, Boston, Massachusetts; VA Boston Healthcare System, West Roxbury, Massachusetts

JOHN E. RECTENWALD, MD, MS
Chief and Associate Professor, Division of Vascular and Endovascular Surgery, The University of Texas Southwestern Medical Center, Dallas, Texas

INDRANI SEN, MBBS
Resident, Vascular and Endovascular Surgery, Mayo Clinic, Rochester, Minnesota

CYNTHIA E.K. SHORTELL, MD
Chief, Division of Vascular and Endovascular Surgery, Chief of Staff, Professor, Department of Surgery, Duke University Medical Center, Durham, North Carolina

MARGARET SMITH, MD
General Surgery Residency, Department of Surgery, University of Michigan, Ann Arbor, Michigan

DEEPAK SUDHEENDRA, MD, FSIR, RPVI
Assistant Professor of Clinical Radiology and Surgery, Department of Radiology, University of Pennsylvania, Perelman School of Medicine, Philadelphia, Pennsylvania

SURESH VEDANTHAM, MD, FSIR
Professor of Radiology and Surgery, Mallinckrodt Institute of Radiology, Washington University in St. Louis, St Louis, Missouri

GLENN WAKAM, MD
General Surgery Residency, Department of Surgery, University of Michigan, Ann Arbor, Michigan

THOMAS WAKEFIELD, MD
James C. Stanley Professor of Vascular Surgery, Department of Surgery, University of Michigan, Ann Arbor, Michigan

Contents

Venous diseases are highly prevalent, mostly caused by valve incompetence and/or obstruction of the vein lumen. Signs and symptoms are diverse and unspecific. Careful clinical assessment and imaging interpretation are crucial to diagnosis. Duplex ultrasound scan is the first choice and often the gold standard imaging technique for this purpose, providing information on the anatomy and function of the veins. This article describes the sonographic anatomic and hemodynamic criteria used for the diagnosis of venous reflux, venous obstruction, and the most frequent complications after interventions in the superficial, perforating, and deep venous systems.

Anticoagulation pharmacy has been dramatically altered with US Food and Drug Administration (FDA) approval of 5 direct oral anticoagulants, 1 novel reversal agent, and a second designated for fast-track approval. Trial data surrounding current trends in anticoagulant choice for venous thromboembolism (VTE), reversal, and bridging are constantly redefining practice. Extended therapy for unprovoked VTE has expanded to include low-dose direct oral anticoagulants, aspirin, and the use of the HERDOO2 system to identify women who can stop anticoagulant therapy without increased risk of recurrent VTE. Trends in thromboprophylaxis include extended-duration low-dose direct oral anticoagulants to prevent VTE in high-risk patients.

Venous thromboembolism (VTE) remains a significant mortal and morbid disease. The major risks have not changed, and many patients present with unprovoked VTE disease. Prevention of VTE in hospitalized patients depends on comprehensive risk factor assessment, with an individual risk score. Proper and timely prophylaxis with mechanical or pharmacologic modalities or both is then effective. Treatment of VTE with parenteral anticoagulation followed by either a direct oral anticoagulant or warfarin is standard to reduce the risk of VTE recurrence and death. Selected cases

anatomic location, presence of disease-free venous architecture, and patient need. Other things being equal, less invasive techniques and disease locations are attempted as first-line therapy. When other options fail and symptoms persist, open venous surgery by means of bypass for obstructive disease and valve repair or replacement for deep venous insufficiency remains a viable option. The basic techniques available and overall success rates of each are considered.

 Video content accompanies this article at http://www.surgical. theclinics.com.

Open saphenous removal, phlebectomy, and venous ligation were historic mainstays of surgical treatment of venous disease. Duplex ultrasound scan has become the standard to diagnose venous insufficiency. Percutaneous modalities have allowed treatments to include thermal and nonthermal endovenous ablation. These treatments vary in preoperative planning, procedural steps, and postprocedural care, but all are safe and effective. An individualized approach should be taken in determining which modality is offered to each patient. Endovenous options, which often are minimally invasive and safely performed in an outpatient setting, allow access to effective treatments with low risk and discomfort.

Ambulatory phlebectomy is a well-known and widely used procedure for residual symptomatic venous disease. Tumescent anesthesia complements the procedure, providing the ability to perform this intervention in a wide range of practice settings. The procedures are well tolerated by most patients, and complications are rare. They include venous thromboembolism, infection, and hematoma and are generally simple to manage. Alternative and emerging techniques of powered phlebectomy and cyanoacrylate glue are providing alternative forms for treatment and will advance the practice further.

Sclerotherapy has wide applicability in treating venous disease at every stage of clinical disease. The various sclerosant drugs and formulations each have unique properties, utilities, and side effects. Treating physicians should be aware of the differences between agents, accounting for disease presentation, vein characteristics, and patient comorbidities when selecting the appropriate sclerosing agents. Successful outcomes rely on proper patient evaluation and assessment for contraindications to sclerotherapy. Thorough patient education regarding realistic expectations with sclerotherapy in terms of symptoms relief, recurrence, and improvement in appearance is of chief importance.

SURGICAL CLINICS
OF NORTH AMERICA

Foreword

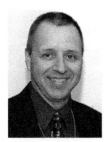

Ronald F. Martin, MD, FACS
Consulting Editor

There is a saying that when you have plenty of oxygen to breathe, you never think about it, and when you don't have enough oxygen to breathe, it is the only thing you think about. In our surgical world, veins may suffer the same ignominy. When it comes to circulation of red cells and tissue perfusion, we are quick to teach students about cardiac pump function, arterial pressure, and even diffusion kinetics, yet we are loathe to teaching much about veins other than a cursory nod to that is how blood gets back somewhere.

Most of our colleagues who are not surgeons do not think of veins the ways that surgeons do. Many of our medical colleagues in primary care think about vein disorders as a cosmetic concern or perhaps symptoms they receive from patients, or our colleague's main question for calling us is to ascertain to whom they can send the patient the disposition out of their queue of matters to address. And while all those concerns have their own validity, they hardly represent the breadth of issues that may occur. Other colleagues of ours look at vein issues as some form of bloodstream access problem that needs to be solved, preferably by someone who is again not them. The ubiquitous use of percutaneously inserted central catheter lines has made that an easier problem to lateral off to someone. Others see veins as merely a source of blood from which to draw fluid to analyze.

To readers of this series, the idea that veins are a physiologically complex structure with a wide variety of maladies that relate directly to their structure and function is no secret. Still, most of our faithful readers do not have to deal with venous disorders or their consequences on a daily basis—or at least we are not aware that we have to. In reality, pretty much all of us who operate are aware that the consequences of venous disorders are omnipresent in our world despite the fact that our interaction with it is relegated to cursory evaluation and standing order sets. From deep venous thrombosis (DVT) and venous thromboembolism prophylaxis to reduction or prevention of bloodstream infection secondary to access devices to simple hemorrhage, surgeons need to be on full-time alert for some venous consequence.

Surg Clin N Am 98 (2018) xiii–xiv
https://doi.org/10.1016/j.suc.2018.01.002
0039-6109/18/© 2018 Published by Elsevier Inc.

surgical.theclinics.com

Perhaps one of the areas where some of our systems really collapse for patients with venous disorders is the chronic nonhealing wound. It is very common to see patients in wound centers who have had just about every known intervention, including arterial angioplasty and sometimes even skin grafts, and no one has properly evaluated the venous drainage, let alone made an attempt to correct it if found to be lacking.

On some level, it is understandable how this oversight occurs. To evaluate veins properly might require equipment such as ultrasound or other gear that requires specialized knowledge to use. In some cases, the problem doesn't seem new or acute and as such escapes concern. But more likely an explanation is that most of our colleagues are simply not tuned in to think about veins as being physiologically as important as other organs.

We must all try to educate others in these matters if we are to help the patients. That said, we must all educate ourselves before we can educate others. Dr Passman and his colleagues have put together for us an excellent compendium of useful and meaningful information that will bring all of us up to speed with what we know about these often-neglected maladies. We are extremely indebted to them for their efforts on our behalf.

As with oxygen, it is better to develop a plan to assure its adequacy when you have plenty than it is to wait until you are in short supply. Whether one is trying to find out how to best prevent DVT or pulmonary embolism, image venous systems, or manage compression of a limb with compromised venous physiology, this issue has excellent and informed content put into context by dedicated experts. I think you will benefit greatly from having this comprehensive resource available to help with a topic that is so often not given its clinical due. As always, we welcome feedback from our readership.

Ronald F. Martin, MD, FACS
Colonel (ret.), United States Army Reserve
Department of Surgery
York Hospital
16 Hospital Drive, Suite A
York, ME 03909, USA

E-mail address:
rmartin@yorkhospital.com

Preface

Current Concepts and Treatments for Venous Disease

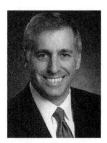

Marc A. Passman, MD
Editor

With expanding interest in venous-related clinical problems, this issue of *Surgical Clinics of North America* features current concepts and advances in treatments for venous disease. The overarching theme of this issue is to highlight evidence-based decision making and evolving techniques toward endovenous options, while reinforcing the foundation of operative options when needed. In this regard, this text is meant to be a comprehensive review of current therapy for venous problems from the perspective of thought leaders in venous disease.

Areas covered include:

Use of reproducible venous duplex ultrasound testing as the cornerstone for diagnosis of acute and chronic venous diseases,

New trends in anticoagulation therapy along with current evidence-based algorithms for pharmacologic prevention and treatment for patients with documented venous thromboembolism,

First-line advanced catheter-directed therapy and traditional operative thrombectomy techniques for appropriate patients with iliofemoral and lower-extremity deep venous thrombosis and pulmonary embolism,

Current indications, techniques, and recommendations for appropriate use of inferior vena cava filters,

Management of superior vena cava syndrome from both endovenous and operative reconstruction perspectives,

Understanding pathophysiology in patients with chronic venous obstruction or insufficiency affecting the lower extremities, and potential for progression to venous ulceration,

Optimal compression and venous ulcer wound care for venous ulcer healing and prevention of recurrence,

Surg Clin N Am 98 (2018) xv–xvi
https://doi.org/10.1016/j.suc.2018.01.001
0039-6109/18/© 2018 Published by Elsevier Inc.

Contemporary treatment of venous outflow obstruction with endovenous stenting and operative reconstruction as options in properly selected patients,

Proper indications and techniques for use of thermal and newer nonthermal endovenous ablation, phlebectomy, and liquid/foam sclerotherapy for patients with superficial venous reflux and varicose veins.

I am proud of the information provided in this issue of *Surgical Clinics of North America* focusing on current concepts and treatments for venous disease and hope that these articles will provide a solid framework for balanced clinical decision making and delivery of quality care for our patients with these challenging venous problems.

Marc A. Passman, MD
Division of Vascular Surgery and
Endovascular Therapy
University of Alabama at Birmingham
1808 7th Avenue South
Birmingham, AL 35233, USA

E-mail address:
mpassman@uabmc.edu

Duplex Ultrasound for the Diagnosis of Acute and Chronic Venous Diseases

Raudel Garcia, MD, RPVI, Nicos Labropoulos, PhD, DIC, RVT*

KEYWORDS

- Duplex ultrasound • Venous reflux • Chronic venous insufficiency
- Acute venous thrombosis • Chronic venous obstruction

KEY POINTS

- Venous diseases are highly prevalent medical conditions, mostly caused by valve incompetence (reflux) and/or obstruction of the vein lumen.
- Duplex ultrasound (DUS) is the first choice and, in many instances, the gold standard imaging technique for the diagnosis of reflux and obstruction.
- DUS is also used for obtaining venous access, guiding venous procedures, determining the immediate outcome of treatment, and short-term and long-term follow-up of patients.
- Cutoff value for venous reflux in the common femoral vein, femoral vein, and popliteal vein is greater than 1000 milliseconds; a lower cutoff (>500 milliseconds) is used in the superficial, perforating, and rest of the deep vein systems.
- Noncompressibility of the veins on axial axis, using grayscale technique, is the most sensitive and specific finding in acute deep vein thrombosis.

INTRODUCTION

Venous disease (VD) is a highly prevalent medical condition in Western countries.[1,2] VD manifests with a variety of signs and symptoms that are caused by obstruction of the vein lumen (acute or chronic) and/or valve incompetence (reflux). The diagnosis of VD, for the most part, relies on correlating the information gathered from patient's history, physical examination, and imaging findings. Contrast venography, impedance plethysmography, duplex ultrasound (DUS), computed tomography venography (CTV), magnetic resonance venography (MRV), and intravascular ultrasound (IVUS) are the main imaging modalities used for the diagnosis of VD.

Disclosure Statement: The authors have nothing to disclose.
Division of Vascular and Endovascular Surgery, Department of Surgery, Stony Brook University Medical Center, 101 Nicolls Road, Stony Brook, NY 11974, USA
* Corresponding author.
E-mail address: nlabrop@yahoo.com

Surg Clin N Am 98 (2018) 201–218
https://doi.org/10.1016/j.suc.2017.11.007
0039-6109/18/© 2017 Elsevier Inc. All rights reserved.

DUS is the imaging method of choice because it is very accurate, noninvasive, cost-effective, and reproducible. DUS is the only imaging modality that provides information on both the anatomy and function of the veins.[3] The treatment strategies for acute vein thrombosis and chronic venous insufficiency (CVI) are based on DUS findings. Additionally, venous DUS is widely used for screening, perioperative guidance, and follow-up. Many other conditions are ruled in or out with DUS (eg, aneurysms, hematomas, cysts, and tumors).

However, an accurate and reliable DUS result depends on the equipment and the protocol used for scanning, as well as the expertise of the technologist performing the study and the physician interpreting the images. Many societies have suggested, to improve patient's care, the use of guidelines and standards for venous DUS equipment, examination protocols, and interpretation.[4–9]

BASIC PRINCIPLES

To achieve an accurate diagnosis, the examiner should be familiar with the indications and limitations of venous DUS. Most DUS studies are performed in patients with suspected acute deep venous thrombosis (DVT), less than 20% reveal abnormalities.[10] Evaluation of CVI, superficial thrombophlebitis, postprocedural assessment of endovenous ablation (EVA), and phlebectomies, as well as, less frequently, venous malformation, aneurysms, and tumors, are among other possible indications. Limitations include obesity, restrictive mobility, severe leg swelling, and the presence of wounds, casts, or dressings.

The patient should be informed about any examination prerequisite (eg, 4–6 hours fasting to evaluate the suprainguinal veins), the maneuvers and techniques involving the study, and the average duration. The Society for Vascular Ultrasound[7] recommends a total time allotment of 75 minutes for performance of bilateral lower extremity venous examination to maximize quality and accuracy, 40 to 60 minutes for direct examination components (equipment optimization and hands-on), and 15 minutes for indirect examination components (obtaining previous examination data; initiating examination worksheet and paperwork; equipment and examination room preparation; patient assessment and positioning, patient communication; postexamination room cleanup; compiling, reviewing, and processing examination data for preliminary and/or formal interpretation; and patient charge and billing activities).

Relevant clinical information, obtained by interviewing the patient or reviewing available medical records, and a focused physical examination are essential elements for a good quality venous DUS. It can help the technologist better target the examination and save valuable scanning time. It also ensures that no pathologic complication is overlooked.[11]

The room and gel should be comfortably warm to prevent vein spasm. For evaluation of CVI, the patient needs to be placed in an upright or reverse Trendelenburg position to better assess the diameter of the veins and valve competence.

Multilinear high-resolution array transducers are used to image superficial veins and any deep structure up to 6-cm depth. Lower frequency (1–5 MHz) curvilinear transducers are preferred for imaging deep veins and obese or edematous patients because of better penetration. The machine settings should be adjusted to acquire high-quality images and reliable blood velocities.[8,12] B-mode images are obtained in transverse and longitudinal axis. The time-gain compensation should be properly set to overcome ultrasound attenuation so that the lumen of the vein appears dark in the absence of stasis and thrombosis. The focal zone is typically positioned at the vein lumen or the deeper wall to maximize lateral resolution. Multiple focal zones can be selected; however, this can slow down the frame rate, therefore degrading temporal resolution. Low-flow settings are recommended for color Doppler and pulse-wave spectral analysis. The scale or pulse repetition frequency should be set at 1500 Hz or lower, but no so low that it causes color bleeding artifact. The wall filter should be at its lowest value. The most accurate velocities are recorded when the Doppler angle (angle of insonation) is set at 0° or parallel to the flow. However, because most veins run parallel to the skin, an angle of less than 60° should be used to optimize results. In general, when recording duration of reflux or waveform patterns, an angle of 0° can be used because it only affects the speed of the blood.

Conventionally, in venous DUS, the blue and red colors represent antegrade (away from the transducer) and retrograde (toward the transducer) blood flow, respectively. Similarly, velocities registered below the baseline, unless the scale is inverted, represent antegrade flow, whereas velocities above the baseline are for retrograde flow (reflux). Retrograde venous flow is defined as physiologic or pathologic, depending on its duration.

DIAGNOSIS OF REFLUX

Venous reflux parameters frequently assessed with DUS include reflux duration, peak velocity, flow volume, and vein diameter. However, only reflux duration with cutoff values greater than 500 milliseconds for the superficial, perforating, deep femoral veins (FVs) and deep calf veins, and greater than 1000 milliseconds for the common FV (CFV), FV, and popliteal vein (POPV) are considered pathologic and of clinical significance.[13] Typically, the apposition of valve leaflets is lengthier in larger veins with fewer valves, therefore different cutoff points are required.

Chronic VD (CVD) is caused by valve incompetence in most patients. Valve incompetence results from localized or multisegmental venous wall dilatation and valve dysfunction, mostly of primary etiologic factors. Venous reflux may also develop as a consequence of valvular damage from previous thrombotic episodes in the superficial and/or the deep veins. Inadequate recanalization after DVT leads to outflow obstruction in many patients and may also be found during a reflux examination. In limbs with CVD, reflux alone exists in 80% of patients, reflux and obstruction are present in 17% of patients, and obstruction alone is found in only 2% of patients. The combination of reflux and obstruction has the highest morbidity.[14,15] Additionally, traumatic venous injuries (mechanical, thermal, or chemical) and arteriovenous fistulas (AVFs) may lead to valvular damage and reflux. Primary and secondary venous reflux accounts for 64% to 79%, and 18% to 28% of all CVD cases, respectively. Venous reflux due to congenital valve agenesis or aplasia in the deep system is found in less than 5% of cases.[16–18] The differentiation between primary and secondary venous reflux is important, and DUS is excellent for this. It allows a clear visualization of the wall and luminal changes and the pattern of reflux. Many patients have asymptomatic thrombosis that is discovered only during the DUS examination.

The pathophysiological events for development of reflux influence the scanning protocols and treatment algorithms in many institutions around the world. The retrograde theory of the origin of reflux explains that reflux starts at the saphenofemoral junction (SFJ) or saphenopopliteal junction (SPJ) and descends, aided by hydrostatic forces, creating progressive venous wall dilatation and valve incompetence sequentially in the truncal veins and its tributaries.[19] Almost all of current varicose vein interventions are based on this concept. However, a competent terminal valve of the SFJ is found in more than 50% of patients with truncal reflux.[9] An antegrade or ascending hypothesis has been proposed,[20] which is fundamentally used by supporters of the ambulatory selective varicose vein ablation under local anesthesia (ASVAL) method.[21,22] The ante-grade hypothesis explains that venous dilatation and reflux begins distally in the supra-fascial saphenous tributaries, creating a dilated and refluxing venous network within the suprafascial space called the varicose reservoir. Eventually, the network becomes larger and creates a filling effect in the saphenous vein that leads to progressive vein wall dilatation in an ascending manner until it reaches the SFJ or SPJ, causing incom-petence at the junction.[23] A diameter reduction of the saphenous vein and elimination of reflux with good durability and excellent clinical outcomes have been reported after ASVAL.[21,22] In this respect, preoperative assessment of reflux abolition in the truncal veins by occluding the refluxing tributaries is suggested (ie, test of reversibility).[24] The origin of venous reflux could be much more complex. A study on healthy volunteers and subjects with early CVD suggests an ascending and/or multicentric progression of reflux, in addition to or separate from gravitational retrograde development.[25]

Most reflux DUS studies are performed in patients with varicose veins (clinical, etio-logic, anatomic, and pathologic [CEAP] class C2) with or without CVI (CEAP class C3–C6). Varicose veins are defined as abnormally dilated ($\geq$3 mm) veins with a tortuous trajectory along the subcutaneous tissue.[26] CVI encompasses more advanced stages of CVD and applies to patients with moderate to severe leg swelling, skin damage, or venous ulcers.[27] Patients with spider and/or reticular veins (CEAP class C1) are usually asymptomatic and they do not need reflux assessment. However, when spider and/or reticular veins are found along the great saphenous vein (GSV) or small saphenous vein (SSV) distribution and the patient desires treatment because of cosmetic reasons, a reflux study should be offered. In this scenario, better outcomes may be achieved by performing EVA of an underlying refluxing saphenous vein. Additionally, a reflux DUS may be indicated in patients with CVD-like symptoms (ie, heaviness, aching, swelling, throbbing pain, itching, night cramps, and/or restless legs) and normal limbs (CEAP class C0) at the physician's discretion, especially if they are aggravated by prolonged standing, relieved with leg elevation and compression therapy, and no other patho-logic complication is suspected.

Proper correlation between the patient's symptoms, clinical stage, and the distribu-tion and anatomic extent of the reflux is crucial for treatment purposes. Typically, pa-tients with C1 and C2 disease have reflux confined to the superficial system. As clinical severity worsens (C3–C6), the prevalence of incompetence in the perforator and deep veins increases. A study conducted to examine patterns of reflux in 465 subjects (594 limbs) belonging to different clinical CVD classes found valve incompetence in 70% of the limbs. Overall, the study revealed an incidence of reflux of 93%, 42%, and 36%, in the superficial, deep, and perforating venous systems, respectively. Superficial reflux only was found in most class 1 subjects, whereas variable combined patterns of reflux were seen more often in those with advanced clinical stages. Isolated deep or perfo-rated incompetence was very uncommon.[28]

Continuous retrograde flow from the groin to the calf is defined as axial reflux and correlates with severity of CVD. Axial reflux could be confined to the superficial or the deep veins, or it could involve any combination of the 3 venous systems (superfi-cial, deep, and/or perforating). Segmental reflux comprises retrograde venous flow in any combination of the 3 venous system with no continuity from the groin to the below the knee veins.[27] Axial reflux is present in most subjects with C6 disease. DUS exam-ination in 83 subjects (93 limbs) with active chronic venous ulcers revealed axial reflux in 79% limbs, and the reflux involved the 3 venous systems in 52% legs. Superficial reflux with or without involvement of other systems was seen in 84 legs (86%), 72 legs (73%) had deep reflux with or without involvement of other systems, and incom-petent perforator veins were identified in 79 limbs (81%).[29]

The GSV, SSV, anterior and posterior accessory saphenous veins, and saphenous tributaries are the most common sites for identification of superficial reflux. Nonsaphenous superficial reflux is detected in 10% of subjects with CVD, more often in multiparous women with more than 2 pregnancies.[30]

Examination Protocol

As previously mentioned, a reflux DUS study is performed with the patient standing and facing toward the examiner. The patient's weight rests on the contralateral limb. The supine position is inappropriate for detection of reflux and measurement of vein diameters. Slight flexion, abduction, and external rotation of the limb being interrogated are recommended. Alternatively, the reverse Trendelenburg position (at least 15°) can be used if the patient cannot stand. The superficial and deep calf veins can be assessed with the patient sitting. Distal compression and release, by manually squeezing the musculature or by using an automatic cuff inflator, is used to evaluate for augmentation, presence, and duration of reflux. The calf veins are examined by squeezing or releasing the midfoot. Active foot plantarflexion provides similar effect in patients with marked leg edema. The Valsalva maneuver is used only in the groin area because its effectiveness in inducing reflux diminishes below that level.

The deep, superficial, and perforating veins at the thigh are examined in this order: first with the patient in erect posture, followed by the calf veins with the patient sitting. The CFVs, SFJs, FVs, and POPVs are evaluated for compressibility in cross-sectional view using B-mode. Color flow and pulse-wave Doppler are used to determine luminal changes, flow direction, augmentation, respiratory phasicity, and reflux.

The GSV is found within the saphenous compartment, which resembles a stylized Egyptian eye in transverse view (**Fig. 1**). Subcutaneous tributaries are easily distinguished and differentiated from the GSV by their course outside the fascial

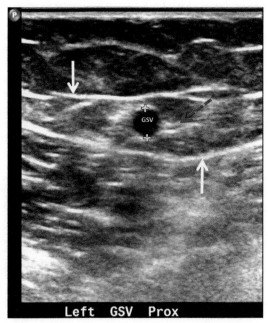

Fig. 1. GSV is seen inside the saphenous canal (saphenous eye). Superficial fascia (*downward arrow*), deep or muscular fascia (*upward arrow*), saphenous ligament (*red arrow*).

compartment. Frequently, the GSV and the anterior accessory GSV (AAGSV) can be found below the SFJ and can be mistakenly interpreted as a duplicated saphenous trunk. The AAGSV lies more anteriorly and lateral to the GSV, aligning with the superficial femoral artery and the FV (alignment sign). The SSV is found in the triangular fascia, surrounded by the crural fascia and the gastrocnemius muscle heads.[9]

Numeric and morphologic variations of the veins are frequent and need to be recorded. Saphenous vein hypoplasia and aplasia are the most common anatomic variations, occurring in varicose limbs more frequently than in healthy ones. The distribution of varicose veins and patterns of reflux in patients with hypoplastic or aplastic vein segments are highly variable and significantly influence surgical management.[31] The saphenous veins are duplicated when both veins are found inside the saphenous compartment. Duplication of the saphenous veins is rare and found in 1.6% to 2% of patients with CVD.[32]

The perforating veins traverse the deep fascia to connect the superficial and deep veins. The deep fascia is dense and echogenic because of its collagen content and is thus easy to visualize on DUS. There are approximately 150 perforator veins in the lower extremity, only 20 of which are of importance in terms of clinically significant reflux. The normal direction of flow is from the superficial to the deep veins through the perforator veins. These veins are examined by transverse and oblique scanning because their long axis is seen in these planes. They are found by following the course of the GSV, the SSV, and their tributaries. Outward flow in these veins is seen only in conjunction with superficial and deep vein reflux.[12]

Superficial, Perforator, and Deep Veins

The GSV is traced in its entire length caudally from the groin to the distal calf by using different views. The vessels in the groin area, imaged in axial axis, resemble Mickey Mouse's face (CFV) and ears (common femoral artery laterally and GSV medially). Two GSV valves (terminal and preterminal) are fairly constant anatomic structures seen on DUS and considered part of the SFJ. It is crucial to identify the source and patterns of reflux because several other veins can be visualized in this area and can affect the management of the patient. Reflux at the SFJ may be detected in continuity with the GSV (**Fig. 2**) and/or the AAGSV. Other contributing veins are found in the lower abdomen and pelvis.

The GSV is examined for reflux, by both color and pulse wave Doppler, at the saphenous arch (between the terminal and preterminal valves) and below it. If reflux is diagnosed, diameters at the junction and along the GSV need to be measured in at least 3 other locations (eg, distal thigh, knee, and proximal calf). The lowest point of reflux should be identified because this is essential for treatment. The depth of the GSV beneath the skin is important in patients in whom endovenous thermal ablation is

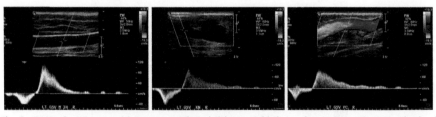

Fig. 2. DUS of a 59-year-old woman with 6 children and bilateral symptomatic CVD. She had large varicose veins in both limbs that were worse on the left. Images show high-velocity, long-duration reflux in the thigh, knee, and calf. GSV was incompetent from SFJ to midcalf with diameters ranging from 4.2 to 7.8 mm. Large tributaries with diameter up to 14 mm had reflux in the lower thigh, knee, and calf.

being considered. The GSV, and most commonly the AAGSV, becomes very tortuous and superficial immediately or few centimeters below the SFJ. In this circumstance, it is important to measure the length of any straight segment from the SFJ to determine the type of procedure to be performed. All refluxing tributaries connecting to the GSV and saphenous varicosities are identified and documented as well. Luminal or venous wall changes due to previous superficial venous thrombosis and/or aneurysmal segments along the saphenous trunk are common and should be recorded.

The SSV is examined starting at the posterior knee with similar approach as it was described for the GSV. A transverse view is used to identify the SSV at its proximal compartment and other major veins of the popliteal fossa. A significant variation of the SSV anatomic termination is found among patients.[9] The SPJ, when present, is assessed for reflux in longitudinal view. Any continuous SSV reflux from the SPJ to the distal calf, as well as the axial diameter of the SSV 3 cm below the SPJ and at the midcalf level needs to be recorded (**Fig. 3**). Other anatomic details needing documentation are the position of the SPJ in relation to the knee crease, the specific connection of the SSV in relation to the POPV circumference, the type of insertion of the gastrocnemius vein, and whether there is an artery accompanying the SSV or the gastrocnemius vein. Alternative sources of reflux are investigated, including communication of the SSV with a popliteal fossa perforator vein, GSV tributaries, pelvic veins traced to the buttock or perineum, or SSV thigh extensions. An intersaphenous vein may be present and is followed in its entire course until it joins the GSV. Often, ascending or descending patterns of reflux in the SSV thigh extension are detected that may explain the physical findings and the patients' symptoms.

Nonsaphenous superficial vein reflux is detected in 10% of all CVD cases. Approximately 90% have varicose veins and lower extremity edema, whereas a more advanced clinical stage is identified in 10% of patients. Most patients have symptoms. The technique to examine these veins is slightly different. Frequently, both linear array and curvilinear transducers are used during the examination. The veins are traced in different directions, from cephalad to caudal and vice versa, in all of the limb aspects. Veins involved include the gluteal, posterolateral thigh perforator, vulvar, lower posterior thigh, popliteal fossa perforator vein, knee perforator, and sciatic nerve veins (**Fig. 4**). Reflux detected at the gluteal and/or vulvar veins is suspicious for pelvic congestion syndrome and may need further investigation.

Perforator veins are grouped based on their topography.[9] Perforators with a cross-sectional diameter at the muscle fascia larger than 3.5 mm are associated with reflux greater than 90% of the times.[33] Not all perforators, either competent or incompetent,

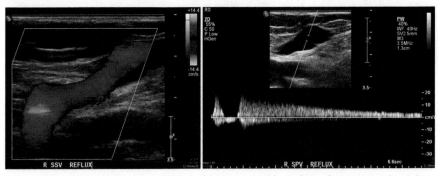

Fig. 3. Ultrasound images of a 38-year-old woman with unilateral symptomatic varicose veins. Both the GSV and SSV had reflux. The images show long-duration reflux at the SPJ and SSV. The SPJ measured 8 mm and the largest SSV diameter is 11 mm.

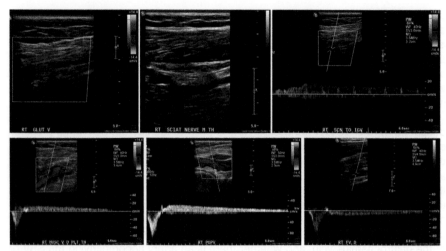

Fig. 4. DUS image of a 49-year-old woman with right lower limb swelling and pain. She had pelvic and right lower limb vein reflux. The image demonstrates prolonged reflux in the POPV. The POPV reflux was in continuity with the right inferior gluteal vein via sciatic nerve veins and muscular veins in the thigh. The right FV was normal.

will be detected with DUS. It is necessary to look for lateral and posterior thigh perforator veins if clinical assessment shows varices in these regions. Refluxing perforator veins larger than 3.5 mm underneath a healed or active venous ulcer are considered pathologic[34] and are, therefore, most commonly discovered at the lower and medial calf (**Fig. 5**). Bidirectional flow in a perforator indicates incompetence of the vein; however, this is only significant when the reflux is elicited during the diastolic phase of a dynamic test (eg, calf muscle relaxation or compression release). Currently, only pathologic perforator veins are treated and, therefore, the interest for other perforator veins is declining.

The deep veins are examined for reflux and/or venous obstruction. Contrary to the superficial system, the reflux cause in these veins is mostly due to previous thrombotic events.[35] Deep reflux may be linked to superficial vein reflux through perforating veins

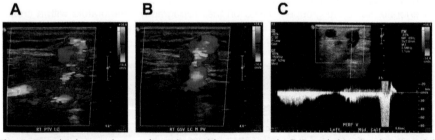

Fig. 5. Doppler images in a male patient with symptomatic CVD and skin discoloration. (*A*) Large lower calf medial incompetent perforator vein. During augmentation, blood moves from superficial to deep veins through the dilated perforator vein (11 mm in diameter). (*B*) After releasing distal compression, there is reflux in the perforator and superficial veins. (*C*) Large reentry perforator vein with enhanced flow measuring 6.3 mm in diameter from a different patient. As seen by the Doppler waveform, there is high flow at rest with large flow augmentation during distal compression. After the compression, there is a short retrograde flow without reflux. The patient had edema and skin discoloration with reflux in GSV and its tributaries. The refluxing blood in the superficial veins renters the deep veins through the perforator veins. Over time, due to the high volume of flow, the perforator veins dilate.

and/or saphenous-deep vein junctions, which could configure recruitment-based deep vein reflux. This type of reflux in the deep veins is usually abolished after effective treatment of the venous incompetence in the superficial system.[23] Reflux detected in the CFV or the POPV below the SFJ or SPJ level, respectively, most likely represent true deep vein reflux. The deep axial and muscular veins in the calf should also be examined for reflux, mainly class C3 to C6 patients with previous DVT.

Pelvic Vein Reflux

Pelvic venous reflux manifests with a variety of signs and symptoms, which most commonly affect multiparous women of reproductive age. Symptoms such as chronic pelvic pain, dyspareunia, and urinary frequency may be associated with vulvar, perineal, gluteal, or lower limb varices. DUS is widely accepted as the first-line test to study these patients. An easy and reproducible method using transabdominal and transperineal windows to examine the pelvic veins was recently published.[36]

The examination is performed after the patient has been fasting overnight. A curvilinear array transducer 2 to 5 MHz is most often used or 1 to 5 MHz in obese patients. The patient is placed in the supine position with head elevation of 30° to examine the inferior vena cava (IVC), left renal vein (LRV), iliac veins, and ovarian veins. The IVC is imaged to detect duplication, hypoplasia or aplasia, obstruction, compression, or collaterals. The renal veins are examined for detection of obstruction, which mostly occurs in the left side by extrinsic compression known as the nutcracker phenomenon. Each iliac vein is assessed for compression or luminal obstruction. The left and right ovarian veins are examined in their full length for detection of reflux. Spontaneous reflux with continuous flow in the left ovarian vein suggests compression of the LRV. If reflux is detected, the axial diameter of the ovarian vein needs to be measured.

To examine the connection of the pelvic floor with the lower extremities, the patient is asked to stand up. The transuterine and periuterine veins (which are also examined using transabdominal approach), and the tributaries of the internal iliac veins are assessed for reflux by placing the probe in the inguinal area first, followed by the perineal space and the gluteal area.

The reflux in the ovarian veins is induced by manual distal compression near the iliac fossa if no spontaneous reflux is seen. In the standing position, the Valsalva maneuver is mainly used for tributaries of the internal iliac vein and the veins extending into the pelvic floor.

DIAGNOSIS OF OBSTRUCTION

Venous obstruction can be caused by extrinsic and/or intrinsic conditions. The most common cause of obstruction is venous thrombosis. Venous thrombosis is frequently associated with more proximal outflow venous obstruction secondary to extrinsic conditions. The veins are most commonly compressed by adjacent arterial vessels, ligaments, and/or bones. Tumors, hematomas, and cysts can also cause extrinsic compression. Long-lasting outflow venous obstruction, postthrombotic and/or extrinsic, gradually leads to ambulatory venous hypertension and the typical signs and symptoms encountered in CVI patients. Diagnosis of these conditions is important because it can alter management. DUS has replaced contrast venography as the first imaging of choice for the diagnosis of the aforementioned conditions. Its sensitivity in this respect is higher than 90%.[37]

For performance of the examination, the patient is placed in a reverse Trendelenburg position with the knee bent and in external rotation. The examination begins below the inguinal ligament at the CFV and the SFJ. The transducer is placed in a transverse orientation to the vein and compression is applied to completely obliterate the normal vein lumen. The transducer is then turned longitudinally to evaluate for flow and augmentation. In the same manner, all the deep veins of the extremity from the groin to the calf are examined in 3-cm to 5-cm intervals. It is important to bear in mind the possibility of variations in venous anatomy. For diagnosis of DVT, only the symptomatic limb is examined. The contralateral CFV is consistently scanned. Unless local signs or symptoms are present, the anterior tibial veins are not routinely examined because of their low incidence of DVT.[38] The saphenous vein trunks are then evaluated.

It is crucial to assess the iliac veins and the IVC when suprainguinal VD is suspected. In this case, however, flow is evaluated chiefly because compression can be difficult and uncomfortable. Asymmetry of flow velocity, waveform, and pattern at rest and during flow augmentation in the CFV indicates proximal obstruction. However, the absence of asymmetry cannot exclude obstruction. Accordingly, when iliocaval obstruction is suspected, the full extent of these veins must be imaged. The presence of stenosis, usually from extrinsic compression, is recognized by the mosaic color (which denotes poststenotic turbulence), abnormal Doppler waveform at the stenotic area, slow flow, spontaneous contrast, and vein dilatation before the stenosis.[39] The reduction in vein diameter can be measured by planimetry to compare the smallest lumen with the normal lumen and by the peak vein velocity ratio (poststenotic or prestenotic). The 4 components that should be examined are visualization, compressibility, flow, and augmentation.

Acute and Recurrent Vein Thrombosis

Venous thromboembolism (VTE) is a major global health problem affecting approximately 1 in 1000 adults annually. VTE encompass a continuum that includes both DVT and pulmonary embolism (PE). Approximately two-thirds of patients with VTE present for care with DVT. Most DVT affects the lower limbs and can be anatomically divided into proximal (POPVs, FVs, deep FVs, and iliac veins) and distal (posterior tibial, peroneal, anterior tibial, gastrocnemius, and soleal). Proximal lower extremity DVT is considered more clinically relevant because of its higher complication rate. Acute PE, the most serious complication of DVT, originates from the proximal veins in approximately 90% of the patients.[40]

The most common symptoms in DVT patients are leg pain, tenderness, and swelling (more specific). Physical examination of the lower limbs may reveal paleness, cyanosis, reddish-purple skin discoloration, pain over the deep veins, pitting edema, palpable cords, and collateral nonvaricose superficial veins. Signs and symptoms of DVT possess a low sensitivity and specificity, therefore a definitive diagnosis requires the assistance of selective imaging modalities.

Ultrasound has become the first-line imaging study in the diagnosis of DVT because of its high sensitivity and specificity, accessibility, and safety. Abnormalities to look for include lack of or no compressibility of the vein, filling defects or no color flow, absence of augmentation, and aphasic or monophasic waveforms on spectral Doppler. Venography, MRV, and CTV are not considered first-choice studies.

The veins are imaged using optimal grayscale technique. Acute thrombi appear mostly anechoic or hypoechoic, and homogeneous. However, the echogenicity of a thrombus cannot be used to determine its age. The veins are dilated and lack compressibility (**Fig. 6**). Smooth and thin walls distinguish acute DVT from chronic postthrombotic changes. The clot may be seen attached to the wall and/or free-floating. A free-floating thrombus is always acute in nature (**Fig. 7**). On color-flow, non-occlusive thrombus is seen as a filling defect of the lumen, whereas complete absence

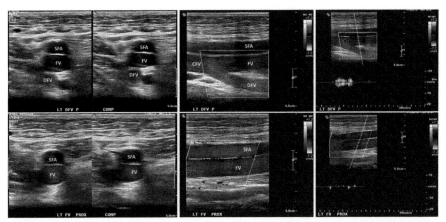

Fig. 6. DUS images of a 66-year-old man with history of prostate cancer treated with radiotherapy, in remission greater than 10 years. He was diagnosed with acute thrombosis of the left GSV (above-the-knee segment) and thrombosed varicosities in the distal thigh more than 3 months ago. He was not treated with anticoagulation. He returned with acute left limb pain and swelling. The DUS images show noncompressibility, absence of color flow, decreased augmentation, and phasicity in the FV and deep FV. Additional images (not shown) revealed thrombus into the left EIV, CFV, POPV, and gastrocnemius veins. EIV, external iliac vein.

of color indicates occlusion. Low-level echoes may be seen in the veins due to sluggish blood flow with visible red blood cells (rouleaux). In this circumstance, Doppler may reveal absence of color. Augmentation by squeezing the calf is often needed to completely fill the vessel with color. Additional criteria for DVT are loss of flow phasicity with respiration and no response to augmentation on spectral Doppler.

Approximately one-quarter of all acute DVT patients may experience a new thrombotic event over the next 5-year period (recurrent DVT).[41] Fresh thrombus may develop in new vein segments or in segments that previously had thrombosis (**Fig. 8**). Identical diagnosis criteria used for acute DVT (described previously) apply for thrombi affecting new vein segments or previously thrombosed segments

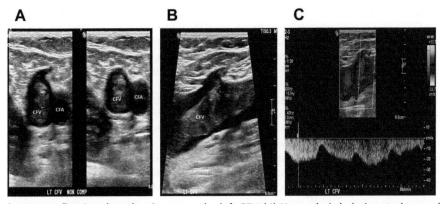

Fig. 7. Free-floating thrombus is seen at the left CFV. (*A*) Hypoechoic halo is noted around the thrombus in the CFV, which is not compressible. (*B*) Hyperechoic thrombus is surrounded by anechoic or hypoechoic areas in the periphery. (*C*) Blood flow channel can be seen between the thrombus and the posterior vein wall. Normal respiratory phasicity within the channel is detected.

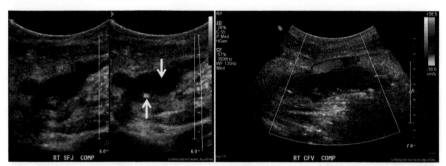

Fig. 8. Ultrasound images of a 57-year-old man with acute swelling and pain in the right lower extremity. He had iliofemoral thrombosis 9 years ago and an IVC filter placed. On the images, recurrent DVT is seen in the CFV. The bright luminal echoes (*upward arrow*) represent chronic luminal changes from the previous thrombosis and the echolucent area (*downward arrow*) is the new thrombus. The vein is not compressible and is dilated. This is a typical picture of recurrent DVT.

exhibiting no residual changes. Suggested sonographic criteria for thrombi involving segments with residual luminal changes include thrombus extending greater than 9 cm in length, increased thrombus thickness greater than or equal to 4 mm, and new noncompressibility of the vein. These criteria are used when baseline ultrasound images are available.[42,43]

Other abnormalities are commonly detected in conjunction with or without DVT. Findings such as enlarged lymph nodes, soft tissue cystic or solid tumors, hematomas, abscesses, muscle tears, joint effusions, and Baker cyst, among others, should be reported. Similarly, waveforms obtained in the CFV and iliac veins may reveal symmetric but very pulsatile flow. This is usually seen in patients with decompensated congestive heart failure or severe tricuspid insufficiency. Such information has significant clinical relevance for the physician in the case.

Chronic Venous Obstruction

Postthrombotic syndrome

Postthrombotic syndrome (PTS) develops in up to one-half of patients after symptomatic DVT. The most important risk factor for PTS is recurrent ipsilateral DVT. Typical symptoms of PTS are leg claudication; swelling; skin damage; and, in more severe cases, venous ulceration. Patients with DVT involving the iliac and CFV tend to develop more severe forms of PTS. PTS not only affects patients physically but also their psychosocial well-being.[44]

About 50% of the proximal veins will have noticeable postthrombotic structural vein changes on DUS.[45] Postthrombotic veins may appear contracted, noncompliant, and partially compressible. The vein walls are usually thickened and reveal very organized, hyperechoic and heterogeneous material attached to it. Multiple irregular and narrow flow channels with collateral vessels are seen with color Doppler (**Fig. 9**). The presence of dilated collateral veins is a sign of obstruction but their absence cannot exclude it. Often the iliac veins are obstructed because they do not recanalize as much as the infrainguinal veins. This is probably due to the large thrombotic burden. Therefore, chronic postthrombotic luminal changes in the iliac veins are frequently seen. Postthrombotic occlusion of the iliac veins has the highest prevalence in patients with venous claudication. Therefore, in such patients, it is mandatory to examine the iliac veins.

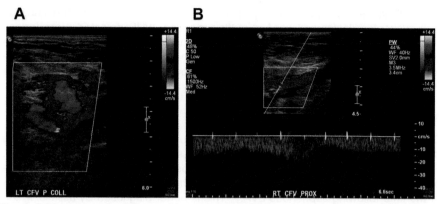

Fig. 9. DUS images of a 52-year-old man with multiple episodes of DVT and PE. He has swelling and skin discoloration in the left lower limb. CFV and iliac veins have chronic obstruction. (*A*) Image shows many collateral veins above the occluded left CFV. (*B*) The right CFV is patent.

Extrinsic compression

Extrinsic venous compression occurs most commonly at 4 different anatomic locations. The resultant outflow venous obstruction may lead to venous hypertension of sudden (thrombosis) and/or gradual onset, and to 4 specific clinical syndromes: (1) nonthrombotic iliac vein lesion is caused by compression of an adjacent iliac artery, (2) venous thoracic outlet syndrome (Paget-Schroetter syndrome) refers chiefly to axillary-subclavian vein thrombosis (effort thrombosis) in patients with a narrow cost-oclavicular space, (3) extrinsic compression of the LRV at the aortomesenteric angle is known as nutcracker syndrome, and (4) POPV compression (popliteal entrapment syndrome type V) results from lateral extension of the origin of the medial head of the gastrocnemius muscle or an anomalous third head of the gastrocnemius muscle.[46] Extrinsic compression of the veins can also occur from tumors, cysts, enlarged lymph nodes, aneurysms, hematoma, and ligaments. The cause of compression is important to recognize because it determines the management of the patient.

DUS, when properly correlated with the patient's history and clinical manifestations, provides valuable information for the diagnosis of venous compression syndrome, therefore it is used as the first diagnostic modality. Acute DVT distal to a stenotic vein segment is easily detected by applying the sonographic criteria described earlier. Criteria have been developed to detect central vein obstruction by DUS. Obstruction is determined by direct planimetric measurements of the luminal diameters, flow velocity changes (ie, peak vein velocity ratio of >2.5, low-flow velocity to absence of flow, and nonphasic flow and reverse flow in the ipsilateral internal iliac or inferior epigastric and other veins), and presence of collateral veins. Planimetric measurements are the primary way to determine stenosis or occlusion. All other findings are used to enhance the diagnostic confidence. In patients with nutcracker syndrome, a higher vein velocity ratio ($\geq$4) is used.[36,39]

IVUS uses a higher frequency transducer to obtain 360° high-resolution images of the vein through a catheter. Currently, there are no hemodynamic criteria to determine which lesion is clinically significant, thus morphologic measurements are used. The cutoff values are an area and/or diameter reduction (by measuring the shortest axis) of the vein greater than 50%. IVUS possesses a higher sensitivity in the detection of clinically relevant venous outflow obstruction compared with conventional venography. In a prospective, multicenter trial Venogram Versus Intravascular Ultrasound for Diagnosing and Treating Iliofemoral Vein Obstruction (VIDIO), Gagne and colleagues[47] compared multiplanar venography with IVUS in 100 subjects with suspected ileofemoral venous outflow disease. IVUS detected more lesions than venography (124 vs 66, $P<.0001$) and was more reliable in terms of the degree of stenosis. The use of IVUS altered the management in most cases. IVUS also identifies intraluminal trabeculations, septations, webs, and wall thickening, which are frequently minimized or missed by venography.

IMAGING AFTER INTERVENTION

DUS after interventions for CVD and/or venous obstruction is routinely performed to determine anatomic or hemodynamic success and to detect complications. Following EVA and/or phlebectomies, DUS is performed to assess for adequate obliteration of the veins and to rule out acute thrombosis. DVT occurs about 1% of the time following saphenous EVA.[48] This is better diagnosed by assessing the veins for compressibility. Protrusion of a thrombus into the lumen of the CFV or the POPV is very unusual (<1%).[49,50] Various acronyms and classification systems to report the extent of the thrombus have been proposed. Postablation superficial thrombus extension (PASTE) is a broader term used for thrombus extending from the saphenous veins to the CFV or the POPV after either thermal or chemical ablation. Endovenous heat-induced thrombosis (EHIT) is specifically used after thermal EVA.[51,52] A thrombus extending up to the junction is called EHIT 1, those into the FV or POPV but occluding less than or more than 50% of the cross-sectional diameter are EHIT 2 and EHIT 3, respectively; and the thrombus is EHIT 4 when it results in complete occlusion (**Fig. 10**).[53]

Patency of an ablated vein and the length of the patent or obstructed segment of the vein should be reported. Saphenous patency for fewer than 4 to 7 days indicates technical failure, whereas late patency after early occlusion suggests recanalization. Anatomic distribution and patterns of reflux of residual and/or recurrence varicosities are also investigated in early and subsequent follow-up ultrasounds. Recurrent reflux at the groin or the popliteal fossa is a frequent problem after high ligation and stripping of the GSV or the SSV, respectively. This can be caused by a too-long residual saphenous stump or, more commonly, by neovascularization. Induction of reflux at the groin to detect neovascularization is performed with the Valsalva maneuver. Two major patterns of reflux connected to the CFV are usually identified. Tortuous multiple small channels are found in more than half of patients, whereas single large channels either with a direct course or a more tortuous one are detected less frequently.[34,54]

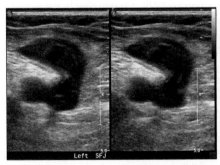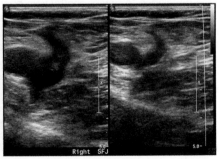

Fig. 10. Images of a 57-year-old woman with EHIT 4 on the left and EHIT 3 on the right after saphenous vein thermal ablations were performed 1 week apart. On the left side, the entire CFV is filled with thrombus and it is noncompressible. On the right side, some thrombus is seen in the CFV, which is partially compressible.

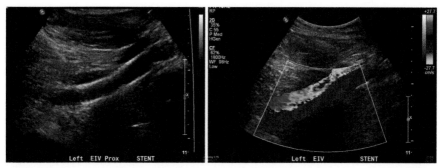

Fig. 11. Ultrasound images of a 60-year-old man with skin damage and chronic postthrombotic iliac vein obstruction. Stents were placed in the left iliac veins. The images demonstrate the stent in the external iliac vein in B-mode and color. The iliac veins are patent with normal flow.

Iatrogenic AVFs following saphenous EVA are rare. Only a few cases have been reported in the literature.[55–57] Thermal injury to the arterial wall in proximity to the ablated saphenous vein and/or direct needle trauma during administration of tumescent anesthesia may cause this complication. AVF, after EVA, have been detected between the common femoral artery and CFV, the superficial femoral artery and the FV, and the GSV and external pudendal artery at the proximal thigh. In the popliteal fossa, an AVF is most commonly found between the SSV and the superficial sural artery. This complication could be associated with early or late recanalization of the saphenous trunks. The diagnosis of an AVF is achieved by detecting low-resistance, high-velocity, and pulsatile flow in the vein.

Furthermore, postintervention DUS is very useful for monitoring success after pelvic coil or chemical embolization for venous reflux in patients with persistent or recurring symptoms. The patency of the veins following angioplasty and venous stenting for outflow venous obstruction is routinely examined by DUS at frequent intervals for extended periods (**Fig. 11**). Stent occlusion due to thrombosis may be detected. Many of these patients are successfully treated with catheter-directed thrombolysis. Less frequently, cannulation complications such as pseudoaneurysms and AVF are found and reported.

REFERENCES

1. Beebe-Dimmer JL, Pfeifer JR, Engle JS, et al. The epidemiology of chronic venous insufficiency and varicose veins. Ann Epidemiol 2005;15(3):175–84.
2. Beckman MG, Hooper WC, Critchley SE, et al. Venous thromboembolism: a public health concern. Am J Prev Med 2010;38(4 Suppl):S495–501.
3. Katz DS, Hon M. Current DVT imaging. Tech Vasc Interv Radiol 2004;7(2):55–62.
4. American College of Radiology website. ACR–AIUM–SPR–SRU practice parameter for the performance of peripheral venous ultrasound examination. 2015 (Resolution 33). Available at: https://www.acr.org/~/media/3FFA49F7E8C34272A0E046CCABE 0219D.pdf. Accessed July 7, 2017.
5. Intersocietal Accreditation Commission website. IAC standards and guidelines for vascular testing accreditation. 2016. Available at: http://www.intersocietal. org/vascular/standards/IACVascularTestingStandards2016.pdf. Accessed July 7, 2017.
6. American College of Phlebology website. Duplex ultrasound imaging of lower extremity veins in chronic venous disease, exclusive of deep venous thrombosis:

guidelines for performance and interpretation of studies. 2012. Available at: http://www.phlebology.org/wp-content/uploads/2014/11/ACP_Imaging_Guidelines _rev1109_a.pdf. Accessed July 7, 2017.

7. Society for Vascular Ultrasound website. Lower extremity venous duplex evaluation (for deep/superficial vein thrombosis). 2014. Available at: http://account.svunet. org/files/positions/svu_venous_guideline2011.pdf. Accessed July 7, 2017.

8. Coleridge-Smith P, Labropoulos N, Partsch H, et al. Duplex ultrasound investigation of the veins in chronic venous disease of the lower limbs: UIP consensus document. Part 1. Basic principles. Eur J Vasc Endovasc Surg 2006;31:83–92.

9. Cavezzi A, Labropoulos N, Partsch H, et al. Duplex ultrasound investigation of the veins in chronic venous disease of the lower limbs—UIP consensus document. Part II. Anatomy. Eur J Vasc Endovasc Surg 2006;31:288–99.

10. Wells PS, Anderson DR, Bormanis J, et al. Value of assessment of pretest probability of deep-vein thrombosis in clinical management. Lancet 1997;350(9094): 1795–8.

11. Necas M. Duplex ultrasound in the assessment of lower extremity venous insufficiency. Australas J Ultrasound Med 2010;13(4):37–45.

12. Leon LR, Labropoulos N. Vascular laboratory: venous duplex scanning. In: Cronenwett JL, Johnston W, editors. Rutherford's vascular surgery. 8th edition. London: Saunders Elsevier; 2014.

13. Labropoulos N, Tiongson J, Pryor L, et al. Definition of venous reflux in lower-extremity veins. J Vasc Surg 2003;38(4):793–8.

14. Labropoulos N, Waggoner T, Sammis W, et al. The effect of venous thrombus location and extent on the development of post-thrombotic signs and symptoms. J Vasc Surg 2008;48(2):407–12.

15. Johnson BF, Manzo RA, Bergelin RO, et al. Relationship between changes in the deep venous system and the development of the postthrombotic syndrome after an acute episode of lower limb deep vein thrombosis: a one- to six-year follow-up. J Vasc Surg 1995;21(2):307–12 [discussion: 313].

16. Kistner RL, Eklof B, Masuda EM. Diagnosis of chronic venous disease of the lower extremities: the "CEAP" classification. Mayo Clin Proc 1996;71(4):338–45.

17. Labropoulos N. CEAP in clinical practice. Vasc Surg 1997;31:224–5.

18. Plate G, Brudin L, Eklof B, et al. Congenital vein valve aplasia. Wold J Surg 1986; 10(6):929–34.

19. Ludbrook J, Beale G. Femoral venous valves in relation to varicose veins. Lancet 1962;1:79–81.

20. Bernardini E, De Rango P, Piccioli R, et al. Development of primary superficial venous insufficiency: the ascending theory. Observational and hemodynamic data from a 9-year experience. Ann Vasc Surg 2010;24(6):709–20.

21. Pittaluga P, Chastanet S, Rea B, et al. Midterm results of the surgical treatment of varices by phlebectomy with conservation of a refluxing saphenous vein. J Vasc Surg 2009;50(1):107–18.

22. Biemans AA, van den Bos RR, Hollestein LM, et al. The effect of single phlebectomies of a large varicose tributary on great saphenous vein reflux. J Vasc Surg Venous Lymphat Disord 2014;2(2):179–87.

23. Lee BB, Nicolaides AN, Myers K, et al. Venous hemodynamic changes in lower limb venous disease: the UIP consensus according to scientific evidence. Int Angiol 2016;35(3):236–352.

24. Gianesini S, Occhionorelli S, Menegatti E, et al. CHIVA strategy in chronic venous disease treatment: instructions for users. Phlebology 2015;30(3):157–71.

25. Labropoulos N, Giannoukas AD, Delis K, et al. Where does venous reflux start? J Vasc Surg 1997;26(5):736–42.
26. Kistner RL, Eklof B. Classification and etiology of chronic venous disease. In: Gloviczki P, editor. Handbook of venous disorders: guidelines of the American Venous Forum. 3rd edition. London: Hodder Arnold; 2009. p. 37–46.
27. Eklof B, Perrin M, Delis KT, et al. Updated terminology of chronic venous disorders: the VEIN-TERM transatlantic interdisciplinary consensus document. J Vasc Surg 2009;49:498–501.
28. Labropoulos N, Delis K, Nicolaides AN, et al. The role of the distribution and anatomic extent of reflux in the development of signs and symptoms in chronic venous insufficiency. J Vasc Surg 1996;23(3):504–10.
29. Danielsson G, Arfvidsson B, Eklof B, et al. Reflux from thigh to calf, the major pathology in chronic venous ulcer disease: surgery indicated in the majority of patients. Vasc Endovascular Surg 2004;38(3):209–19.
30. Labropoulos N, Tiongson J, Pryor L, et al. Nonsaphenous superficial vein reflux. J Vasc Surg 2001;34(5):872–7.
31. Caggiati A, Mendoza E. Segmental hypoplasia of the great saphenous vein and varicose disease. Eur J Vasc Endovasc Surg 2004;28(3):257–61.
32. Kockaert M, de Roos KP, van Dijk L, et al. Duplication of the great saphenous vein: a definition problem and implications for therapy. Dermatol Surg 2012;38(1):77–82.
33. Sandri JL, Barros FS, Pontes S, et al. Diameter-reflux relationship in perforating veins of patients with varicose veins. J Vasc Surg 1999;30:867–74.
34. Gloviczki P, Comerota AJ, Dalsing MC, et al. The care of patients with varicose veins and associated chronic venous diseases: clinical practice guidelines of the Society for Vascular Surgery and the American Venous Forum. J Vasc Surg 2011;53(5 Suppl):2S–48S.
35. Labropoulos N, Leon M, Nicolaides AN, et al. Venous reflux in patients with previous deep venous thrombosis: correlation with ulceration and other symptoms. J Vasc Surg 1994;20(1):20–6.
36. Labropoulos N, Jasinski PT, Adrahtas D, et al. A standardized ultrasound approach to pelvic congestion syndrome. Phlebology 2017;32(9):608–19.
37. Meissner MH, Moneta G, Burnand K, et al. The hemodynamics and diagnosis of venous disease. J Vasc Surg 2007;46(Suppl S):4S–24S.
38. Labropoulos N, Webb KM, Kang SS, et al. Patterns and distribution of isolated calf deep vein thrombosis. J Vasc Surg 1999;30:787–91.
39. Labropoulos N, Borge M, Pierce K, et al. Criteria for defining significant central vein stenosis with duplex ultrasound. J Vasc Surg 2007;46(1):101–7.
40. Saeger W, Genzkow M. Venous thromboses and pulmonary emboli in postmortem series: Probable causes by correlations of clinical data and basic diseases. Pathol Res Pract 1994;190:394–9.
41. Prandoni P, Lensing AW, Cogo A, et al. The long-term clinical course of acute deep venous thrombosis. Ann Intern Med 1996;125(1):1–7.
42. Linkins LA, Pasquale P, Paterson S, et al. Change in thrombus length on venous ultrasound and recurrent deep vein thrombosis. Arch Intern Med 2004;164(16):1793–6.
43. Linkins LA, Stretton R, Probyn L, et al. Interobserver agreement on ultrasound measurements of residual vein diameter, thrombus echogenicity and Doppler venous flow in patients with previous venous thrombosis. Thromb Res 2006;117(3):241–7.
44. Kahn SR. The post-thrombotic syndrome: progress and pitfalls. Br J Haematol 2006;134(4):357–65.

45. Kearon C. Natural history of venous thromboembolism. Circulation 2003;107(23 Suppl 1):I22–30.
46. White JM, Comerota AJ. Venous compression syndromes. Vasc Endovascular Surg 2017;51(3):155–68.
47. Gagne PJ, Tahara R, Fastabend C, et al. Venogram versus intravascular ultrasound for diagnosing and treating iliofemoral vein obstruction (VIDIO): report from a multicenter, prospective study of iliofemoral vein interventions. J Vasc Surg Venous Lym Dis 2016;4(1):136.
48. Khilnani NM, Grassi CJ, Kundu S, et al. Multi-society consensus quality improvement guidelines for the treatment of lower-extremity superficial venous insufficiency with endovenous thermal ablation from the Society of Interventional Radiology, Cardiovascular Interventional Radiological Society of Europe, American College of Phlebology, and Canadian Interventional Radiology Association. J Vasc Interv Radiol 2010;21:14–31.
49. Hingorani A, Ascher E, Markevich N, et al. Deep venous thrombosis after radiofrequency ablation of greater saphenous vein: a word of caution. J Vasc Surg 2004;40:500–4.
50. Marsh P, Price BA, Holdstock J, et al. Deep vein thrombosis (DVT) after venous thermoablation techniques: rate of endovenous heat-induced thrombosis (EHIT) and classical DVT after radiofrequency and endovenous laser ablation in a single center. Eur J Vasc Endovasc Surg 2010;40:521–7.
51. Wright D, Morrison N, Recek C, et al. Post ablation superficial thrombus extension (PASTE) into the common femoral vein as a consequence of endovenous ablation of the great saphenous vein. Acta Phlebologica 2010;11(3):59–64.
52. Dexter D, Kabnick L, Berland T, et al. Complications of endovenous lasers. Phlebology 2012;27(Suppl 1):40–5.
53. Khilnani NM. Duplex ultrasound evaluation of patients with chronic venous disease of the lower extremities. AJR Am J Roentgenol 2014;202(3):633–42.
54. van Rij AM, Jones GT, Hill GB, et al. Neovascularization and recurrent varicose veins: more histologic and ultrasound evidence. J Vasc Surg 2004;40(2):296–302.
55. Timperman PE. Arteriovenous fistula after endovenous laser treatment of the short saphenous vein. J Vasc Interv Radiol 2004;15:625–7.
56. Rudarakanchana N, Berland T, Chasin C, et al. Arteriovenous fistula after endovenous ablation for varicose veins. J Vasc Surg 2012;55:1492–4.
57. Theivacumar NS, Gough MJ. Arterio-venous fistula following endovenous laser ablation for varicose veins. Eur J Vasc Endovasc Surg 2009;38(2):234–6.

New Trends in Anticoagulation Therapy

Margaret Smith, MD[a], Glenn Wakam, MD[a], Thomas Wakefield, MD[b],
Andrea Obi, MD[c],*

KEYWORDS

- Direct oral anticoagulants • Venous thromboembolism • Deep venous thrombosis
- VTE chemoprophylaxis • VTE extended therapy • Anticoagulation
- Perioperative bridging

KEY POINTS

- Based on ease of dosing and large noninferiority trials, direct oral anticoagulant agents should be considered as the first-line therapy for the treatment of venous thromboembolism.
- New strategies for treatment of unprovoked venous thromboembolism now exist: prophylactic dose rivaroxaban or apixaban, aspirin, and the HERDOO2 scoring system to identify women at low risk of recurrence.
- Betrixaban is the newest DOAC to gain approval from the US Food and Drug Administration with an indication for extended thromboprophylaxis in high-risk medical patients.
- Selective, rather than routine, bridging of anticoagulants should occur in the setting of atrial fibrillation and prosthetic heart valves.

INTRODUCTION

In the last several years, anticoagulation pharmacology has been dramatically altered in the United States with approval from the US Food and Drug Administration of 5 new direct oral anticoagulant (DOAC) agents. In 2012, the American College of Chest Physicians (AACP) recommended treatment of acute venous thromboembolism (VTE) with vitamin K antagonists (VKAs), while recognizing a major shift on the horizon: "Given the paucity of currently available data and that new data are rapidly emerging, we give a weak recommendation in favor of vitamin K antagonists and

The authors have nothing to disclose.
[a] General Surgery Residency, Department of Surgery, University of Michigan, 2207 Taubman Center, 1500 East Medical Center Drive, Ann Arbor, MI 48109-5867, USA; [b] Section of Vascular Surgery, Department of Surgery, University of Michigan, 5463 Cardiovascular Center, 1500 East Medical Center Drive, Ann Arbor, MI 48109-5867, USA; [c] Section of Vascular Surgery, Department of Surgery, University of Michigan, 5372 Cardiovascular Center, 1500 East Medical Center Drive, Ann Arbor, MI 48109-5867, USA
* Corresponding author.
E-mail address: easta@med.umich.edu

Surg Clin N Am 98 (2018) 219–238
https://doi.org/10.1016/j.suc.2017.11.003
0039-6109/18/© 2017 Elsevier Inc. All rights reserved.

LMWH therapy over dabigatran and rivaroxaban."[1] By the time the updated ACCP guidelines were released in 2016, DOACs were a routine part of the prevention and treatment of VTE. With the advent of a new drug class, an explosion of clinical studies is underway to determine the usefulness of each medication for a myriad of indications.

In this article, we explore some of the most rapidly developing, exciting, and important areas of change for the practicing clinician. These include new details on how to choose the best anticoagulant for VTE treatment, considerations for extended anticoagulation for the prevention of recurrent VTE, developments in extended thromboprophylaxis for patients at high risk for VTE, and data and trends in perioperative bridging. Within 2017 alone, 2 useful clinical prediction trials emerged from large studies: the SAMe-TT$_2$R$_2$ score for predicting the quality of anticoagulation with VKA and the HERDOO2 score (Hyperpigmentation, Edema, or Redness in either leg; D-dimer level 250 µg/L or greater; Obesity with body mass index $\geq$30 kg/m^2; or Older age [$\geq$65 years]) for identifying women at low risk of recurrent VTE. Within this same time period, a fifth DOAC (Betrixaban, Bevyxxa, Portola Inc., South San Francisco, CA) underwent the FDA approval process, adding to the array of available anticoagulants. We have designed the following sections to place newer studies in the context of historical data to allow for a perspective on how this information may be practically incorporated into every day practice.

Anticoagulant Choice for Venous Thromboembolism

Approved in 1954, VKAs (warfarin, coumadin) for more than one-half of a century, had been the mainstay of therapy for thrombotic diseases. Given the established safety profile of VKAs, as well as the efficacy in reducing the risk for fatal pulmonary embolism and recurrent thrombosis, they represent the gold standard by which every new agent now must be compared. There are several shortcomings associated with VKAs: they require monitoring, the metabolism of the drug is affected by diet and other medications, and they have a defined bleeding risk of 5% to 6% per year,[2] which cannot be mitigated by targeting a lower International Normalized Ratio.[3,4] Until recently, few alternatives existed. The other commonly prescribed anticoagulants before the emergence of DOACs were the low-molecular-weight heparins (LMWHs). Despite the downside of subcutaneous administration (necessitating daily or twice daily home injections), rather than an oral route, the LMWHs had several advantages: dosing was weight based and predictable, routine laboratory monitoring did not need to occur, and efficacy was similar to VKAs. In a pooled analysis of LMWH and VKAs in the treatment of VTE, the rate of fatal pulmonary embolism during treatment of DVT was 0.4% and of pulmonary embolism was 1.5%; the rates were similarly low after the cessation of anticoagulation.[5] In certain patient populations, LMWH proved superior to VKAs; for instance, in patients with malignancy, treatment with LMWH decreased the risk of recurrent VTE by about 50% at 6 months to 1 year compared with warfarin, without a difference in bleeding rates.[6] In the HOME-LITE trial, tinzaparin (an LMWH), was superior to warfarin for the prevention of postthrombotic syndrome, development of leg ulcers, and treatment satisfaction.[7]

Although VKAs and LMWH remain viable options for the treatment of VTE, in the last few years there has been a rapid development of a significant body of scientific evidence supporting the use of DOACs in VTE. The 2 categories of DOACs are the direct Xa inhibitors and direct thrombin inhibitors. Currently, of the direct Xa inhibitors apixaban, rivaroxaban, and edoxaban have all been FDA approved for the treatment of VTE. Dabigatran is the sole approved direct thrombin inhibitor. The DOACs are appealing because they are all administered orally, have fixed doses that do not need to be adjusted based on weight, and there is no need for monitoring. Two major initial clinical concerns regarding the DOACs were efficacy and safety, and reversibility in the event of major bleeding. In the last 10 years, all of these DOACs each have at least 1 large randomized, controlled trial demonstrating noninferiority in the treatment of VTE compared with VKAs.[8–11] Furthermore, in every study there was no increased incidence of bleeding in patients who used DOACs compared with standard VTE therapy. Of all of the DOACs, apixaban alone demonstrated a superior reduction in bleeding (major bleeding and clinically relevant nonmajor bleeding) compared with VKAs.

One of the appealing aspects of VKAs (and to a lesser extent LMWH), is the ability to be quickly reversed by protamine (for heparin and to a lesser degree LMWH), fresh frozen plasma, or prothrombin complex concentrate, if indicated clinically. In addition, there is an available laboratory test (International Normalized Ratio for VKAs and anti-Xa level for heparin and LMWH) to quantify the adequacy of reversal. Historically, the same had not been true for the DOACs, with reversal being limited to supportive measures, prothrombin complex concentrate, or selective dialysis.[12] Although the issue of reversibility has not been resolved fully, progress was achieved with the FDA approval of idarucizumab (Praxbind) in October 2015. Idarucizumab is a monoclonal antibody that binds to dabigatran and can reverse its anticoagulant effects within minutes.[13] Two other agents currently in development include andexanet alfa and aripazine. Andexanet alfa is recombinant factor Xa protein that acts as a decoy for all factor Xa inhibitors, including DOACs, LMWHs, and fondaparinux.[14] Clinical trials have shown the andexanet alfa can effectively reverse the anticoagulant effect of DOACs by about one-half without any known thrombotic events in healthy patients.[15] Currently, Prospective, Open-Label Study of Andexanet Alfa in Patients Receiving a Factor Xa Inhibitor Who Have Acute Major Bleeding (ANNEXA-4; NCT02329327), a phase III open-label study, is ongoing to evaluate the use of the medication in patients with ongoing major bleeding, with an estimated completion date of 2022. The final reversal agent progressing in development with FDA fast track designation for hemorrhage is aripazine (PER-977, Ciraparantag, Perosphere Inc., Danbury, CT). It is a water-soluble, catatonic molecule available in intravenous formulation that noncovalently binds to and reverses the anticoagulation of all anticoagulation agents (LMWH, UFH, factor Xa inhibitors, dabigatran) in both animal models and healthy volunteers.[15] In total, at least 5 phase I or II trials have been completed or are ongoing to evaluate the usefulness of aripazine for anticoagulant reversal.

As a result of the multitude of evidence showing both the effectiveness and safety of DOACs, in 2016 the AACP recommended DOACs as the first-line treatment for acute VTE over VKAs in patients who do not have an associated cancer (grade 2B).[16] In patients with cancer who develop acute VTE, LMWH remains the recommended first-line treatment. Although guidelines recommend DOACs over VKA in non–malignancy-related VTE, there are several scenarios that would preclude the use of DOACs; for example, patients with mechanical heart valves, patients who cannot afford the cost of the medication, and patients with impaired renal function. Given that all of the comparison studies showed noninferiority, in many cases either a DOAC or a VKA is acceptable. However, recent work by Kataruka and colleagues[17] has shown that certain patients are at much higher risk of treatment failure with VKAs than others. They applied the scoring system SAMe-TT$_2$R$_2$ (**Fig. 1**), which had been previously successfully validated for use in atrial fibrillation, and demonstrated that patients with a high score were significantly more likely to experience adverse events and recurrent VTE on VKA therapy than those with a low score. As the anticoagulation field continues

Clinical equipose regarding VKA or DOAC selection

Calculate SAMe TT_2R_2

	Variables	Points
S	Sex (female)	1
A	Age (<60 y)	1
Me[a]	Medical problems (>2 co-morbidities)	1
T	Treatments (medications known to interact with VKAs)	1
T_2	Tobacco use	2
R_2	Race (non-Caucasian)	2

Score 0 or 1 Acceptable for VKA	Score ≥2 Consider alternate anticoagulant (DOAC or LMWH)
• Time in therapeutic range >60% • Recurrent VTE risk 1.5/100 patient years • Adverse events 4.5/100 patient years	• Time in therapeutic range <60% • Recurrent VTE risk 4.2/100 patient years • Adverse events 7.9/100 patient years

Fig. 1. In the event of clinical equipoise regarding selection of vitamin K agonists (VKAs) or direct oral anticoagulant (DOAC) agents for the treatment of venous thromboembolism (VTE), the SAMe-TT_2R_2 score can be used to predict individuals likely to have adverse events, VTE recurrence, and poor time in the therapeutic range with VKA treatment. [a] Medical co-morbidities include diabetes, hypertension, renal disease, hepatic disease, pulmonary disease, congestive heart failure, coronary artery disease, peripheral vascular disease, or previous stroke. LMWH, low-molecular-weight heparin.

to expand with increased agents and changing guidelines, it will be important for providers to critically decide which anticoagulation treatment would be best for each individual patient (**Table 1**).

Extended Anticoagulation Treatment to Reduce the Risk of Recurrent Venous Thromboembolism

The recommended duration of anticoagulation for the treatment of provoked proximal and symptomatic distal VTE is 3 months (grade 1B). Extended therapy traditionally is considered under the following circumstances:

- Previous VTE event;
- Thrombophilias associated with a high risk of recurrence; and
- Unprovoked (idiopathic) VTE.

Virtually all authorities agree that for a second idiopathic VTE, anticoagulant therapy should be continued owing to the high recurrence risk well past 3 months in those patients with low and moderate bleeding risks (grades 1B, 2B).[16] For patients with diagnosed hereditary thrombophilias, those that are associated with a higher risk of VTE recurrence include protein C or protein S deficiency (especially with a family history), antithrombin deficiency, homozygous factor V Leiden, homozygous prothrombin 20210 gene mutation, and multiple thrombophilias in the same patient. Factor V Leiden heterozygous mutation alone does not confer an increased risk; however, when combined with prothrombin 20210 gene mutation recurrence is increased and

Table 1
Dosing and considerations for various anticoagulant choices

	Dosing	Half-Life	Considerations
Apixaban	10 mg BID ×7 d Then 5 mg BID (2.5 mg BID for long-term therapy)	7–11 h	• Superior to standard therapy with no increase in bleeding • Twice daily dosing • No renal adjustment
Rivaroxaban	15 mg BID ×3 wk Then 20 mg/d	12 h	• Once daily regimen • May need to be renal adjusted • Increase in GI bleeding compared with warfarin
Dabigatran	LMWH for 5–10 d 150 mg BID	8–15h	• Poor choice in renal dysfunction • Requires heparin bridge • Increase in GI bleeding compared with warfarin • Up to 10% have dyspepsia • Avoid in patients with significant CAD
Edoxaban	LMWH for 5–10 d 60 mg/d 30 mg/d with ≤60 kg or CrCl 15–50	10–14 h	• Once daily dosing • Requires heparin bridge • Needs to be renal adjusted • Increase in GI bleeding compared with warfarin
Warfarin	Variable dosing titrate to goal INR	~40 h	• Reliable and predictable reversal • Can use SAMe-TT$_2$R$_2$ to predict poor candidates • Requires bridging • Requires frequent monitoring • Has many interactions with food and other medications

Abbreviations: BID, 2 times a day; CAD, coronary artery disease; CrCl, creatinine clearance; GI, gastrointestinal; INR, International Normalized Ratio; LMWH, low-molecular-weight heparin.

prolonged anticoagulant therapy is recommended. Among acquired thrombophilias, the presence of antiphospholipid antibodies and active cancer mandate extended therapy.[18]

Idiopathic first-time VTE remains a difficult clinical scenario, because one must balance the competing risks and implications of recurrent VTE and major bleeding. D-Dimer and repeat duplex testing have both been advocated as useful tests to determine risk of recurrence with cessation of anticoagulation among these patients. D-Dimer is measured approximately 1 month after stopping oral anticoagulation. If elevated, this suggests that active thrombosis is occurring and the rate of recurrence is 15% compared with 6.2% with a normal D-dimer. This risk can be mitigated with resumption of anticoagulation, which reduces the VTE rate to 2.9%.[16,19] The use of repeat serial lower extremity ultrasound examination to determine the state of the thrombosed veins has been studied, with the assumption that if the veins are occluded with fibrotic scar tissue, flow will be sluggish and the risk of recurrent VTE increased. The usefulness of this test is less certain, because this approach used a very difficult quantification scheme, which is difficult to reproduce in day-to-day clinical practice.

Two major new advances that have come about in recent years include the validation of the HERDOO2 score and low-dose anticoagulant and antiplatelet therapies for the prevention of recurrent VTE. Recently, the HERDOO2 score was developed and validated prospectively. This identified women at low risk of recurrence after unprovoked VTE who may safely discontinue anticoagulants after short-term (standard) treatment. Women receive 1 point for (a) hyperpigmentation, edema, or redness in either leg, (b) VIDAS (bioMérieux, Marcy-l'Étoile, France) D-dimer of 250 μg/L or greater, (c) obesity (body mass index of ≥30), and (d) older age (≥65 years). Patients with 0 or 1 point were considered low risk for recurrent VTE and discontinued long-term anticoagulation therapy (**Fig. 2**). Women who were defined as low risk and discontinued therapy had a 3.0% risk of recurrent VTE per patient year, compared with an 8.1% risk in high-risk women who discontinued anticoagulants (see **Fig. 2**).[20] This clinical algorithm should be easily adopted in day-to-day clinical practice.

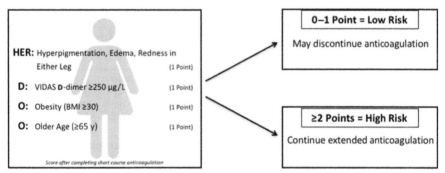

Fig. 2. In women with first-time unprovoked VTE, the HERDOO2 score can identify those that are at low risk of recurrent VTE after initial standard anticoagulant therapy and can safely stop anticoagulation. HERDOO2, Hyperpigmentation, Edema, or Redness in either leg; D-dimer level 250 μg/L or greater; Obesity with body mass index ≥30 kg/m²; or Older age (≥65 years).

The advent of the DOACs has also reopened the possibility of low-dose anticoagulation for the prevention of recurrent thrombosis as a method of improving the risk–benefit profile by decreasing the bleeding risks associated with anticoagulant therapy. Previous studies with low-dose VKAs failed to demonstrate an improvement in bleeding profile and has been largely abandoned in clinical practice.[21] Interestingly, aspirin has recently been investigated as an alternative to mitigate bleeding risk. Several studies, including the International Collaboration of Aspirin Trials for Recurrent Venous Thromboembolism (INSPIRE) trial (a collaboration of the Warfarin and Aspirin [WARFASA] and Aspirin to Prevent Recurrent Venous Thromboembolism [ASPIRE] trials, **Table 2**) have demonstrated a reduced risk of VTE recurrence by more than one-third in patients treated with aspirin compared with placebo.[22,23] More recently, both treatment and thromboprophylactic doses of rivaroxaban and apixaban have been shown to be more effective in prevention of VTE recurrence with no increased risk of bleeding compared with placebo or aspirin (see **Table 2**).[24,25] Although evidence exists that lower dose anticoagulants may effectively reduce VTE recurrence, the most effective therapy with the safest treatment profile and lowest cost is still being debated.

Extended Venous Thromboembolism Prophylaxis for Patients at High Risk

Extended DVT prophylaxis refers to chemoprophylaxis that is continued beyond the initial in-hospital 5 to 14 days, for up to 35 days. This concept reflects an important

Table 2
Recent trials evaluating different extended duration therapies for prevention of recurrent VTE

Study Name	N	Study Drug	Primary Efficacy Endpoint	Primary Safety Endpoint	Summary
INSPIRE	1224	ASA 100 mg once a day for 2 y (vs placebo)	Recurrent VTE 7.5%/y placebo vs 5.1%/y ASA, $P = .008$	Major bleeding 0.4%/y placebo vs 0.4%/y ASA, $P = .67$	ASA after anticoagulant treatment reduces the overall risk of recurrent VTE without increasing the risk of bleeding
EINSTEIN CHOICE	3396	Rivaroxaban 20 mg once a day or 10 mg once a day for 12 mo (vs ASA 100 mg once a day for 12 mo)	Composite of symptomatic, recurrent fatal or nonfatal VTE or unexplained death for which PE could not be excluded Treatment dose (20 mg) 1.5% (study) vs 4.4% (ASA; HR, 0.34; 95% CI, 0.20–0.59; $P<.001$) Thromboprophylactic dose (10 mg) 1.2% (study) vs 4.4% (ASA; HR, 0.26; 95% CI, 0.14–0.47; $P<.001$)	Major bleeding Treatment dose (20 mg) 0.5% (study) vs 0.3% (ASA; HR, 2.01; 95% CI, 0.50–8.04; $P = .32$) Thromboprophylactic dose (10 mg) 0.4% (study) vs 0.3% (ASA; HR, 1.64; 95% CI, 0.39–6.84; $P = .50$)	Rivaroxaban (both treatment and prophylactic dose) was superior to ASA in the prevention of recurrent VTE, with no difference in bleeding risk. The study was not powered to show noninferiority of prophylactic dose vs treatment dose.
AMPLIFY EXTEND	2486	Apixaban 2.5 mg BID or 5 mg BID for 12 mo (vs placebo)	Composite of symptomatic recurrent VTE or death from any cause Treatment dose (5 mg) 4.2% (study) vs 11.6% (placebo; RR, 0.36; 95% CI, 0.25–0.53) Thromboprophylactic dose (2.5 mg) 3.8% (study) vs 11.6% (placebo; RR, 0.33; 95% CI, 0.22–0.48)	Major bleeding Treatment Dose (5 mg) 0.1% (study) vs 0.5% (placebo; RR, 0.25; 95% CI, 0.03–2.24) Thromboprophylactic dose (2.5 mg) 0.2% (study) vs 0.5% (placebo; RR, 0.49; 95% CI, 0.09–2.64)	Extended anticoagulation with either treatment dose or prophylactic dose apixaban is superior to placebo in the prevention of recurrent VTE, with no increase in bleeding rates compared with placebo.

Abbreviations: ASA, aspirin; BID, 2 times a day; CI, confidence interval; HR, hazard ratio; RR, relative risk; VTE, venous thromboembolism.

fact about the epidemiology of VTE: namely, that many VTE events occur after the index hospitalization.[26] Analysis of large administrative databases indicates that for both recently hospitalized surgical patients[27] and medical patients,[28] approximately 56% of VTE occur after discharge. Over the last decade, considerable progress has been made in identifying high-risk surgical cohorts and mitigating risk. Most recently, an effort has been made toward decreasing postdischarge VTE in medical patients.

Extended thromboprophylaxis for elective cancer operations

The highest incidence of VTE after inpatient surgery is in the 2 to 3 weeks after the procedure,[29] suggesting that thromboprophylaxis in this vulnerable period after hospital discharge could be beneficial. The Enoxaparin and Cancer (ENOXACAN) I study identified that 15% of patients undergoing elective cancer operations with 10 days of LMWH prophylaxis suffer from VTE.[30] Subsequently, the ENOXACAN II trial demonstrated a 60% relative risk reduction in VTE after abdominal or pelvic cancer surgery, without an increased risk of bleeding.[31] Therefore, the first group in which extended VTE prophylaxis was advocated for was those undergoing major operations with the additional risk factor of malignancy. The current ACCP guidelines (grade IB) and American Society of Clinical Oncology clinical practice guidelines suggest that these patients undergoing abdominal or pelvic surgery for cancer, who are not otherwise at high risk for a major bleeding complications, should be treated with extended duration pharmacologic prophylaxis for 4 weeks.[32,33] Most recently, extended antithrombotic prophylaxis was shown to have a 91% relative risk reduction among patients undergoing laparoscopic colorectal cancer resection.[34]

Extended thromboprophylaxis for orthopedic procedures

Similar to operations for malignancy, orthopedic procedures have been historically associated with a high rate of postoperative VTE; up to 15% to 30% before 1980, and modern-day estimates of 4.3% out to 35 days.[35] The use of LMWH has been associated with about a 60% decrease in VTE. The median date of VTE diagnosis after major orthopedic surgery is 7 days for total knee arthroplasty and 17 days for total hip arthroplasty (THA), which has been an impetus for testing the usefulness of extended VTE prophylaxis in this patient population.[36] The current ACCP guidelines suggest "extending thromboprophylaxis in the outpatient setting for up to 35 days from the day of surgery rather than only 10 to 14 day (Grade 2B)."[37] This recommendation was given on the basis of compiled data from 7 studies evaluating placebo compared with extended prophylaxis with LMWH (largely in patients undergoing THA), demonstrating a decrease in 9 fewer symptomatic VTE per 1000 patients without an increase in major bleeding.

From 2007 to 2011, a remarkable number of trials evaluating the use of DOACs for 6 to 10 days and extended (28–39 days) thromboprophylaxis in orthopedic surgery patients was undertaken. In the Oral Dabigatran Versus Enoxaparin for Thromboprophylaxis After Primary Total Hip Arthroplasty (RE-NOVATE) II trial, dabigatran was found to be noninferior to LMWH in patients undergoing THA, with a similar bleeding rate.[38] In the Apixaban Dose Orally Vs. ANtiCoagulation with Enoxaparin 3 (ADVANCE-3)[39] and REnal Cell cancer treatment with Oral RAD001 given Daily (RECORD-1)[40] trials, extended duration apixaban and rivaroxaban were found to be superior to extended duration LMWH for VTE risk reduction among patients undergoing THA, with a similar safety profile. Despite these trials, the American Association of Orthopedic Surgery leaves the decision up to the surgeon and patient regarding the use of extended thromboprophylaxis. The reasoning is that, contrary to the ACCP guidelines, the emphasis is placed on "critical" endpoints (pulmonary embolism, major bleeding, and mortality) rather than "noncritical" endpoints (symptomatic DVT, any DVT, and proximal DVT), and extended prophylaxis is more effective in these noncritical endpoints.[41] The result is a widely variable practice across developed countries with regard to the type and duration of VTE thromboprophylaxis after orthopedic operations.

Extended thromboprophylaxis in acutely medically ill patients

Within the last several years, there have been a flurry of studies aimed at decreasing the postdischarge risk of VTE among medical patients. These include the Extended Prophylaxis for Venous ThromboEmbolism in Acutely Ill Medical Patients With Prolonged Immobilization (EXCLAIM),[42] A Diabetes Outcome Progression Trial (ADOPT),[43,44] Multicenter, Randomized, Parallel Group Efficacy and Safety Study for the Prevention of Venous Thromboembolism in Hospitalized Acutely Ill Medical Patients Comparing Rivaroxaban with Enoxaparin (MAGELLAN),[45] and Acute Medically Ill VTE (Venous Thromboembolism) Prevention with Extended Duration Betrixaban (APEX) trials.[44] The summary of these trials is presented in **Table 3**. Taken together, these trials have evaluated the usefulness of prophylactic enoxaparin, apixaban, rivaroxaban, and betrixaban in acutely ill patients for an extended period of 28 to 35 days compared with standard therapy. With the exception of the APEX trial (betrixaban), every extended regimen has had a higher risk of major bleeding, which offsets a decreased VTE risk. A pooled metaanalysis of all 4 trials, encompassing 28,000 patients found a decrease in VTE and symptomatic DVT, but an increase in major bleeding.[46] The number needed to treat for VTE was 239 and number needed to harm for major bleeding was 247, suggesting that the general use of extended thromboprophylaxis in this patient population should not be undertaken. Of all the agents, betrixaban lacked the bleeding profile and decreased the relative risk of VTE by 24%. The study used a smaller "enriched" cohort (patients with elevated D-dimer) as a method of decreasing heterogeneity and demonstrating efficacy. However, this measure failed to demonstrate statistical significance ($P = .054$), despite apparent significance in the larger, unselected study population (see **Table 3**). In June 2017, betrixaban received FDA approval for extended prophylaxis in medically ill patients. Whether it will be widely adopted into clinical practice is still uncertain. The A Study of Rivaroxaban (JNJ-39039039) on the Venous Thromboembolic Risk in Post-Hospital Discharge Patients (MARINER) trial (NCT02111564) is a current, ongoing trial evaluating thromboprophylaxis with rivaroxaban in selected medically ill patients based on the IMPROVE VTE risk score and D-dimer.[47] This study may further define how best to treat this patient population.

Perioperative Bridging

Historically, all but the lowest risk patients with an indication for anticoagulation such as VTE, atrial fibrillation, prosthetic heart valve, or left ventricular assist device were managed preoperatively with an anticoagulant "bridge," to avoid the risk of thromboembolism (TE). The VKA would be discontinued 5 days before the proposed procedure and either intravenous heparin or LMWH subcutaneous administered from when the International Normalized Ratio was subtherapeutic (<2.0 or <2.5 depending on the indication), until 6 to 12 hours before the procedure. Anticoagulation was then immediately resumed with both a bridging agent and the VKA typically 12 to 24 hours after the procedure, or whenever it was felt safe to do so based on the procedure being performed. In modern times, this method remains true for high-risk patients under anticoagulant therapy for recent VTE, but a major paradigm shift has occurred for atrial fibrillation.

Table 3
Trials evaluating extended thromboprophylaxis in the medically ill

Study Name	N	Study Drug	Primary Efficacy Endpoint	Primary Safety Endpoint	Summary
ADOPT	6528	Apixaban 2.5 mg BID for 30 d (vs enoxaparin 6–14 d)	30-d composite of death related to VTE, PE, symptomatic DVT, or asymptomatic proximal leg DVT 2.7% (study) vs 3.1% (placebo; RR, 0.87; 95% CI, 0.62 to 1.23; P = .44)	Major bleeding 0.47% (study) vs 0.17% (placebo); RR, 2.58; 95% CI, 1.02 to 7.24; P = .04)	Extended thromboprophylaxis with apixaban was not superior to a shorter course with enoxaparin. Apixaban was associated with significantly more major bleeding events.
APEX	7513	Betrixaban 80 mg once daily for 35 d (vs enoxaparin 10 d)	Asymptomatic proximal DVT and symptomatic VTE Patients with elevated D-dimer: 6.9% (study) vs 8.5% (placebo; RR, 0.81; 95% CI, 0.66 to 0.98; P = .054) Overall population[a]: 5.3% (study) vs 7.0% (placebo; RR, 0.76; 95% CI, 0.63 to 0.92; P = .0006)	Major bleeding 0.7% (study) and 0.6% placebo (RR, 1.19; 95% CI, 0.67 to 2.12; P = .55)	Among the prespecified cohort (patients will elevated D-dimer), no significant difference. In the overall population, exploratory analysis suggests a benefit in VTE reduction in the treatment group without an increased risk of bleeding complications.
EXCLAIM	5963	Enoxaparin 40 mg once daily for 28 d (vs enoxaparin 10 d)	VTE (symptomatic/asymptomatic DVT, symptomatic/fatal PE) 2.5% (study) vs 4.0% (placebo; absolute risk difference −1.53%; 95% CI -2.54% to −0.52%)	Major bleeding events 0.8% (study) vs 0.3% (placebo; absolute risk difference 0.51%; 95% CI, 0.12% to 0.89%)	Use of extended duration enoxaparin reduced VTE rates but had higher major bleeding events compared with placebo.
MAGELLAN	8101	Rivaroxaban 10 mg once a day for 35 d (vs enoxaparin 10 d)	Asymptomatic proximal or symptomatic VTE 4.4% (study) vs 5.7% (placebo; RR, 0.77; 95% CI, 0.62 to 0.96; P = .02)	Composite of major or clinically relevant nonmajor bleeding 4.1 (study) vs 1.7% (placebo) P<.001	Rivaroxaban was noninferior to enoxaparin for standard duration thromboprophylaxis. Extended duration rivaroxaban reduced the risk of VTE, but was associated with an increased risk of bleeding.

Abbreviations: BID, 2 times a day; CI, confidence interval; DVT, deep venous thrombosis; PE, pulmonary embolism; RR, relative risk; VTE, venous thromboembolism.
[a] Exploratory analysis according to trial design.

Bridging in the setting of atrial fibrillation

Nearly 1 in 6 patients treated with warfarin for atrial fibrillation undergo invasive procedures each year. Previous guidelines for bridging anticoagulation were primarily founded on observational studies, with the question of necessity of bridging therapy largely unanswered in the literature. More recently, the randomized controlled trial Perioperative Bridging Anticoagulation in Patients with Atrial Fibrillation (BRIDGE) addressed the question of bridging requirements in patients with atrial fibrillation on VKA therapy and found routine bridging of low- and moderate-risk patients to be harmful. Specifically, forgoing bridging anticoagulation was shown to be noninferior to bridging therapy in the prevention of TE (0.4% versus 0.3%), and the incidence of major bleeding was 3.2% in bridged patients compared with 1.3% in the nonbridged group.[48] Although the current body of evidence demonstrates that bridging anticoagulation of low- and moderate-risk patients with atrial fibrillation leads to increased rates of bleeding with no clear evidence of minimizing TE events, it must be noted that the majority of trials have underrepresented high-risk patients with atrial fibrillation (CHADS$_2$ score of ≥ 5), patients with mechanical heart valves, and those with recent venous or arterial thrombosis. Changes to anticoagulation practices should, therefore, be extrapolated to these populations with caution. Overall, most authorities now suggest patients with atrial fibrillation at low risk of TE who require oral anticoagulant therapy interruption temporarily discontinue anticoagulation without use of bridging therapies. In patients at high risk of TE, anticoagulation may be temporarily discontinued, but bridging therapy should be assessed individually based on bleeding and TE risk and remains strongly encouraged by some organizations including the American College of Cardiology (ACC; grade 2C evidence).[49,50]

Bridging in the setting of mechanical heart valves

Until recently, mechanical heart valves were considered to be at very high risk of TE with recommendations for perioperative bridging in all patients requiring oral anticoagulant therapy interruption. More recent studies demonstrate a perioperative risk of TE in patients with mechanical heart valves to be approximately 1%, with previous estimates likely influenced by a larger proportion of very high-risk valves (eg, cage-ball, tilting disk).[51] To date, there have been no randomized, controlled trials evaluating "bridging" versus "no bridging" in patients with prosthetic heart valves, and results from trials including only atrial fibrillation patients should be generalized cautiously. However, based on the results of the BRIDGE trial, the American Heart Association/ American College of Cardiology 2017 Updates on Bridging Therapy for Prosthetic Valves modified the class of recommendation supporting bridging anticoagulation from class I to IIa. Noting increasing concerns of bridging anticoagulation exposing patients to increased rates of bleeding with no reduction in the risk of TE, the recommendations now support bridging on an individualized basis, accounting for the risk of both TE and bleeding.[52] Ongoing studies, including the A Double Blind Randomized Control Trial of Post-Operative Low Molecular Weight Heparin Bridging Therapy Versus Placebo Bridging Therapy for Patients Who Are at High Risk for Arterial Thromboembolism (PERIOP-2) trial, are evaluating the need for bridging therapy in patients at moderate risk with a mechanical heart valve.

Bridging in the setting of direct oral anticoagulant agent therapy

Similarly, the introduction of DOACs for the treatment of atrial fibrillation and VTE introduced the practice of avoiding bridging owing to the short half-life. Initially, it was thought that dabigatran would require 3 to 4 days of cessation, and the direct Xa inhibitors 2 to 3 days of cessation based on half-life.[26] However, since their FDA approval, additional data from the Randomized Evaluation of Long Term Anticoagulation Therapy with Dabigatran Etexilate (RE-LY) trial and Dresden DOAC registry, among others, have better quantified the perioperative bleeding and thrombosis risks associated with DOAC use. Additionally, there are a subset of low-risk procedures for which it has been found safe to continue uninterrupted DOAC use.

In patients where anticoagulation interruption is required perioperatively, the management of DOACs aims to minimize or eliminate residual anticoagulant effect at the time of surgery. For procedures with a moderate bleeding risk, dabigatran, rivaroxaban, and apixaban should be held 1 day before surgery. This corresponds to 2 to 3 half-lives elapsing before surgery with possible 12% to 25% residual anticoagulant effect at the time of surgery. For high-risk bleeding procedures and major operations, DOACs should be held 2 days before surgery, allowing 4 to 5 half-lives to elapse and a residual anticoagulant effect of less than 10% (**Table 4**). Importantly, the specific duration of time for these medications to be held is significantly impacted by patient renal function, with recommendations to discontinue DOACs for greater periods of time in patients with even moderate renal impairment.[53,54]

The rapid offset and onset of action of DOACs negates the need for perioperative bridging. Additionally, in trials where patients have received bridging anticoagulation for DOAC interruption, increased rates of bleeding with no benefit in TE risk have been shown. Interruptions in anticoagulation occurred frequently in the RE-

Table 4 Bridging and reversal strategy for DOACs						
Agent	Mechanism of Action	No. of Days to Hold for Minor Procedures	No. of Days to Hold for Major Procedures	Reversal Agent	Alternative Treatment Option	Bridging Therapy Required
Apixaban	Factor Xa inhibitor	1 (2 doses)	2 (4 doses)	Unavailable	• 4-Factor PCC (*Kcentra*) • Factor VIIa • Tranexamic acid • Hemodialysis	No
Rivaroxaban	Factor Xa inhibitor	1 (1 dose)	2 (2 doses)	Unavailable	• 4-Factor PCC (*Kcentra*) • Factor VIIa • Tranexamic acid	No
Dabigatran	Direct thrombin inhibitor	1 (2 doses)[a]	2 (4 doses)[b]	Idarucizumab	• 4-Factor PCC (*Kcentra*) • Factor VIIa • Tranexamic acid	No
Edoxaban	Factor Xa inhibitor	1 (1 dose)	2 (2 doses)	Unavailable	• 4-Factor PCC (*Kcentra*) • Factor VIIa • Tranexamic acid	No

Abbreviations: DOAC, direct oral anticoagulant (agent); PCC, prothrombin complex concentrate.
[a] Hold for 2 d in renal insufficiency.
[b] Hold for 4 d in renal insufficiency.

Table 5	
Low bleeding risk procedures not requiring therapy interruption	
Category	**Procedure**
Dental	• Dental Extraction (1–2 teeth) • Endodontic procedure (root canal) • Subgingival scaling or cleaning
Ophthalmology	• Cataract surgery
Cardiology	• Diagnostic coronary angiography • Pacemaker insertion • Internal defibrillator placement
Dermatology	• Superficial Procedures (biopsy)
Gastroenterology	• Gastroscopy or colonoscopy with or without mucosal biopsy
Other selected procedures	• Thoracocentesis • Paracentesis • Arthrocentesis • Bone marrow biopsy

LY trial. In that study, 15.4% of dabigatran-treated patients whose anticoagulation was interrupted periprocedurally were bridged, with increased rates of major bleeding in the bridged group compared with nonbridged (6.5% vs 1.8%; odds ratio, 3.68) and no difference in rates of TE (0.5% vs 0.3%).[48] Although most experts agree that given DOACs' pharmacokinetics, no preoperative bridging is required, given the rapid onset and lack of reversal agents, in rare cases patients may require postoperative bridging therapy for high-risk patients who have delayed the reinitiation of DOACs.[50]

Procedures in which continuing anticoagulation may be lower risk than bridging therapy
Procedures with moderate to high bleeding risk often require interruption of oral anticoagulant therapy, even in high-risk patients. However, for certain low bleeding risk procedures, uninterrupted VKA therapy was found to have a lower risk of bleeding than therapy interruption with bridging.[55] Prospective data regarding uninterrupted anticoagulation with DOACs is limited; however, many suggest continued therapy for procedures with low bleeding risk based on the experience with VKA therapy (**Table 5**).[50,53,56] Alternatively, given the lack of prospective data with uninterrupted therapy and lack of widely accessible reversal agents, some recommend continuing medications until the day of surgery and performing the procedure at the time of the drug's trough level to achieve an overall decreased anticoagulant effect without significant disruption of therapy.[54]

SUMMARY

After one-half of a decade of incremental gains and, in some areas, stagnation of forward progress, anticoagulation pharmacology has abruptly become a rapidly developing, expansive, and progressive field. The standard of care is quickly evolving, and even for an experienced clinician, the onslaught of newly approved medications and studies is difficult to interpret and implement in the context of day to day practice. We have identified the most recent trends in anticoagulation in the context of current standard of care (**Table 6**). It is our hope that this may serve as a practical guide.

	Current (or Historical) Standard of Care	New Trend
Table 6 **New trends in anticoagulation**		
Anticoagulant choice	LMWH/VKA first line	DOACs 1st line SAMeT2R2 to identify patients at high risk of VKA failure.
Extended duration therapy for unprovoked VTE	Prolonged anticoagulation with no testing, or D-dimer or duplex to determine duration of anticoagulation Long-term full-dose anticoagulation with VKAs	HERDOO score to identify low-risk women who can avoid long-term anticoagulation. Long-term prophylactic dosing with rivaroxaban or apixaban or ASA.
Extended thromboprophylaxis	Extended duration prophylaxis for open abdominal/pelvic cancer operations only	Include laparoscopic cancer resection. Betrixaban for extended thromboprophylaxis in the medically ill.
Bridging	Routine bridging for atrial fibrillation and prosthetic valves Always hold anticoagulation for invasive procedures Hold DOACs 2–4 d	No bridging for CHADS2 ≤ 2; selective bridging for prosthetic valves. Select procedures safer to continue anticoagulation. Hold DOACs 1–2 d

Abbreviations: ASA, aspirin; DOAC, direct oral anticoagulant (agent); HERDOO2, Hyperpigmentation, Edema, or Redness in either leg; D-dimer level 250 μg/L or greater; Obesity with body mass index ≥30 kg/m^2; or Older age (≥65 years); LMWH, low-molecular-weight heparin; VKA, vitamin K agonist; VTE, venous thromboembolism.

Anticoagulant Choice

Whether these new trends become widely adopted remains uncertain. Certainly, the prescription of DOACs for the treatment of VTE has become widespread, but whether daily use of the SAMe-TT_2R_2 score is as readily adopted, as say the CHADS2 score for atrial fibrillation, remains uncertain. In fact, in most cases, there will be overriding comorbidities or patient preference that will drive the selection of an anticoagulant. In our own practice, the SAMe-TT_2R_2 score serves to identify patients at high risk of low time in the therapeutic range, and thereby allow for shorter term and more frequent follow-up.

Extended duration therapy for unprovoked venous thromboembolism

Similarly, the validation of the HERDOO2 score for the identification of low-risk women who may safely discontinue anticoagulation after a standard course after unprovoked VTE represents a new clinical scoring system, with an uncertain fate in terms of clinical implementation. A similar scoring system incorporating men and elderly patients would represent a much needed major advancement in the management of first time unprovoked VTE. Although apixaban and rivaroxaban have shown net clinical benefit for prevention of recurrent VTE, the issue of cost remains. Even with insurance coverage, it becomes an ethical question of social responsibility—is the risk reduction so great as to offset the cost to society? Aspirin, although not as effective, does offer risk reduction and is inexpensive. In practice, the patients likely to benefit from aspirin are those at high bleeding risk who have a contraindication (such as end-stage renal disease) to DOACs (or who cannot afford them).

Extended thromboprophylaxis
Although much money and effort was expended in the early DOAC trials (RECORD, ADVANCE), proving extended duration thromboprophylaxis was efficacious in reducing VTE, these have yet to be adopted into clinical practice. This is likely because of the priority placed by orthopedic surgeons on avoiding bleeding complications, and that the trials used LMWH (rather than placebo) as comparison group. Similarly, APEX trial resulted in approval of betrixaban for thromboprophylaxis in the medically ill, but owing to study design limitation, resulting in failure to meet the primary efficacy endpoint, it is uncertain as to whether this strategy will be widely adopted. With so many available FDA-approved DOACs, it remains certain that any other newcomers to the field will similarly have to expand into indications outside of primary nonvalvular atrial fibrillation and VTE treatment to gain approval, such as laparoscopic cancer resection. This may prove to be beneficial, because there are still gains to be made in thromboprophylaxis.

Bridging
Although TE is always a feared risk in patients stopping anticoagulation, the BRIDGE trial was the first rigorous trial to bring to light the very tangible risks associated with bridging therapy. Although it is accepted that the recurrent TE risk decreases over time, there is no predictive algorithm or similar trial with VTE patients to clearly delineate the risk–benefit profile of bridging and these data are very much needed. Other advancements in this area include the exploration of procedures in which it is safe to continue anticoagulation and the discovery that safety of shorter interruptions of DOACs before invasive procedures.

Future directions
The fact remains that, despite an incredible number of trials and drug development over the last decade, there are a multitude of unanswered questions and studies to be done. For instance, there are, as of yet, no compelling data regarding the use of DOACs in cancer patients, representing a large group of individuals relegated to daily or twice daily LMWH injections. A substantial number of ongoing randomized control trials, largely involving rivaroxaban and apixaban, will answer this question in the upcoming years. As the APEX study inadvertently highlighted, we still have much to learn about selection of the highest risk medical patients who would benefit from extended thromboprophylaxis. Furthermore, even with perfect in-hospital compliance with thromboprophylaxis, development of VTE is in some cases inevitable, a fact that should prompt us all not become complacent with the current anticoagulation options. As hematologist and thrombosis researcher Dr Robert Flaumenhaft has stated, "inhibiting thrombosis without inducing bleeding is the holy grail of anticoagulant therapy… there are no commercially available anticoagulants that achieve that goal." Much of decision making regarding anticoagulation therapy centers around risk and benefit; such an agent would absolve much of the imperfect and complicated decision making that occurs daily. Until such an ideal agent is discovered, we can envision that a male version of the HERDOO2 scoring system and a similarly designed BRIDGE trial for VTE patients would offer useful clinical information. Finally, as newer expensive anticoagulants paired with even more expensive reversal agents enter the market, the issue of cost effectiveness has begun to permeate the medical literature; suggesting that the modern-day doctor cannot function in isolation as a steward for his or her patient's

well-being, but must take into consideration the social and economic constraints surrounding such choices.

REFERENCES

1. Kearon C, Akl EA, Comerota AJ, et al. Antithrombotic therapy for VTE disease: antithrombotic therapy and prevention of thrombosis, 9th ed: American College of Chest Physicians Evidence-Based Clinical Practice Guidelines. Chest 2012; 141(2 Suppl):e419S–96S. Available at: http://www.ncbi.nlm.nih.gov/pubmed/22315268.
2. Schulman S, Rhedin AS, Lindmarker P, et al. A comparison of six weeks with six months of oral anticoagulant therapy after a first episode of venous thromboembolism. Duration of Anticoagulation Trial Study Group. N Engl J Med 1995; 332(25):1661–5. Available at: http://www.ncbi.nlm.nih.gov/entrez/query.fcgi?cmd=Retrieve&db=PubMed&dopt=Citation&list_uids=7760866.
3. Ridker PM, Goldhaber SZ, Glynn RJ. Low-intensity versus conventional-intensity warfarin for prevention of recurrent venous thromboembolism. N Engl J Med 2003;349(22):2164–7 [author reply: 7]. Available at: http://www.ncbi.nlm.nih.gov/pubmed/14658125.
4. Kearon C, Ginsberg JS, Kovacs MJ, et al. Comparison of low-intensity warfarin therapy with conventional-intensity warfarin therapy for long-term prevention of recurrent venous thromboembolism. N Engl J Med 2003;349(7):631–9. Available at: http://www.ncbi.nlm.nih.gov/pubmed/12917299.
5. Douketis JD, Kearon C, Bates S, et al. Risk of fatal pulmonary embolism in patients with treated venous thromboembolism. JAMA 1998;279(6):458–62. Available at: http://www.ncbi.nlm.nih.gov/entrez/query.fcgi?cmd=Retrieve&db=PubMed&dopt=Citation&list_uids=9466640.
6. Lee AY, Levine MN, Baker RI, et al. Low-molecular-weight heparin versus a coumarin for the prevention of recurrent venous thromboembolism in patients with cancer. N Engl J Med 2003;349(2):146–53. Available at: http://www.ncbi.nlm.nih.gov/pubmed/12853587.
7. Hull RD, Pineo GF, Brant R, et al, LITE Trial Investigators. Home therapy of venous thrombosis with long-term LMWH versus usual care: patient satisfaction and post-thrombotic syndrome. Am J Med 2009;122(8):762–9.e3. Available at: http://www.ncbi.nlm.nih.gov/pubmed/19635277.
8. EINSTEIN Investigators, Bauersachs R, Berkowitz SD, Brenner B, et al. Oral rivaroxaban for symptomatic venous thromboembolism. N Engl J Med 2010;363(26): 2499–510. Available at: https://www.ncbi.nlm.nih.gov/pubmed/21128814.
9. Schulman S, Kearon C, Kakkar AK, et al, RE-COVER Study Group. Dabigatran versus warfarin in the treatment of acute venous thromboembolism. N Engl J Med 2009;361(24):2342–52. Available at: https://www.ncbi.nlm.nih.gov/pubmed/19966341.
10. Hokusai VTEI, Buller HR, Decousus H, et al. Edoxaban versus warfarin for the treatment of symptomatic venous thromboembolism. N Engl J Med 2013; 369(15):1406–15. Available at: https://www.ncbi.nlm.nih.gov/pubmed/23991658.
11. Agnelli G, Buller HR, Cohen A, et al. Oral apixaban for the treatment of acute venous thromboembolism. N Engl J Med 2013;369(9):799–808. Available at: https://www.ncbi.nlm.nih.gov/pubmed/23808982.
12. Knepper J, Horne D, Obi A, et al. A systematic update on the state of the novel anticoagulants and a primer on reversal and bridging. J Vasc Surg Venous Lymphat

Disord 2013;1(4):418–26. Available at: https://www.ncbi.nlm.nih.gov/pubmed/26992768.

13. Pollack CV Jr, Reilly PA, Eikelboom J, et al. Idarucizumab for Dabigatran Reversal. N Engl J Med 2015;373(6):511–20. Available at: https://www.ncbi.nlm.nih.gov/pubmed/26095746.

14. Siegal DM, Curnutte JT, Connolly SJ, et al. Andexanet Alfa for the Reversal of Factor Xa Inhibitor Activity. N Engl J Med 2015;373(25):2413–24. Available at: https://www.ncbi.nlm.nih.gov/pubmed/26559317.

15. Crowther M, Crowther MA. Antidotes for novel oral anticoagulants: current status and future potential. Arterioscler Thromb Vasc Biol 2015;35(8):1736–45. Available at: https://www.ncbi.nlm.nih.gov/pubmed/26088576.

16. Kearon C, Akl EA, Ornelas J, et al. Antithrombotic Therapy for VTE Disease: CHEST Guideline and Expert Panel Report. Chest 2016;149(2):315–52. Available at: https://www.ncbi.nlm.nih.gov/pubmed/26867832.

17. Kataruka A, Kong X, Haymart B, et al. SAMe-TT2R2 predicts quality of anticoagulation in patients with acute venous thromboembolism: the MAQI2 experience. Vasc Med 2017;22(3):197–203. Available at: https://www.ncbi.nlm.nih.gov/pubmed/28145152.

18. Gabriel F, Portoles O, Labios M, et al, RIETE Investigators. Usefulness of thrombophilia testing in venous thromboembolic disease: findings from the RIETE registry. Clin Appl Thromb Hemost 2013;19(1):42–7. Available at: https://www.ncbi.nlm.nih.gov/pubmed/22327823.

19. Palareti G, Cosmi B, Legnani C, et al. D-dimer testing to determine the duration of anticoagulation therapy. N Engl J Med 2006;355(17):1780–9. Available at: https://www.ncbi.nlm.nih.gov/pubmed/17065639.

20. Rodger MA, Le Gal G, Anderson DR, et al. Validating the HERDOO2 rule to guide treatment duration for women with unprovoked venous thrombosis: multinational prospective cohort management study. BMJ 2017;356(j1065). Available at: https://www.ncbi.nlm.nih.gov/pubmed/28314711.

21. Kearon C, Gent M, Hirsh J, et al. A comparison of three months of anticoagulation with extended anticoagulation for a first episode of idiopathic venous thromboembolism. N Engl J Med 1999;340(12):901–7. Available at: http://www.ncbi.nlm.nih.gov/entrez/query.fcgi?cmd=Retrieve&db=PubMed&dopt=Citation&list_uids=10089183.

22. Simes J, Becattini C, Agnelli G, et al, INSPIRE Study Investigators (International Collaboration of Aspirin Trials for Recurrent Venous Thromboembolism). Aspirin for the prevention of recurrent venous thromboembolism: the INSPIRE collaboration. Circulation 2014;130(13):1062–71. Available at: https://www.ncbi.nlm.nih.gov/pubmed/25156992.

23. Becattini C, Agnelli G, Schenone A, et al. Aspirin for preventing the recurrence of venous thromboembolism. N Engl J Med 2012;366(21):1959–67. Available at: https://www.ncbi.nlm.nih.gov/pubmed/22621626.

24. Weitz JI, Lensing AWA, Prins MH, et al. Rivaroxaban or Aspirin for Extended Treatment of Venous Thromboembolism. N Engl J Med 2017;376(13):1211–22. Available at: https://www.ncbi.nlm.nih.gov/pubmed/28316279.

25. Agnelli G, Buller HR, Cohen A, et al, AMPLIFY-EXT Investigators. Apixaban for extended treatment of venous thromboembolism. N Engl J Med 2013;368(8):699–708. Available at: https://www.ncbi.nlm.nih.gov/pubmed/23216615.

26. Spencer FA, Lessard D, Emery C, et al. Venous thromboembolism in the outpatient setting. Arch Intern Med 2007;167(14):1471–5. Available at: http://www.

ncbi.nlm.nih.gov/entrez/query.fcgi?cmd=Retrieve&db=PubMed&dopt=Citation&list_uids=17646600.

27. White RH, Zhou H, Romano PS. Incidence of symptomatic venous thromboembolism after different elective or urgent surgical procedures. Thromb Haemost 2003;90(3):446–55. Available at: http://www.ncbi.nlm.nih.gov/entrez/query.fcgi?cmd=Retrieve&db=PubMed&dopt=Citation&list_uids=12958614.

28. Amin AN, Varker H, Princic N, et al. Duration of venous thromboembolism risk across a continuum in medically ill hospitalized patients. J Hosp Med 2012; 7(3):231–8. Available at: https://www.ncbi.nlm.nih.gov/pubmed/22190427.

29. Sweetland S, Green J, Liu B, et al, Million Women Study Collaborators. Duration and magnitude of the postoperative risk of venous thromboembolism in middle aged women: prospective cohort study. BMJ 2009;339:b4583. Available at: https://www.ncbi.nlm.nih.gov/pubmed/19959589.

30. Efficacy and safety of enoxaparin versus unfractionated heparin for prevention of deep vein thrombosis in elective cancer surgery: a double-blind randomized multicentre trial with venographic assessment. ENOXACAN Study Group. Br J Surg 1997;84(8):1099–103. Available at: http://www.ncbi.nlm.nih.gov/entrez/query.fcgi?cmd=Retrieve&db=PubMed&dopt=Citation&list_uids=9278651.

31. Bergqvist D, Agnelli G, Cohen AT, et al, ENOXACAN II Investigators. Duration of prophylaxis against venous thromboembolism with enoxaparin after surgery for cancer. N Engl J Med 2002;346(13):975–80. Available at: https://www.ncbi.nlm.nih.gov/pubmed/11919306.

32. Gould MK, Garcia DA, Wren SM, et al. Prevention of VTE in nonorthopedic surgical patients: antithrombotic therapy and prevention of thrombosis, 9th ed: American College of Chest Physicians Evidence-Based Clinical Practice Guidelines. Chest 2012;141(2 Suppl):e227S–77S. Available at: https://www.ncbi.nlm.nih.gov/pubmed/22315263.

33. Lyman GH, Bohlke K, Falanga A, American Society of Clinical Oncology. Venous thromboembolism prophylaxis and treatment in patients with cancer: American Society of Clinical Oncology clinical practice guideline update. J Oncol Pract 2015; 11(3):e442–4. Available at: https://www.ncbi.nlm.nih.gov/pubmed/25873061.

34. Vedovati MC, Becattini C, Rondelli F, et al. A randomized study on 1-week versus 4-week prophylaxis for venous thromboembolism after laparoscopic surgery for colorectal cancer. Ann Surg 2014;259(4):665–9. Available at: http://www.ncbi.nlm.nih.gov/pubmed/24253138.

35. Falck-Ytter Y, Francis CW, Johanson NA, et al. Prevention of VTE in orthopedic surgery patients: antithrombotic therapy and prevention of thrombosis, 9th ed: American College of Chest Physicians Evidence-Based Clinical Practice Guidelines. Chest 2012;141(2 Suppl):e278S–325S. Available at: https://www.ncbi.nlm.nih.gov/pubmed/22315265.

36. White RH, Romano PS, Zhou H, et al. Incidence and time course of thromboembolic outcomes following total hip or knee arthroplasty. Arch Intern Med 1998; 158(14):1525–31. Available at: https://www.ncbi.nlm.nih.gov/pubmed/9679793.

37. Guyatt GH, Akl EA, Crowther M, et al, American College of Chest Physicians Antithrombotic Therapy and Prevention of Thrombosis Panel. Executive summary: antithrombotic therapy and prevention of thrombosis, 9th ed: American College of Chest Physicians Evidence-Based Clinical Practice Guidelines. Chest 2012;141(2 Suppl):7S–47S. Available at: https://www.ncbi.nlm.nih.gov/pubmed/22315257.

38. Eriksson BI, Dahl OE, Huo MH, et al, RE-NOVATE II Study Group. Oral dabigatran versus enoxaparin for thromboprophylaxis after primary total hip arthroplasty (RE-

NOVATE II*). A randomised, double-blind, non-inferiority trial. Thromb Haemost 2011;105(4):721–9. Available at: https://www.ncbi.nlm.nih.gov/pubmed/21225098.

39. Lassen MR, Gallus A, Raskob GE, et al, ADVANCE-3 Investigators. Apixaban versus enoxaparin for thromboprophylaxis after hip replacement. N Engl J Med 2010;363(26):2487–98. Available at: https://www.ncbi.nlm.nih.gov/pubmed/21175312.

40. Eriksson BI, Borris LC, Friedman RJ, et al. Rivaroxaban versus enoxaparin for thromboprophylaxis after hip arthroplasty. N Engl J Med 2008;358(26):2765–75. Available at: https://www.ncbi.nlm.nih.gov/pubmed/18579811.

41. Nikolaou VS, Desy NM, Bergeron SG, et al. Total knee replacement and chemical thromboprophylaxis: current evidence. Curr Vasc Pharmacol 2011;9(1):33–41. Available at: https://www.ncbi.nlm.nih.gov/pubmed/21044024.

42. Hull RD, Schellong SM, Tapson VF, et al, EXCLAIM (Extended Prophylaxis for Venous ThromboEmbolism in Acutely Ill Medical Patients With Prolonged Immobilization) study. Extended-duration venous thromboembolism prophylaxis in acutely ill medical patients with recently reduced mobility: a randomized trial. Ann Intern Med 2010;153(1):8–18. Available at: https://www.ncbi.nlm.nih.gov/pubmed/20621900.

43. Goldhaber SZ, Leizorovicz A, Kakkar AK, et al, ADOPT Trial Investigators. Apixaban versus enoxaparin for thromboprophylaxis in medically ill patients. N Engl J Med 2011;365(23):2167–77. Available at: https://www.ncbi.nlm.nih.gov/pubmed/22077144.

44. Cohen AT, Harrington RA, Goldhaber SZ, et al, APEX Investigators. Extended Thromboprophylaxis with Betrixaban in Acutely Ill Medical Patients. N Engl J Med 2016;375(6):534–44. Extended. Available at: https://www.ncbi.nlm.nih.gov/pubmed/27232649.

45. Cohen AT, Spiro TE, Buller HR, et al. Extended-duration rivaroxaban thromboprophylaxis in acutely ill medical patients: MAGELLAN study protocol. J Thromb Thrombolysis 2011;31(4):407–16. Available at: https://www.ncbi.nlm.nih.gov/pubmed/21359646.

46. Dentali F, Mumoli N, Prisco D, et al. Efficacy and safety of extended thromboprophylaxis for medically ill patients. A meta-analysis of randomised controlled trials. Thromb Haemost 2017;117(3):606–17. Available at: https://www.ncbi.nlm.nih.gov/pubmed/28078350.

47. Raskob GE, Spyropoulos AC, Zrubek J, et al. The MARINER trial of rivaroxaban after hospital discharge for medical patients at high risk of VTE. Design, rationale, and clinical implications. Thromb Haemost 2016;115(6):1240–8. Available at: https://www.ncbi.nlm.nih.gov/pubmed/26842902.

48. Douketis JD, Healey JS, Brueckmann M, et al. Perioperative bridging anticoagulation during dabigatran or warfarin interruption among patients who had an elective surgery or procedure. Substudy of the RE-LY trial. Thromb Haemost 2015;113(3):625–32. Available at: https://www.ncbi.nlm.nih.gov/pubmed/25472710.

49. Rechenmacher SJ, Fang JC. Bridging anticoagulation: primum non nocere. J Am Coll Cardiol 2015;66(12):1392–403. Available at: https://www.ncbi.nlm.nih.gov/pubmed/26383727.

50. Doherty JU, Gluckman TJ, Hucker WJ, et al. 2017 ACC expert consensus decision pathway for periprocedural management of anticoagulation in patients with nonvalvular atrial fibrillation: a report of the American College of Cardiology Clinical Expert Consensus Document Task Force. J Am Coll Cardiol 2017;69(7):871–98. Available at: https://www.ncbi.nlm.nih.gov/pubmed/28081965.

51. Wysokinski WE, McBane RD 2nd. Periprocedural bridging management of anti-coagulation. Circulation 2012;126(4):486–90. Available at: https://www.ncbi.nlm.nih.gov/pubmed/22825410.

52. Nishimura RA, Otto CM, Bonow RO, et al. 2017 AHA/ACC Focused Update of the 2014 AHA/ACC Guideline for the Management of Patients With Valvular Heart Disease: a report of the American College of Cardiology/American Heart Association Task Force on Clinical Practice Guidelines. Circulation 2017;135(25):e1159–95. Available at: https://www.ncbi.nlm.nih.gov/pubmed/28298458.

53. Baron TH, Kamath PS, McBane RD. Management of antithrombotic therapy in patients undergoing invasive procedures. N Engl J Med 2013;368(22):2113–24. Available at: https://www.ncbi.nlm.nih.gov/pubmed/23718166.

54. NOACS/DOACS. Peri-operative management. Whitby, ON, Canada: Thrombosis Canada; 2017. p. 1–7. Available at: http://thrombosiscanada.ca/wp-content/uploads/2017/09/22_NOACs-DOACs-Peri-Operative-Management-2017Jul26.pdf.

55. Birnie DH, Healey JS, Wells GA, et al. Pacemaker or defibrillator surgery without interruption of anticoagulation. N Engl J Med 2013;368(22):2084–93. Available at: https://www.ncbi.nlm.nih.gov/pubmed/23659733.

56. Raval AN, Cigarroa JE, Chung MK, et al. Management of patients on non-vitamin K antagonist oral anticoagulants in the acute care and periprocedural setting: a scientific statement from the American Heart Association. Circulation 2017;135(10):e604–33. Available at: https://www.ncbi.nlm.nih.gov/pubmed/28167634.

Evidence-Based Therapies for Pharmacologic Prevention and Treatment of Acute Deep Vein Thrombosis and Pulmonary Embolism

Ben Jacobs, MD, Peter K. Henke, MD*

KEYWORDS

- Venous thromboembolism • Pulmonary embolism • Deep vein thrombosis
- Anticoagulation • Thrombolysis • Risk prediction

KEY POINTS

- DVT and pulmonary embolism remain a significantly morbid and mortal problem in the world.
- A useful classification of DVT is those with temporally related risks and those without, so-called unprovoked, because the latter has higher risk of recurrence.
- The key to prevention of VTE is adequate and specific risk assessment, and appropriate timely prophylaxis.
- The standard therapy for VTE is rapid anticoagulation with LMWH or fondaparinux followed by a direct oral anticoagulant or warfarin.
- Appropriately selected patients with iliofemoral DVT may benefit from catheter-directed pharmacomechanical thrombolysis.

INTRODUCTION

Deep vein thrombosis (DVT) represents a significant burden of disease in North America.[1–3] The long-term sequela of DVT is the post-thrombotic syndrome, characterized by chronic, potentially severe, lower extremity swelling and skin ulceration. DVT also has potentially life-threatening sequela in the form of pulmonary embolism, which can be rapidly fatal, with debilitating long-term sequelae of its own, including heart failure and pulmonary hypertension. Together, DVT and pulmonary embolism encompass venous thromboembolic (VTE) disease. Despite continued improvements in prevention, diagnosis, and treatment of VTE, its incidence has remained steady in recent decades.

The authors have nothing to disclose.
Section of Vascular Surgery, Department of Surgery, University of Michigan, 1500 East Medical Center Drive, Ann Arbor, MI 48109, USA
* Corresponding author.
E-mail address: henke@umich.edu

Surg Clin N Am 98 (2018) 239–253
https://doi.org/10.1016/j.suc.2017.11.001
0039-6109/18/© 2017 Elsevier Inc. All rights reserved.

surgical.theclinics.com

DVT of the lower extremity is divided into categories based on anatomic distribution of the thrombus: iliocaval, iliofemoral, or femoropopliteal. Clinicians often forgo these more precise terms in favor of the more general "proximal" and "distal" DVT.

EPIDEMIOLOGY AND RISK FACTORS

When considering the epidemiology of DVT, it is important to consider two general classes of patient: those in the community and those in the hospital. In the past two decades VTE rates have remained stable or slightly increased. Generally speaking, annual VTE incidence ranges roughly from 100 to 200 events per 100,000 person-years, as estimated from the Olmsted County, Minnesota database.[4] African-Americans have the highest incidence, followed by white persons, with the lowest incidence found in Asian-Americans and Hispanics.

Recurrence of VTE is common, and occurs in roughly 30% of patients at 10 years. Risk of recurrence is greatest within the first 6 to 12 months after initial diagnosis. Independent predictors of recurrence for the most part map to risk factors for initial VTE, including male sex, increasing age, higher body mass index, malignancy, genetic hypercoagulable states, and leg paresis or paralysis from neurologic diseases or injury. Importantly, idiopathic, or unprovoked, VTE carries an increased risk of recurrence.[5] Certain factors predisposing to the development of initial VTE are associated with a lower risk of recurrence. These include development of VTE during pregnancy or peripartum, hormonal therapies including oral contraceptives, and gynecologic surgery.

Numerous risk factors have been identified for VTE (**Box 1**). Risk factors are conceptualized as either patient-specific or disease-specific.

Patient-Specific Risk Factors

Several patient-specific factors influence the risk of VTE, including age, body mass index, gender, genetic hypercoagulability, or coronary artery disease. Personal history

---

Box 1
Risk factors for venous thromboembolism

Patient-specific risk factors

Age

Body mass index

Sex

Genetic hypercoagulability

Personal history of VTE

Family history of VTE

Pregnancy

Disease-specific risk factors

Malignancy

Trauma

Major surgery

Inflammatory bowel disease

Sepsis

Rheumatic disease

of VTE is the strongest patient-specific risk factor. Around 25% of patients developing DVT have a personal history of the disease.[6,7] Patients of any age can develop DVT, although increasing age is a strong risk factor for occurrence. There is a 30-fold increase in DVT risk between patients aged 30 and those aged 80.[8] At ages younger than 45 years, VTE more commonly affects females; this predominance disappears after that age, and VTE is more common in males at older ages. The effect of age on DVT incidence may represent increasing biologic predisposition with aging and collinearity of age with development of other risk factors.[9]

Disease-Specific Risk Factors

The most significant disease-specific risk factors are active malignancy and major surgery.[2,10,11] About 30% of new diagnoses of VTE occur in the setting of malignancy. Indeed, VTE-related mortality is second only to infection as cause of death in patients with cancer.[12]

A 70-fold increase in risk has been identified in hospitalized patients over the general population, and roughly one-third of patients admitted to hospitals in the United States are at risk for VTE while inpatient.[13] Surgery drastically increases the risk of VTE in the perioperative period, remaining elevated up to 12 weeks after an operation. This is true across a broad range of common and uncommon operations.[11,14–16] Risk varies considerably by type of operation performed,[17] with the highest risks associated with orthopedic and oncologic surgeries, and a low risk associated with outpatient operations, such as laparoscopic cholecystectomy and breast surgery.[11,17,18]

Traumatic injury, especially when followed by critical illness, is strongly associated with the development of VTE.[1] The presence of venous varicosities has unclear effects on risk, but has been shown in some studies to confer an increased risk of VTE.[19] VTE also is associated with many specific disease states, including inflammatory bowel disease, sepsis, bacteremia, and rheumatic disease, and pregnancy.

PATHOPHYSIOLOGY

VTE is a multifactorial disease. The traditional understanding of the pathogenesis of VTE has been based in Virchow triad: blood stasis, injury to the endothelium, and hypercoagulable state. Scientific developments of the past few decades have demonstrated that Virchow triad represents a somewhat oversimplified construct, but it remains an excellent framework for conceptualizing the roles of the various players in the hemostatic and thrombotic processes. Indeed, the complex interrelationships between these factors are broadly categorized as relating to endothelial damage and activation, fluid dynamics in the valve pocket and vessel lumen, and hypercoagulable state, although hypercoagulability is now believed to result from baseline states (eg, genetic predisposition) and from disease-specific states relating to systemic and local activation of inflammatory cascades. Activation and inhibition of the coagulation and inflammatory cascades are paired, and linked at multiple points. This likely arises from the evolutionary necessity for these systems to work in tandem for the maintenance of bodily integrity in injury and fighting of infection.

Normal hemostasis begins immediately on endothelial disruption. The initial cells involved are platelets and the endothelium. Ultimately, coagulation proceeds through a series of serine proteases, culminating in the creation of thrombin, which cleaves soluble fibrinogen to insoluble fibrin. Physiologic hemostasis is protective, and the response of the hemodynamic and inflammatory mechanisms to tissue injury. However, pathologic thrombosis occurs independently of direct tissue injury, when these systems are activated inappropriately in response to some stress. Turbulent flow in the valve pockets of the deep veins creates a hypoxic stress, leading to inappropriate endothelial activation and development of microthromboses at these locations.[20] Endothelium exposed to local hypoxia upregulates expression of P-selectin, which in turn initiates platelet activation and adherence of tissue-factor bearing microparticles and leukocytes.[1] In most patients these microthrombi are transient, when countervailing mechanisms dissolve the thrombus before a clinical effect is seen. However, in patients in whom these mechanisms are dysregulated, these microthrombi progress to acute thrombosis of the deep veins.

PREVENTION OF VENOUS THROMBOEMBOLISM

VTE is one of the most common preventable diseases, and as such, it represents a significant challenge. The importance of efforts to prevent VTE has been emphasized by numerous institutions and societies.[21] Several risk assessment models have been created for assessment of VTE risk. The most commonly used and well validated is the Caprini score (**Fig. 1**), which performs well in many types of surgical patients.[16,22–24] For example, the 2005 Caprini score has been integrated into the electronic medical record at the University of Michigan Hospitals and Health System and associated with increased prophylaxis compliance.[25,26] Risk is estimated by calculation of a score after assessment of the patient for 40 individual risk factors. Risk factors are given

Venous Thromboembolism
Risk Factor Assessment

Please Choose All That Apply

Each Risk Factor Represents 1 Point
- ☐ Age 41–60 y
- ☐ Minor surgery planned (<45 min)
- ☐ History of prior major surgery (<1 mo)
- ☐ Varicose veins
- ☐ History of inflammatory bowel disease
- ☐ Swollen legs (current)
- ☐ Obesity (BMI >25)
- ☐ Acute myocardial infarction (<1 mo)
- ☐ Congestive heart failure (<1 mo)
- ☐ Sepsis (<1 mo)
- ☐ Serious lung disease including pneumonia (<1 mo)
- ☐ Abnormal pulmonary function (COPD)
- ☐ Medical patient currently at bed rest
- ☐ Other risk factors[c] _____

Each Risk Factor Represents 2 Points
- ☐ Age 61–74 y
- ☐ Major surgery (>45 min)[a]
- ☐ Arthroscopic surgery (>45 min)[a]
- ☐ Laparoscopic surgery (>45 min)[a]
- ☐ Previous or present malignancy
- ☐ Central venous access
- ☐ Immobilizing leg plaster cast (<1 mo)
- ☐ Patient confined to bed (>72 h)

For Women Only: Each Risk Factor Represents 1 Point
- ☐ Oral contraceptives or hormone replacement therapy
- ☐ Pregnancy or postpartum (<1 mo)
- ☐ History of unexplained stillborn infant, recurrent spontaneous abortion (≥3), premature birth with toxemia or growth-restricted infant

Each Risk Factor Represents 3 Points
- ☐ Age 75 y or more
- ☐ History of DVT/PE
- ☐ Family history of DVT/PE[b]
- ☐ Positive Factor V Leiden
- ☐ Positive Prothrombin 20210A
- ☐ Elevated serum homocysteine
- ☐ Positive Lupus anticoagulant
- ☐ Elevated anticardiolipin antibodies
- ☐ Heparin-induced thrombocytopenia (HIT)
- ☐ Other congenital or acquired thrombophilia
- ☐ If yes:
     Type _____

Each Risk Factor Represents 5 Points
- ☐ Elective major lower extremity arthroplasty
- ☐ Hip, pelvis or leg fracture (<1 mo)
- ☐ Stroke (<1 mo)
- ☐ Multiple trauma (<1 mo)
- ☐ Acute spinal cord injury (paralysis)(<1 mo)

Total Risk Factor Score =

Fig. 1. Caprini score worksheet for Venous Thromboembolism risk factor assessment.

different point values, based on known variations in risk with certain comorbidities or disease states, such as cancer or a personal history of VTE.

The use of risk-stratification is predicated on evidence for the effectiveness of pharmacoprophylaxis. The utility of individualized risk stratification in general, and the 2005 Caprini score specifically, is that it identifies high-risk patients and also identifies patients who will benefit from a targeted intervention to decrease VTE risk with chemoprophylaxis.[27,28] Meta-analyses in surgical patients as a whole also have suggested this.[29,30]

Pharmacologic Prevention

Heparin and low-molecular-weight heparin

Unfractionated heparin (UFH) and low-molecular-weight heparin (LMWH) are the most commonly used prophylactic agents for DVT (**Table 1**). LMWH and UFH have shown efficacy for prevention of DVT in a variety of patients, with LMWH showing superiority in some trials for patients with cancer and trauma patients.[31] Dosing is either once or twice daily, and is adjusted for patient factors, such as obesity or renal insufficiency.

Direct oral anticoagulants for venous thromboembolic disease prevention

The direct oral anticoagulants (DOACs) have been investigated for VTE prophylaxis in several patient populations. Lassen and colleagues[32] showed that rivaroxiban was noninferior to LMWH in patients undergoing hip and knee arthroplasty. Dabigatran has also been shown to be noninferior in these patients.[33] Apixaban was similarly shown noninferior for VTE prophylaxis.[34]

DIAGNOSIS OF VENOUS THROMBOEMBOLISM

The diagnosis of DVT has been the subject of intense research over the past several decades. Because clinical presentation is not always reliable, several additional tests are usually necessary to establish a definitive diagnosis of DVT.

Clinical Presentation

The clinical presentation of DVT is varied, and patients can present anywhere along a range from asymptomatic to critically ill. The most commonly associated symptoms are edema greater in one leg than the other, leg discomfort, erythema, and fever. Homan sign (pain on forced dorsiflexion of the foot) is not reliable for the diagnosis of DVT and should not be used. Patients in rare cases present with phlegmasia cerulean dolens, in which the affected leg is tense, pulseless, and severely tender. These

Table 1
Venous thromboembolism prophylaxis recommendations for Caprini Risk Score

Caprini Score	Risk Level	Prophylaxis Recommendation
0	Very low	Early ambulation
1–2	Low	Mechanical prophylaxis (sequential compression)
3–4	Moderate	Chemoprophylaxis (mechanical prophylaxis optional) Heparin, 5000 units SC TID Low-molecular-weight heparin, 30 units SC BID Low-molecular-weight heparin, 40 units SC QD
≥5	High	Chemoprophylaxis *and* mechanical prophylaxis Heparin, 5000 units SC TID Low-molecular-weight heparin, 30 units SC BID Low-molecular-weight heparin, 40 units SC QD

Abbreviation: SC, subcutaneous.

Box 2
Postoperative laboratory monitoring

Fibrinogen level <100 mg/dL

Half the tissue plasminogen activator dose

2 units cryoprecipitate STAT

Repeat fibrinogen 1 hour after completion of cryoprecipitate infusion

Fibrinogen level <50 mg/dL

Stop tissue plasminogen activator

2 units cryoprecipitate STAT

Repeat fibrinogen 1 hour after completion of cryoprecipitate infusion

---

patients have compromised arterial inflow to the leg because of elevated venous pressures and represent a true surgical emergency.

Prediction Scores

Because clinical presentation and physical examination are unreliable in DVT, much work has been done in the creation and validation of prediction scores to aid in the diagnosis of DVT. The most commonly used is the Well score (**Box 2**). It combines several patient factors with a score of 1 point each to allow for stratification of patients into low-, intermediate-, or high-risk groups. There is a subjective component to the score, in which negative 2 points are given for an alternative diagnosis that seems as or more likely than DVT.

Patients with a low-likelihood Well score should be evaluated with biomarker measurement, whereas those with a high likelihood of DVT should undergo diagnostic ultrasound (**Fig. 2**). The American College of Chest Physicians (ACCP) Guidelines currently make a grade 2B recommendation that choice of diagnostic test for VTE be guided first by estimation of the patient's pretest probability.[35]

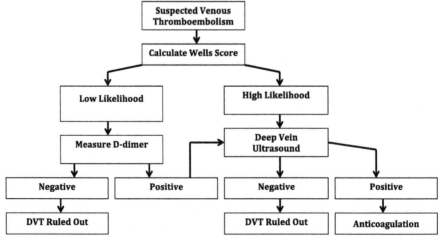

Fig. 2. Suspected venous thromboembolism flow chart.

Biomarkers

The most commonly used biomarker for the diagnosis of DVT is D-dimer, a degradation product of fibrin. The advantage of D-dimer is its high sensitivity but low specificity, which means that it makes an excellent "rule out," but not "rule in" test. Importantly, D-dimer is elevated by several other physiologic and pathologic states, including pregnancy, trauma, recent surgery, and malignancy. These factors decrease the specificity of D-dimer in precisely those patients at greatest risk for DVT. Moreover, there is variation in the diagnostic accuracy of each of the several types of D-dimer assay, and different methods are in use in different hospital systems.[36] The accuracy of D-dimer is significantly improved when used in combination with a clinical prediction score, such as the Well score.

Soluble P-selectin is currently under investigation as a complement to D-dimer.[37] Although P-selectin is not in wide clinical use, new evidence continues to lend support to the use of P-selectin as a "rule-in" test.[38] It has been shown to provide a greater specificity for the diagnosis of DVT than D-dimer and has performed well in patients with malignancy. When simple assays for P-selectin are more widely available, it likely will provide a high level of diagnostic accuracy when used in combination with the Well score and D-dimer.

Ultrasound

Ultrasound has supplanted venography as the gold standard for the diagnosis of DVT.[39] The ACCP Guidelines recommend use of ultrasound as the initial test in those patients in whom there is a high suspicion of DVT or a low suspicion of DVT, but who have a comorbid condition known to increase the D-dimer in the absence of thrombosis. In those patients with a low suspicion for DVT, in whom D-dimer is positive, ultrasound should be the next diagnostic maneuver. Ultrasound is preferred over venography with a grade 1B recommendation. Ultrasound is, however, limited by operator dependency and variable patterns of availability at odd hours in some hospital systems.

Venography

Contrast venography is an invasive test and has been supplanted as the gold standard for DVT diagnosis by compression ultrasound. The invasive nature of venography, its greater expense, hypersensitivity reactions and nephrotoxicity from contrast agents, and the high diagnostic performance of compression ultrasound have contributed to this change in practice. The ACCP does make exception in the 2012 Guidelines regarding the use of venography in patients in a situation where the patient or provider places a greater weight on avoiding the consequences of treating a false-positive result or avoiding the inconvenience of serial ultrasounds in certain patients.

TREATMENT OF VENOUS THROMBOEMBOLISM
Initial Therapy

All patients are initiated on full parenteral anticoagulation on diagnosis. Other, non-pharmacologic therapies include compression and early ambulation. Guidelines recommend initiation of anticoagulation before definitive diagnosis in patients with an intermediate or high likelihood of VTE. UFH can be used during this period, according to established nomograms based on weight, and most often for inpatients. For patients with a low suspicion of VTE, no presumptive therapy is needed while awaiting the results of diagnostic tests. Moreover, patients with initial diagnostic test suggesting a distal (calf-vein) DVT, without risk factors for extension and without severe symptoms, can be followed with serial ultrasound imaging for the first 2 weeks without starting anticoagulant therapy (grade 2C). If there is no extension of the clot after 2 weeks, no therapeutic intervention is necessary (grade 1B).[40]

The choice of initial parenteral therapy is a LMWH, fondaparinux, and followed by a vitamin K antagonist (VKA) or one of the DOACs. If VKA is the chosen anticoagulant, it is begun on the day of diagnosis concurrently with LMWH. Guidelines for patients being treated as an outpatient recommend beginning with a warfarin dose of 10 mg, followed by international normalized ratio (INR) measurements each day for the first 2 days, followed by INR measurement at longer intervals once the initial dose has stabilized.[40] The INR goal for these patients is between 2.0 and 3.0.

LMWH and fondaparinux should be avoided in patients with renal insufficiency, or the dose should be adjusted appropriately. LMWH does not require laboratory monitoring, in general. In many cases, decision to choose LMWH over VKA is made based on patient comfort, cost, and access to routine testing.

The latest recommendations of the 2016 ACCP update (**Table 2**) are to use a DOAC over VKA in patients without cancer (grade 2B).[41] Evidence for their use in cancer has been regarded as insufficient, because cancer has been an exclusion criterion in many currently published trials.[40] However, in a post hoc analysis of two trials using dabigatran for VTE treatment, efficacy was found similar to warfarin.[42] The benefits of DOACs are their use without regular INR monitoring, the decreased likelihood of dietary effects on dosing and pharmacokinetics, and generally lower bleeding risk. Dabigatran has been demonstrated to be noninferior for patients with acute DVT in several studies, and has demonstrated a lower bleeding risk than warfarin. Apixaban was shown to reduce the risk of recurrent DVT with extended use, without a concomitant increase in bleeding risk in patients so treated.

Duration of Therapy

Three months of oral anticoagulant therapy are recommended for all initial episodes of VTE, except in the case of patients with known, uncured malignancy, in which case anticoagulation is continued until the patient is cancer free (**Fig. 3**).[41] In patients in whom there is a low or moderate bleeding risk, with unprovoked iliofemoral DVT, the ACCP Guidelines recommend continuation of anticoagulation longer than 3 months (grade 2B).[41] Once completed, the VKA can simply be stopped; there is no need to gradually taper the dose. High-bleeding-risk patients should have only 3 months of anticoagulation.

Continuation of anticoagulation after the first 3 months is made based on D-dimer level at the end of treatment.[43] A prolonged elevation of D-dimer after treatment of initial DVT has been shown to predict recurrence with a hazard ratio of 2.27 ($P = .02$).[44] There is unclear benefit to aspirin after initial 3 months, although it is recommended in patients at moderate risk for recurrence, whereas those at a high risk for recurrence should continue anticoagulation therapy.[45]

Reversal Agents

Agents for reversal of anticoagulation are presented in **Table 3**. LMWH is reversed by aripazine or protamine. Warfarin is best reversed with prothrombin complex concentrate (PCC), according to most recent guidelines, supplanting fresh frozen plasma as the preferred reversal agent.[46] PCC is available in three-factor or four-factor forms. Four-factor PCC is generally preferred because three-factor PCC has low amounts of factor VII and thus also requires administration of fresh frozen plasma to reverse VKAs completely. Until recently, no specific reversal agent was available for the

Table 2
Summary of American College of Chest Physicians 2016 antithrombotic therapy for VTE guidelines: key recommendations and updates

Recommendation	Grade
Choice of anticoagulant	
Patients with proximal DVT or PE without cancer should receive 3 mo of therapy with NOAC or VKA, rather than with low-molecular-weight heparin.	1B
In patients with VTE without cancer, choice of anticoagulant therapy should be 3 mo with a NOAC, rather than with WKA.	2B
In patients with VTE with cancer, choice of anticoagulant therapy should be 3 mo with low-molecular-weight heparin, rather than NOAC or VKA.	2C
Duration of treatment	
Patients with DVT or PE provoked by surgery or a nonsurgical transient risk factor should receive 3 mo of therapy.	1B
Patients with unprovoked proximal DVT or PE with a low to moderate bleeding risk should receive extended anticoagulant therapy; no scheduled stop date.	2B
Patients with unprovoked proximal DVT or PE with a high bleeding risk should receive 3 mo of anticoagulant therapy, rather than with no scheduled stop date.	1B
In patients with unprovoked proximal DVT, aspirin is recommended after stopping anticoagulation for patients in whom there is no contraindication.	2B
Treatment of isolated distal DVT	
Patients with isolated distal DVT with no risk factors for extension (cancer, >5 cm in length, >7 mm diameter, multiple veins) should undergo surveillance ultrasound at 2 wk.	2C
Patients treated for isolated distal DVT should receive NOAC or VKA for 3 mo, as with proximal DVT.	1B
Treatment of recurrent VTE	
Patients with recurrent VTE while undergoing treatment with VKA or NOAC therapy should be switched to LMWH, for a period of at least 1 mo.	2C
Patients with a recurrent VTE while compliant with LMWH, should have dose increased by one-quarter to one-third.	2C
Other recommendations	
In patients with acute DVT of the leg, compression stockings are not recommended for the prevention of post-thrombotic syndrome.	2B
In patients with subsegmental PE, anticoagulation should be used only in those with a high risk of recurrent VTE. Patients with low risk can undergo surveillance.	2C
In patients with acute PE without hypotension, recommend against systemic thrombolytic therapy, except in those who deteriorate after anticoagulation has begun.	1B, 2C
In patients with acute PE, systemic thrombolytic therapy is preferred over catheter-directed thrombolysis.	2C
In patients with chronic thromboembolic pulmonary hypertension, recommend pulmonary thromboendarterectomy if expert treatment is available.	2C

Abbreviation: PE, pulmonary embolism.

DOACs. PCC has shown efficacy in the reversal of rivaroxiban, but not dabigatran.[47] A monoclonal antibody idarucizumab (Praxbind) was recently approved by the Food and Drug Administration for reversal of dabigatran.[48] Hemodialysis is a secondary option for reversal of dabigatran.[49] A new reversal agent for the oral anti-Xa inhibitors called andexenet alfa is currently under investigation.[50]

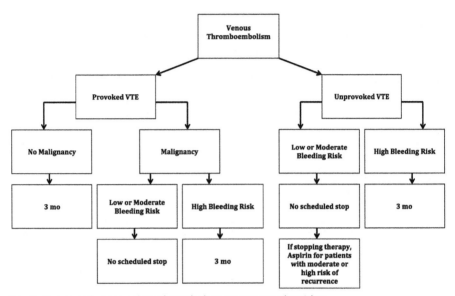

Fig. 3. Suggested venous thromboembolism treatment algorithm.

INTERVENTIONAL TREATMENT OF PROXIMAL DEEP VEIN THROMBOSIS

A possible benefit to early thrombus removal, generally by pharmacomechanical therapy, exists in properly selected patients to decrease the development of post-thrombotic syndrome. Current guidelines from the Society for Vascular Surgery and American Venous Forum recommend a strategy of early thrombus removal in patients with a first episode of iliofemoral DVT in whom thrombus has been present for fewer than 14 days and with a low risk of hemorrhagic complications (**Fig. 4**).[51]

Catheter-Directed Thrombolysis

Catheter-directed thrombolysis (CDT) is the preferred treatment of iliofemoral DVT in patients without a contraindication, such as bleeding, recent stroke within 2 months, known intracranial malignancy, aneurysm or arteriovenous malformation, active duodenal ulcer, or recent major trauma.[51]

Several trials have shown benefit to CDT for eligible patients (**Fig. 4**). A Cochrane review of randomized controlled trials of CDT found that in patients undergoing CDT there was significantly decreased likelihood of developing post-thrombotic syndrome, but with concomitant increased risk for hemorrhagic complications. The relative risk

Table 3
Reversal agents for anticoagulants

Heparin	Warfarin	Dabigatran	Rivaroxaban	Apixaban	Edoxaban
Protamine	Fresh frozen plasma PCC (four-factor PCC is preferred)	Idarucizumab– monoclonal antibody to dabigatran Hemodialysis	PCC (partially reversed activity in *in vitro* studies)	No specific antidote	No specific antidote

Andexanet: reversal agent for rivaroxaban, apixaban, edoxaban, and heparins; currently in phase 3 trials.
Ciraparantag: reversal agent for dabigatran, rivaroxaban, apixaban, edoxaban, and heparins; currently in phase 2 trials.

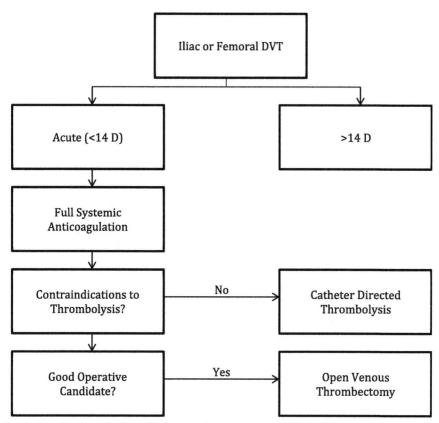

Fig. 4. Benefits to early thrombus removal.

for hemorrhagic complications was 2.23 in the CDT group (confidence interval, 1.41–3.52; P<.01). Generally, patients are considered eligible for lysis if the thrombus is fewer than 14 to 21 days old.

When CDT is performed, a catheter is first placed under ultrasound guidance, and a wire is guided through the thrombus and an infusion catheter is introduced, through which venography is performed and infusion of lytic agent can proceed. The pulse spray technique, in which a bolus dose of lytic agent is manually injected directly into the thrombus, has been shown to be more effective than infusion alone.[52] The results of studies of benefit for mechanical combined with pharmacologic lysis have been inconclusive.[53] The infusion is continued postoperatively in an intensive care unit setting to monitor for hemorrhagic complications and serial laboratory measurements including hemoglobin and hematocrit, platelets, fibrinogen, D-dimer and INR. Recombinant tissue plasminogen activator is run at a rate of 0.5 to 1 mg/h, along with UFH at a rate of 500 units/h. The University of Michigan algorithm for monitoring and dosing is presented in **Box 2**. Infusion continues for 2 to 4 days, during which time the patient is returned daily to the operating suite for repeat venography.

Open Venous Thrombectomy

Open venous thrombectomy, as described by Meissner and coworkers,[51] is another option for early thrombus removal in patients with contraindications to CDT. In a hybrid operating room, contrast venography is obtained to evaluate the inferior vena cava and iliac veins. The common femoral vein is exposed through a groin incision along with the saphenofemoral junction, the takeoff of the profunda femoral vein. Longitudinal venotomy is created in the femoral vein just distal to the saphenofemoral junction, and proximal and distal clot are removed directly with the use of Fogarty balloons. The venotomy is closed and, in some cases, followed by the creation of an arteriovenous fistula from the proximal superficial femoral artery to a transected saphenous to prevent early rethrombosis.

THE FUTURE

Current tools, such as individual VTE risk assessment, institution of appropriate VTE prophylaxis, and rapid therapy for established VTE, will greatly diminish the incidence of this disease and its sequlae. The DOACs have the potential to reduce variations in anticoagulation efficacy, and complications associated with warfarin, but the patient needs to be compliant with taking the medicine. Invasive approaches to DVT management should find their niche, and likely in properly selected low-bleeding-risk patients. Better biomarkers and therapies that affect coagulation without inhibiting hemostasis are the next frontier.

REFERENCES

1. Geerts WH, Code KI, Jay RM, et al. A prospective study of venous thromboembolism after major trauma. N Engl J Med 1994;331(24):1601–6.
2. Agnelli G, Bolis G, Capussotti L, et al. A clinical outcome-based prospective study on venous thromboembolism after cancer surgery: the @RISTOS project. Ann Surg 2006;243(1):89–95.
3. Heit JA, Silverstein MD, Mohr DN, et al. Risk factors for deep vein thrombosis and pulmonary embolism: a population-based case-control study. Arch Intern Med 2000;160(6):809–15.
4. Heit JA. Epidemiology of venous thromboembolism. Nat Rev Cardiol 2015;12(8): 464–74.
5. Prandoni P, Noventa F, Ghirarduzzi A, et al. The risk of recurrent venous thromboembolism after discontinuing anticoagulation in patients with acute proximal deep vein thrombosis or pulmonary embolism. A prospective cohort study in 1,626 patients. Haematologica 2007;92(2):199–205.
6. Piccioli A, Prandoni P, Goldhaber SZ. Epidemiologic characteristics, management, and outcome of deep venous thrombosis in a tertiary-care hospital: the Brigham and Women's Hospital DVT registry. Am Heart J 1996;132(5):1010–4.
7. Nordstrom M, Lindblad B, Bergqvist D, et al. A prospective study of the incidence of deep-vein thrombosis within a defined urban population. J Intern Med 1992; 232(2):155–60.
8. Rosendaal FR. Thrombosis in the young: epidemiology and risk factors. A focus on venous thrombosis. Thromb Haemost 1997;78(1):1–6.
9. Anderson FA Jr, Wheeler HB, Goldberg RJ, et al. The prevalence of risk factors for venous thromboembolism among hospital patients. Arch Intern Med 1992; 152(8):1660–4.
10. Osborne NH, Wakefield TW, Henke PK. Venous thromboembolism in cancer patients undergoing major surgery. Ann Surg Oncol 2008;15(12):3567–78.
11. Sweetland S, Green J, Liu B, et al. Duration and magnitude of the postoperative risk of venous thromboembolism in middle aged women: prospective cohort study. BMJ 2009;339:b4583.

12. Khorana AA, Francis CW, Culakova E, et al. Thromboembolism is a leading cause of death in cancer patients receiving outpatient chemotherapy. J Thromb Haemost 2007;5(3):632–4.

13. Anderson FA Jr, Zayaruzny M, Heit JA, et al. Estimated annual numbers of US acute-care hospital patients at risk for venous thromboembolism. Am J Hematol 2007;82(9):777–82.

14. Pannucci CJ, Basta MN, Fischer JP, et al. Creation and validation of a condition-specific venous thromboembolism risk assessment tool for ventral hernia repair. Surgery 2015;158(5):1304–13.

15. Quera R, Shanahan F. Thromboembolism: an important manifestation of inflammatory bowel disease. Am J Gastroenterol 2004;99(10):1971–3.

16. Bahl V, Hu HM, Henke PK, et al. A validation study of a retrospective venous thromboembolism risk scoring method. Ann Surg 2010;251(2):344–50.

17. White RH, Zhou H, Romano PS. Incidence of symptomatic venous thromboembolism after different elective or urgent surgical procedures. Thromb Haemost 2003; 90(3):446–55.

18. Lindberg F, Bergqvist D, Rasmussen I. Incidence of thromboembolic complications after laparoscopic cholecystectomy: review of the literature. Surg Laparosc Endosc 1997;7(4):324–31.

19. Muller-Buhl U, Leutgeb R, Engeser P, et al. Varicose veins are a risk factor for deep venous thrombosis in general practice patients. Vasa 2012;41(5):360–5.

20. Esmon CT. Basic mechanisms and pathogenesis of venous thrombosis. Blood Rev 2009;23(5):225–9.

21. Rathbun S. Cardiology patient pages. The Surgeon General's call to action to prevent deep vein thrombosis and pulmonary embolism. Circulation 2009;119(15): e480–2.

22. Pannucci CJ, Obi A, Alvarez R, et al. Inadequate venous thromboembolism risk stratification predicts venous thromboembolic events in surgical intensive care unit patients. J Am Coll Surgeons 2014;218(5):898–904.

23. Obi AT, Pannucci CJ, Nackashi A, et al. Validation of the Caprini venous thromboembolism risk assessment model in critically ill surgical patients. JAMA Surg 2015;150(10):941–8.

24. Shuman AG, Hu HM, Pannucci CJ, et al. Stratifying the risk of venous thromboembolism in otolaryngology. Otolaryngol Head Neck Surg 2012;146(5):719–24.

25. Caprini JA. Risk assessment as a guide for the prevention of the many faces of venous thromboembolism. Am J Surg 2010;199(1 Suppl):S3–10.

26. Arcelus JI, Candocia S, Traverso CI, et al. Venous thromboembolism prophylaxis and risk assessment in medical patients. Semin Thromb Hemost 1991;17(Suppl 3):313–8.

27. Bahl V, Shuman AG, Hu HM, et al. Chemoprophylaxis for venous thromboembolism in otolaryngology. JAMA Otolaryngol Head Neck Surg 2014;140(11): 999–1005.

28. Pannucci CJ, Dreszer G, Wachtman CF, et al. Postoperative enoxaparin prevents symptomatic venous thromboembolism in high-risk plastic surgery patients. Plast Reconstr Surg 2011;128(5):1093–103.

29. Pannucci CJ, Swiston J, Macdonald B, et al. The 2005 Caprini score predicts both baseline VTE risk and effectiveness of chemoprophylaxis: a meta-analysis of 13,412 surgical patients. Orlando (FL): American Venous Forum; 2016.

30. Pannucci CJ, MacDonald JK, Ariyan S, et al. Benefits and risks of prophylaxis for deep venous thrombosis and pulmonary embolus in plastic surgery: a systematic

review and meta-analysis of controlled trials and consensus conference. Plast Reconstr Surg 2016;137(2):709–30.

31. Jacobs BN, Cain-Nielsen AH, Jakubus JL, et al. Unfractionated heparin versus low molecular weight heparin for venous thromboembolism prophylaxis in trauma. J Trauma Acute Care Surg 2017;83(1):151–8.

32. Lassen MR, Gent M, Kakkar AK, et al. The effects of rivaroxaban on the complications of surgery after total hip or knee replacement: results from the RECORD programme. J Bone Joint Surg Br 2012;94(11):1573–8.

33. Eriksson BI, Dahl OE, Huo MH, et al. Oral dabigatran versus enoxaparin for thromboprophylaxis after primary total hip arthroplasty (RE-NOVATE II*). A randomised, double-blind, non-inferiority trial. Thromb Haemost 2011;105(4):721–9.

34. Goldhaber SZ, Leizorovicz A, Kakkar AK, et al. Apixaban versus enoxaparin for thromboprophylaxis in medically ill patients. N Engl J Med 2011;365(23): 2167–77.

35. Bates SM, Jaeschke R, Stevens SM, et al. Diagnosis of DVT: antithrombotic therapy and prevention of thrombosis, 9th ed: American College of Chest Physicians evidence-based clinical practice guidelines. Chest 2012;141(2 Suppl): e351S–418S.

36. Stein PD, Hull RD, Patel KC, et al. D-dimer for the exclusion of acute venous thrombosis and pulmonary embolism: a systematic review. Ann Intern Med 2004;140(8):589–602.

37. Jacobs B, Obi A, Wakefield T. Diagnostic biomarkers in venous thromboembolic disease. J Vasc Surg Venous Lymphat Disord 2016;4(4):508–17.

38. Vandy FC, Stabler C, Eliassen AM, et al. Soluble P-selectin for the diagnosis of lower extremity deep venous thrombosis. J Vasc Surg Venous Lymphatic Disord 2013;1(2):1117–25.

39. Kearon C, Julian JA, Newman TE, et al. Noninvasive diagnosis of deep venous thrombosis. McMaster diagnostic imaging practice guidelines initiative. Ann Intern Med 1998;128(8):663–77.

40. Guyatt GH, Akl EA, Crowther M, et al. Executive summary: antithrombotic therapy and prevention of thrombosis, 9th ed: American College of Chest Physicians evidence-based clinical practice guidelines. Chest 2012;141(2 Suppl):7S–47S.

41. Kearon C, Akl EA, Ornelas J, et al. Antithrombotic therapy for VTE disease: CHEST guideline and expert panel report. Chest 2016;149(2):315–52.

42. Schulman S, Goldhaber SZ, Kearon C, et al. Treatment with dabigatran or warfarin in patients with venous thromboembolism and cancer. Thromb Haemost 2015;114(1):150–7.

43. Kearon C, Spencer FA, O'Keeffe D, et al. D-dimer testing to select patients with a first unprovoked venous thromboembolism who can stop anticoagulant therapy: a cohort study. Ann Intern Med 2015;162(1):27–34.

44. Palareti G, Cosmi B, Legnani C, et al. D-dimer to guide the duration of anticoagulation in patients with venous thromboembolism: a management study. Blood 2014;124(2):196–203.

45. Wakefield TW, Obi AT, Henke PK. An aspirin a day to keep the clots away: can aspirin prevent recurrent thrombosis in extended treatment for venous thromboembolism? Circulation 2014;130(13):1031–3.

46. Khorsand N, Kooistra HA, van Hest RM, et al. A systematic review of prothrombin complex concentrate dosing strategies to reverse vitamin K antagonist therapy. Thromb Res 2015;135(1):9–19.

47. Eerenberg ES, Kamphuisen PW, Sijpkens MK, et al. Reversal of rivaroxaban and dabigatran by prothrombin complex concentrate: a randomized, placebo-controlled, crossover study in healthy subjects. Circulation 2011;124(14):1573–9.

48. Pollack CV Jr, Reilly PA, van Ryn J, et al. Idarucizumab for dabigatran reversal - full cohort analysis. N Engl J Med 2017;377(5):431–41.

49. Kaatz S, Kouides PA, Garcia DA, et al. Guidance on the emergent reversal of oral thrombin and factor Xa inhibitors. Am J Hematol 2012;87(S1):S141–5.

50. Lu G, Hollenbach SJ, Baker DC, et al. Preclinical safety and efficacy of andexanet alfa in animal models. J Thromb Haemost 2017;15(9):1747–56. Available at: https://www.ncbi.nlm.nih.gov/pubmed/?term=Preclinical+safety+and+efficacy+of+andexanet+alfa+in+animal+models2017.

51. Meissner MH, Gloviczki P, Comerota AJ, et al. Early thrombus removal strategies for acute deep venous thrombosis: clinical practice guidelines of the Society for Vascular Surgery and the American Venous Forum. J Vasc Surg 2012;55(5): 1449–62.

52. Yamada N, Ishikura K, Ota S, et al. Pulse-spray pharmacomechanical thrombolysis for proximal deep vein thrombosis. Eur J Vasc Endovascular Surg 2006; 31(2):204–11.

53. Baker R, Samuels S, Benenati JF, et al. Ultrasound-accelerated vs standard catheter-directed thrombolysis–a comparative study in patients with iliofemoral deep vein thrombosis. J Vasc Interv Radiol 2012;23(11):1460–6.

Catheter-Directed Therapy Options for Iliofemoral Venous Thrombosis

Deepak Sudheendra, MD, FSIR, RPVI[a],*, Suresh Vedantham, MD, FSIR[b]

KEYWORDS

- Deep vein thrombosis • Pulmonary embolism • Postthrombotic syndrome
- May Thurner syndrome • Iliac vein compression

KEY POINTS

- Proximal deep venous thrombosis (DVT) is linked to a 50% risk of pulmonary embolism and postthrombotic syndrome.
- Catheter-directed thrombolysis (CDT) can be a useful adjunct to anticoagulant therapy for carefully selected patients with proximal acute DVT.
- CDT combined with mechanical thrombectomy allows for greater thrombus removal and decreased use of thrombolytics.
- An individualized approach to patient selection, with careful assessment of the risk for bleeding, is recommended.
- Risk of acute kidney injury from hemoglobinuria during pharmacomechanical thrombectomy can be reduced with periprocedural hydration, alkalinization of urine, and diuresis.

INTRODUCTION

Venous thromboembolism (VTE), which includes deep venous thrombosis (DVT) and pulmonary embolism (PE), is the third leading cause of cardiovascular death behind heart attack and stroke.[1] Up to one-third of patients diagnosed with VTE will die within 1 month of diagnosis, and nearly 25% of patients with PE will have sudden death as the presenting symptom.[2] Furthermore, VTE remains the leading cause of preventable hospital death.[3,4] Despite these sobering statistics, little is known by the general public about VTE and its long-term sequelae, including chronic thromboembolic pulmonary hypertension and the postthrombotic syndrome (PTS).

Disclosure Statement: Dr D. Sudheendra is a consultant for Boston Scientific and Teleflex. Dr S. Vedantham's institution receives research support from BSN Medical and Cook Medical for studies he conducts.
[a] Department of Radiology, University of Pennsylvania, Perelman School of Medicine, 1 Silverstein, 3400 Spruce Street, Philadelphia, PA 19104, USA; [b] Mallinckrodt Institute of Radiology, Washington University in St. Louis, 510 South Kingshighway, Box 8131, St Louis, MO 63110, USA
* Corresponding author.
E-mail address: Deepak.Sudheendra@uphs.upenn.edu

Surg Clin N Am 98 (2018) 255–265
https://doi.org/10.1016/j.suc.2017.11.012
0039-6109/18/© 2017 Elsevier Inc. All rights reserved.

DVT is classified as distal (involving the calf veins) or proximal (involving the popliteal and/or more proximal veins) in nature. Although distal DVT tends to have a more benign disease course, proximal DVT is linked to an estimated 50% risk of PE and nearly 50% risk of PTS.[5,6] PTS, which consists of a medley of chronic symptoms including pain, leg swelling, skin discoloration, and sometimes progression to venous ulcers, is most commonly associated with iliofemoral DVT (which is defined as DVT involving the iliac and/or common femoral vein, with or without involvement of other veins) in particular. As a result, patients presenting with iliofemoral DVT have traditionally been considered the patients who may be most likely to experience long-term benefit from endovascular thrombus removal.

Presently, the standard of care for acute DVT is systemic anticoagulation. The purpose of systemic anticoagulation is to prevent thrombus propagation, thereby reducing the incidence of PE. However, it is the body's endogenous fibrinolytic system that plays the primary role in thrombus resolution. Even with systemic anticoagulation, the massive clot burden in iliofemoral DVT is overwhelming for the body's fibrinolytic system and usually results in incomplete clot dissolution. The remaining thrombus burden can predispose the patient to recurrent thrombosis and PTS secondary to ambulatory venous hypertension, which develops from the combination of venous obstruction and venous valvular dysfunction.

Endovascular treatment options with catheter-directed thrombolysis (CDT) and pharmacomechanical catheter-directed thrombolysis (PCDT) are often used for iliofemoral DVT to lessen the thrombus burden and expedite symptom resolution. They are also hypothesized to minimize valvular damage and thereby reduce the incidence and severity of PTS.

CLINICAL EVALUATION AND PATIENT SELECTION

Anticoagulation remains the standard of care for DVT treatment. CDT is a more aggressive treatment option requiring a thorough clinical evaluation and proper patient selection to ensure good outcomes and minimize complications. Although the vast majority of patients can be treated in a nonurgent manner, patients with a threatened limb (ie, phlegmasia cerulea dolens) warrant emergent thrombolysis and/or surgical thrombectomy for limb salvage.

Several factors must be considered in determining a suitable candidate for thrombolysis (**Fig. 1**). These factors include the following:

Age and Extent of Thrombus

Knowing the approximate age of the thrombus is critical in determining whether CDT or pharmacomechanical thrombectomy will be effective. At present, this assessment generally relies mainly on a careful medical history to document the onset date of symptoms. Noninvasive imaging with ultrasound (US) or computed tomography (CT) can lend additional information on whether the DVT is acute/subacute or chronic in nature. Thrombus that is acute ($\leq$14 days) has the highest likelihood of responding to thrombolytic therapy compared with older thrombus, which has become more organized and in some cases calcified.[7] In the authors' experience, there is no established role for thrombolytic therapy for chronic thrombus except in some situations of acute on chronic DVT. For extension of thrombus into the inferior vena cava (IVC) or free floating thrombus in the IVC, some practitioners consider the use of an IVC filter. However, the authors do not recommend this as a routine practice because available studies suggest that PE is rare with CDT. If an IVC filter is planned, the risks and benefits should be discussed with the patient.

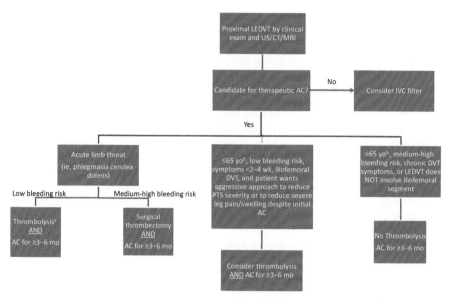

Fig. 1. Management algorithm for patients with acute proximal LEDVT. AC, anticoagulation; LEDVT, lower extremity deep vein thrombosis; PTS, postthrombotic syndrome; yo, years old. [a]Patients older than 65 years were shown to have a higher risk of bleeding from thrombolysis (as per ATTRACT study results). [b]Thrombolysis should be reserved as first-line treatment to speed symptom relief and reduce PTS in patients who want aggressive treatment (given ATTRACT study results).

Age of the Patient

Younger, healthier patients are more likely to benefit from aggressive therapy. Studies of thrombolytic therapy for multiple indications have shown that the risk of major bleeding is significantly higher for patients older than 65 years.[8]

Anatomic Abnormalities

Anatomic considerations that may increase the risk of the procedure, extend the duration of the procedure, necessitate further discussion of risk with the patient, or require more expertise include iliac vein compression (ie, May Thurner syndrome) and IVC stenosis and/or thrombosis.[9-11]

Presence of an Inferior Vena Cava Filter

The presence of an IVC filter is important in procedural planning because it will often need to be removed to prevent future complications (ie, filter fracture, IVC thrombosis) and recurrent DVT.[12] Removal of the filter may require complex IVC filter retrieval techniques necessitating referral to a more experienced center.

Patient Comorbidities Including Bleeding Diathesis

Absolute contraindications to CDT or pharmacomechanical thrombectomy include active bleeding or known bleeding diathesis; recent surgery, obstetric delivery, major trauma, or cerebrovascular event; the presence of a lesion that could bleed in a critical site (eg, central nervous system); and the presence of a contraindication to anticoagulation. Relative contraindications include pregnancy, uncontrolled hypertension, and congestive heart failure.[8] Patients with chronic renal insufficiency may be at a higher risk for acute kidney injury from iodinated contrast administration and hemoglobinuria from mechanical thrombectomy; in some instances, renal protective agents may be considered for use before and during the procedure.[13]

PREPROCEDURE DIAGNOSTIC IMAGING

Noninvasive imaging with duplex US is the most common imaging modality used to diagnose DVT. However, US has limitations in evaluating the extent of DVT above the inguinal ligament because of body habitus or overlying bowel gas. CT or magnetic resonance venography may be used to quantify the extent of DVT and more importantly evaluate for other abnormalities such as structural lesions (ie, iliac vein compression from May Thurner syndrome), anatomic variation (ie, duplicated IVC), tumor compression, or caval thrombosis from an IVC filter. Cross-sectional imaging may also assist in determining the optimal access points for performing CDT.[14]

PREPROCEDURE PATIENT DISCUSSION AND PREPARATION

An honest and open discussion with the patient and their family about the risks and benefits of catheter-directed therapy options is essential given that these modalities are outside the standard of care. The risk of major hemorrhagic complications (3%–10%) should be discussed, including the risk of fatal or intracranial bleeding (0.5%).[15–17] In the Catheter directed Venous Thrombolysis in Acute Iliofemoral Vein Thrombosis (CaVenT) study, the risk of major bleeding was 3%, which suggests that careful patient selection is crucial in minimizing hemorrhagic complications.[17] Patients should be made aware that additional procedures may be needed in the future, and that currently available stents are permanent devices that are used off-label and for which there are limited data on long-term fate. In addition, there is the possibility that thrombolysis may be unsuccessful. Of paramount importance is that patients understand that anticoagulation will be needed for at least 6 months or possibly lifelong and that these procedures are not a replacement for anticoagulation. Although the goal of CDT or PCDT is to improve DVT symptoms and potentially minimize the long-term complications of PTS, it must be made clear that PTS may not be completely avoided and that the impact of CDT/PCDT on long-term outcome is still under study. Finally, adjunct therapies such as the use of compression stockings may be recommended to improve symptomatic swelling only with no potential benefit in preventing PTS.[18]

VENOUS ACCESS

Depending on the extent of DVT, the patient may be placed in either the supine or the prone position. Common sites of access include the internal jugular, common femoral, greater/smaller saphenous, popliteal, or calf veins. Preprocedural bedside US evaluation is important to determine the proper access site for thrombolysis. If possible, access should be obtained below the lowest point of occlusive thrombus and not within a thrombosed segment of vein. In order to minimize potential bleeding complications and inadvertent arterial injury, real-time US guidance should always be used. Once access has been established, the following steps may be performed as outlined in later discussion for CDT.

Catheter-Directed Thrombolysis

CDT involves the delivery of a thrombolytic agent through a multi-side-hole infusion catheter positioned within the occluded vein. This technique enables a higher concentration of thrombolytic agent to be delivered locally within the thrombus while minimizing the systemic dose. At present, no fibrinolytic is approved by the US Food and Drug Administration for DVT therapy. Tissue plasminogen activator (TPA), the most commonly used agent, may be used at 0.01 mg/kg/h, not to exceed 1.0 mg/h. Treatment of unilateral iliofemoral DVT typically requires 24 to 30 hours of infusion.[15] After CDT, venography is performed to assess for thrombus resolution and exclude any underlying structural abnormalities that may contribute to DVT formation. Adjunctive maneuvers such as balloon maceration and/or mechanical thrombectomy can be performed to enhance thrombus removal (**Fig. 2**).

Catheter-Directed Thrombolysis Technique

CDT can be performed alone or in conjunction with mechanical thrombectomy. Because of the logistics involved with CDT, a firm understanding of the procedure is necessary by the medical and nursing staff to ensure that complications are avoided. Listed is a generalized technique for CDT:

1. Real-time US-guided access, ideally below the lowest point of occlusive thrombus
2. Lower extremity venogram performed to define thrombus extent
3. 0.035 hydrophilic guidewire and 4-F or 5-F catheter advanced through thrombus and into IVC. IVC venogram performed to evaluate for caval anomalies and patency
4. Multi-side-hole infusion catheter placed over wire with side-holes within the entire thrombosed segment
5. Recombinant TPA (eg, alteplase) infused through the catheter at 0.01 mg/kg/h not to exceed 1.0 mg/h. If both legs are being lysed, 0.5 mg/h of thrombolytic is used in each catheter for a total of 1.0 mg/h
6. Unfractionated heparin (UFH), usually targeted to subtherapeutic range, for example, activated partial thromboplastin time (aPTT) targeted 1.2–1.7 times (control) is started through the side arm of the access sheath (preferred) or through a peripheral intravenous line. If full-dose unfractionated heparin is used based on patient-specific considerations, close monitoring to prevent the partial thromboplastin time from becoming supratherapeutic is essential to avoid bleeding. Alternatively, full-dose, twice-daily injections of low-molecular-weight heparin (LMWH) may be used.
7. The patient is transferred to an intensive care unit or monitored bed for close observation, including every hour neurovascular checks to evaluate for any change in mental status that could signify a potential intracranial or other major hemorrhage. If the patient has severe head/neck pain or change in mental status, thrombolysis is stopped and an STAT noncontrast head CT scan is obtained. If nonintracranial major bleeding is suspected, thrombolysis is stopped and targeted clinical evaluation is performed urgently. Excellent communication between the physician team and nursing staff is paramount.
8. Hemoglobin and aPTT (if the patient is on unfractionated heparin) is checked every 6 hours while the patient is undergoing thrombolysis. Fibrinogen may also be checked, but it has not been established that doing so is associated with reduced bleeding complications.
9. To prevent acute kidney injury from potential hemoglobinuria caused by mechanical thrombectomy, aggressive fluid hydration with a goal urine output of 50 cc/h is performed overnight.

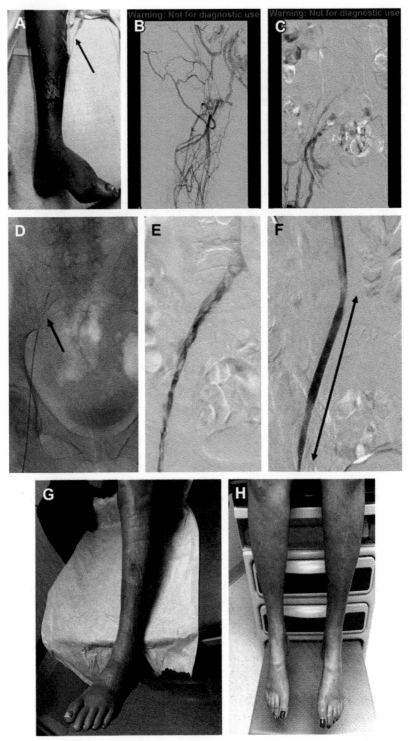

Fig. 2. A 62-year-old woman after pheochromocytoma resection presents with extensive subacute left iliofemoral DVT. (*A*) Photograph of the left leg at presentation shows

10. Repeat venography is performed. Depending on the amount and location of any residual thrombus, CDT may be continued or mechanical thrombectomy may be used to remove residual thrombus.

Pharmacomechanical Catheter-Directed Thrombolysis

PCDT has been used to accelerate thrombolysis and decrease the amount of thrombolytic used compared with conventional CDT. Devices for which case series have been published include the AngioJet Rheolytic Thrombectomy System (Boston Scientific, Marlborough, MA, USA), and the Arrow-Trerotola Percutaneous Thrombectomy device (Teleflex, Wayne, PA, USA). When used in aspiration mode, the AngioJet device uses the Bernoulli-Venturi effect to create a negative pressure gradient that results in thrombus being drawn into the catheter, where it is then fragmented and aspirated. Also, in power pulse-spray mode, dilute TPA can be sprayed under high pressure throughout the thrombus and allowed to dwell for approximately 30 minutes after which thrombus aspiration is performed. The Arrow-Trerotola Percutaneous Thrombectomy device does not aspirate thrombus but has a rotational mechanism that fragments thrombus, enabling its use to debulk thrombus in conjunction with CDT.[19]

Pharmacomechanical Catheter-Directed Thrombolysis Technique

The many variations of PCDT are beyond the scope of this article. To summarize, mechanical thrombectomy may be performed in conjunction with CDT or alone as a single-session PCDT for acute iliofemoral DVT (**Fig. 3**). Common side effects of mechanical thrombectomy that the physician must be aware of include hemoglobinuria and bradycardia if using the AngioJet device. Hemoglobinuria occurs as a result of intravascular hemolysis by the AngioJet catheter, resulting in the release of large amounts of free hemoglobin. Aggressive periprocedural hydration, urine alkalinization, and diuresis can reduce the occurrence of renal damage. Bradycardia during thrombectomy is usually self-limiting with temporary cessation of device activation; the mechanism of action is not well understood. One theory is that adenosine is released as a result of intravascular hemolysis and may result in transient bradycardia. A more plausible but still not substantiated theory is that stretch receptor activation in the right heart from cyclical high-pressure gradients by the device may play a more important role.[20] However, it is recommended that atropine be readily available should the patient become symptomatic from the bradycardia. Hemoglobinuria and bradycardia are not commonly seen with other thrombectomy devices.

---

significant swelling, erythema, and cellulitis (*double arrow*). Infusion catheter is in left popliteal vein (*arrow*). (*B*) Initial venogram from left popliteal vein access in the prone position shows occlusive thrombus in the left femoral and common femoral veins. A small amount of flow in the left external and common iliac veins is present. (*C*) Venogram after overnight CDT shows marginal thrombus reduction with small amount of flow in the external and common iliac veins. (*D*) Pharmacomechanical thrombectomy with AngioJet Rheolytic thrombectomy device (not shown) performed along with mechanical thrombectomy with Arrow-Trerotola thrombectomy device (*arrow*). (*E*) Significant improvement in flow in left iliac veins with persistent residual chronic thrombus. (*F*) An 18 mm × 9 cm Wallstent (*double arrow* shows length of stent) placed and angioplastied to 16 mm to increase length of stent. (*G*) Photograph of left lower extremity at 1-month follow-up shows improvement in swelling and cellulitis. (*H*) Photograph of left lower extremity at 4-year follow-up shows no evidence of recurrent DVT. (*Courtesy of* [D] Boston Scientific, Marlborough, MA and Teleflex, Wayne, PA; and [F] Boston Scientific, Marlborough, MA.)

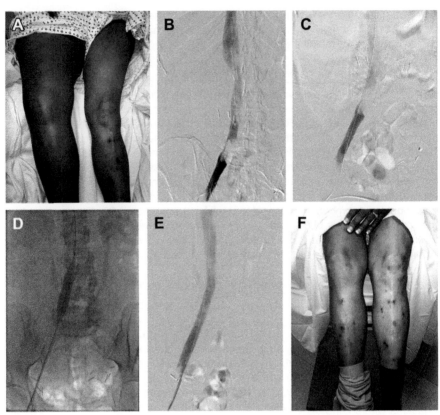

Fig. 3. A 54-year-old woman with recurrent urothelial cancer and right lower-extremity common iliac vein DVT. (*A*) Photograph of the right leg at presentation shows significant swelling. (*B*) Initial venogram from a right greater saphenous vein access shows occlusive thrombus in the right common iliac vein extending into the distal IVC. (*C*) Residual chronic thrombus of the right iliac vein is seen after pharmacomechanical thrombectomy with TPA (alteplase) and the AngioJet Rheolytic thrombectomy device (not shown). (*D, E*) A 16 mm × 9 cm Wallstent placed for maceration of chronic thrombus and for compressive effect of recurrent tumor on the iliac vein. (*F*) Photograph of legs 1 month after pharmacomechanical thrombolysis and stent placement shows resolution of initial swelling.

Stent Placement

Underlying venous stenoses that are uncovered after standard or PCDT are often treated with stenting. However, indications for stenting are not entirely clear, resulting in a wide range of stenting practices. According to current guidelines, stenoses in iliocaval vessels are appropriate for stent placement.[21] Femoral-popliteal stenoses are generally treated with angioplasty alone. The patency of stents in the venous system for acute DVT patients who have stent placement is excellent with 87% primary patency and 89% secondary patency at 1 year. Stent patency in nonthrombotic cases is extremely favorable with up to a 96% primary patency and 99% secondary patency at 1 year.[22–24] For acute DVT patients, stent placement is generally avoided across the inguinal ligament to prevent potential stent fracture and in-stent restenosis; however, for established PTS, stenting into the common femoral vein is often needed to maximize inflow.

CLINICAL RESULTS AND LITERATURE REVIEW

One rigorously conducted randomized controlled trial has shown improved thrombus reduction and reduced rates of PTS following CDT for proximal DVT. In the CaVenT trial, a 14.4% absolute reduction in PTS rate was seen in patients with iliac or femoral treated with infusion CDT compared with patients receiving anticoagulation alone at 24-month follow-up (41% vs 56%, $P = $ .047).[15,17,25] However, there was no difference in 2-year health-related quality of life. Questions about the applicability of the CaVenT study to US practice relate to its small-medium size, lack of use of mechanical thrombectomy devices, and its performance in a geographically limited area (Southern Norway). The BERNUTIFUL (BERN Ultrasound-enhanced Thrombolysis for Iliofemoral Deep Vein Thrombolysis) trial compared US-assisted CDT (Ekowave catheter, EKOS Corporation, Bothell, WA, USA) for iliofemoral DVT versus standard CDT. However, no significant difference in important clinical outcomes, including thrombus load reduction and PTS, was found between the US-assisted CDT and conventional CDT groups.[26,27]

POSTPROCEDURE CARE AND FOLLOW-UP

After CDT or PCDT, the patient should remain on bed rest for 2 to 4 hours to allow for hemostasis. Sequential compression devices are encouraged to stimulate the calf muscle pump system. The patient is also encouraged to drink plenty of fluids in order to minimize the effects of hemoglobinuria. By the next day, the patient is encouraged to ambulate. Twenty to 30 mm Hg thigh-high compression stockings are recommended to help with lower-extremity edema. The patient should be discharged with a defined plan for anticoagulant therapy that is consistent with their risk of recurrence, and a follow-up office visit in 1 month with US or cross-sectional imaging to evaluate for deep venous and/or stent patency. Appropriate referral to hematology is warranted in patients with an unprovoked DVT or possible thrombophilia.

SUMMARY

CDT and PCDT are endovascular techniques that enable rapid recanalization of acute iliofemoral DVT, at the price of an increased risk of early bleeding. Although the long-term outcomes of these techniques continue to be studied, they are likely to be beneficial for selected patient groups provided careful pretreatment assessment and close monitoring are performed.

REFERENCES

1. Goldhaber SZ, Bounameaux H. Pulmonary embolism and deep vein thrombosis. Lancet 2012;379(9828):1835–46.
2. Beckman MG, Hooper WC, Critchley SE, et al. Venous thromboembolism: a public health concern. Am J Prev Med 2010;38(4 Suppl):S495–501.
3. Lindblad B, Eriksson A, Bergqvist D. Autopsy-verified pulmonary embolism in a surgical department: analysis of the period from 1951 to 1988. Br J Surg 1991; 78(7):849–52.
4. Sandler DA, Martin JF. Autopsy proven pulmonary embolism in hospital patients: are we detecting enough deep vein thrombosis? J R Soc Med 1989; 82(4):203–5.
5. Kahn SR, Shrier I, Julian JA, et al. Determinants and time course of the postthrombotic syndrome after acute deep venous thrombosis. Ann Intern Med 2008; 149(10):698–707.

6. Kahn SR, Shbaklo H, Lamping DL, et al. Determinants of health-related quality of life during the 2 years following deep vein thrombosis. J Thromb Haemost 2008; 6(7):1105–12.

7. Mewissen MW, Seabrook GR, Meissner MH, et al. Catheter-directed thrombolysis for lower extremity deep venous thrombosis: report of a national multicenter registry. Radiology 1999;211(1):39–49.

8. Vedantham S, Sista AK, Klein SJ, et al. Quality improvement guidelines for the treatment of lower-extremity deep vein thrombosis with use of endovascular thrombus removal. J Vasc Interv Radiol 2014;25(9):1317–25.

9. O'Sullivan GJ. The role of interventional radiology in the management of deep venous thrombosis: advance therapy. Cardiovasc Intervent Radiol 2011;34(3): 445–61.

10. O'Sullivan GJ, Semba CP, Bittner CA, et al. Endovascular management of iliac compression (May-Thurner) syndrome. J Vasc Interv Radiol 2000;11(7):823–36.

11. Bass JE, Redwine MD, Kramer LA, et al. Spectrum of congenital anomalies of the inferior vena cava: cross-sectional imaging findings. Radiographics 2000;20(3): 639–52.

12. PREPIC Study Group. Eight-year follow-up of patients with permanent vena cava filters in the prevention of pulmonary embolism: the PREPIC (Prevention du Risque d'Embolie Pulmonaire par Interruption Cave) randomized study. Circulation 2005;112(3):416–22.

13. Dukkipati R, Yang EH, Adler S, et al. Acute kidney injury caused by intravascular hemolysis after mechanical thrombectomy. Nat Clin Pract Nephrol 2009;5:112–6.

14. Kanne JP, Lalani TA. Role of computed tomography and magnetic resonance imaging for deep venous thrombosis and pulmonary embolism. Circulation 2004; 109(12 suppl 1):115–21.

15. Enden T, Kløw NE, Sandvik L, et al. Catheter-directed thrombolysis vs. anticoagulant therapy alone in deep vein thrombosis: results of an open randomized, controlled trial reporting on short-term patency. J Thromb Haemost 2009;7(8): 1268–75.

16. Elsharawy M, Elzaya E. Early result of thrombolysis vs anticoagulation in iliofemoral venous thrombosis: a randomized clinical trial. Eur J Vasc Endovasc Surg 2002;24(3):209–14.

17. Enden T, Haig Y, Kløw NE, et al. Long-term outcome after additional catheter-directed thrombolysis versus standard treatment for acute iliofemoral deep vein thrombosis (the CaVenT study): a randomized controlled trial. Lancet 2012; 379(9810):31–8.

18. Kahn SR, Shapiro S, Wells PS, et al. Compression stockings to prevent post-thrombotic syndrome: a randomized placebo-controlled trial. Lancet 2014; 383(9920):880–8.

19. Park KM, Moon IS, Kim JI, et al. Mechanical thrombectomy with Trerotola compared with catheter-directed thrombolysis for treatment of acute iliofemoral deep vein thrombosis. Ann Vasc Surg 2014;28(8):1853–61.

20. Jeyabalan G, Saba S, Baril DT, et al. Bradyarrhythmias during rheolytic pharmacomechanical thrombectomy for deep vein thrombosis. J Endovasc Ther 2010; 17(3):416–22.

21. Mahnken AH, Thomson K, de Haan M, et al. CIRSE standards of practice guidelines on iliocaval stenting. Cardiovasc Intervent Radiol 2014;37(4):889–97.

22. Hartung O, Loundou AD, Barthelemy P, et al. Endovascular management of chronic disabling ilio-caval obstructive lesions: long-term results. Eur J Vasc Endovasc Surg 2009;38(1):118–24.

23. Xue GH, Huan XZ, Ye M, et al. Catheter-directed thrombolysis and stenting in the treatment of iliac vein compression syndrome with acute iliofemoral deep vein thrombosis: outcome and follow-up. Ann Vasc Surg 2014;28(4):957–63.
24. Sharifi M, Bay C, Mehdipour M, et al. TORPEDO Investigators. Thrombus obliteration by rapid percutaneous endovenous intervention in deep venous occlusion (TORPEDO) trial: midterm results. J Endovasc Ther 2012;19(2):273–80.
25. Razavi MK, Jaff MR, Miller LE. Safety and effectiveness of stent placement for iliofemoral venous outflow obstruction: systematic review and meta-analysis. Circ Cardiovasc Interv 2015;8(10):e002772.
26. Engelberger RP, Spirk D, Willenberg T, et al. Ultrasound-assisted versus conventional catheter-directed thrombolysis for acute iliofemoral deep vein thrombosis. Circ Cardiovasc Interv 2015;8(1):e002027.
27. Engelberger RP, Stuck A, Spirk D, et al. Ultrasound-assisted versus catheter-directed thrombolysis for acute iliofemoral deep vein thrombosis: 1-year follow-up data of a randomized-controlled trial. J Thromb Haemost 2017;15(7): 1351–60.

Advances in Operative Thrombectomy for Lower Extremity Venous Thrombosis

Matthew C. Koopmann, MD, Robert B. McLafferty, MD*

KEYWORDS

- Thrombectomy • Vein • Iliac • Femoral • Venous • Thrombosis • Surgery • Open

KEY POINTS

- Open thrombectomy is considered when thrombus removal is indicated but thrombolysis is contraindicated.
- Open thrombectomy can reduce postthrombotic syndrome and venous reflux versus anticoagulation alone.
- Contemporary operative venous thrombectomy uses a hybrid approach with open thrombectomy for thrombus removal and ilio-caval stenting to treat residual outflow stenosis.

INTRODUCTION: NATURE OF THE PROBLEM

Lower extremity deep venous thrombosis (LEDVT) affects men and women of all ages and is a leading cause of morbidity and mortality in the United States. The mainstay of therapy for acute LEDVT is medical: systemic anticoagulation, leg compression, and early ambulation. Anticoagulation is safe and effective at reducing the rates of pulmonary embolism and recurrent venous thromboembolic events after acute LEDVT. However, anticoagulation does not remove the thrombus and restore venous patency. Residual thrombus can lead to chronic venous obstruction as well as valve dysfunction and reflux. These complications, in turn, cause venous hypertension, which can ultimately lead to the postthrombotic syndrome, a debilitating and costly condition comprising pain, heaviness, edema, varicose veins, hyperpigmentation, inflammation, and ulceration. In a cohort of patients followed after a first episode of deep venous thrombosis (DVT), the cumulative incidence of any postthrombotic syndrome at 5 years was 28.0% and the incidence of severe symptoms was 9.3%.[1]

Early thrombus removal, in conjunction with anticoagulation, can restore venous patency, preserve venous valve function, and may reduce the incidence of

The authors have nothing to disclose.
Department of Surgery, Veterans Affairs Portland Health Care System, Oregon Health & Sciences University, 3710 Southwest US Veterans Hospital Road, P3-OC, Portland, OR 97239, USA
* Corresponding author.
E-mail address: robert.mclafferty@va.gov

postthrombotic syndrome. The Society for Vascular Surgery (SVS) and the American Venous Forum (AVF) 2012 guidelines[2] for early thrombus removal in acute LEDVT give the following indications for early thrombus removal:

- First episode of acute iliofemoral DVT
- Symptoms less than 14 days in duration
- Low risk of bleeding
- Limb-threatening venous ischemia (phlegmasia cerulea dolens)
- Patients are ambulatory with
  - Good functional capacity
  - Acceptable life expectancy

Patients with symptoms of greater than 14 days may have inferior results, although the results of the Catheter-Directed Venous Thrombolysis in Acute Iliofemoral Vein Thrombosis (CaVenT) trial suggest that thrombus removal in patients with symptoms less than 21 days is advantageous.[3,4]

Strategies for early thrombus removal include

- Catheter-based therapies
  - Pharmaco-mechanical (preferred)
  - Pharmacologic
- Open thrombectomy

The SVS-AVF 2012 guidelines recommend catheter-directed therapies over open thrombectomy, as they are less invasive with fewer potential surgical complications.[2] However, in patients with a contraindication to thrombolytic agents, but who can receive anticoagulation, open thrombectomy should be considered if indications for thrombus removal are met and patients are good operative risks.

SURGICAL TECHNIQUE
Preoperative Planning

The initial diagnosis of iliofemoral LEDVT is clinical, based on the history and physical examination findings of unilateral leg swelling. A thorough history focusing on the duration of symptoms remains important in determining if it has been greater than 14 to 21 days since the onset. Although venous duplex is sensitive and specific for LEDVT, the extent of iliac vein thrombus may be difficult to determine by duplex alone. Computed tomography or magnetic resonance venography should be performed to confirm the diagnosis of iliofemoral thrombosis and determine the extent of thrombus to guide operative thrombectomy. In particular, the extension of thrombosis into the inferior vena cava needs to be evaluated to determine if embolic protection with a filter is needed before thrombectomy.

As soon as the diagnosis of LEDVT is made, appropriate hematologic laboratory testing should be completed and patients should immediately be anticoagulated in the therapeutic range with unfractionated heparin. A blood type and crossmatch should be obtained and available for transfusion if patients are anemic. Intraoperative blood salvage may be considered as well. General anesthesia is preferred, but local anesthesia and sedation can also be used.[5] A hybrid operative suite with fixed imaging capabilities is desirable, but the procedure can also be performed in a standard operating room with a mobile C-arm with digital subtraction angiography capabilities.

Preparation and Patient Positioning

The patients are placed on a fluoroscopic table that will allow imaging from the feet to the neck. The ipsilateral groin is clipped; the abdomen, both groins, and the circumferential ipsilateral leg are prepared using chlorhexidine-alcohol skin prep. One arm should be tucked to allow free passage of the C-arm. The right neck may need to be used for internal jugular vein access and this should be coordinated with the anesthesia team before sterile preparation and draping.

Surgical Approach

Step 1: exposure, vessel control, and venotomy
A vertical incision is made on the groin for exposure.[5] Although a horizontal or oblique incision may promote better wound healing, especially in obese patients with pannus, the vertical incision allows for more extensive exposure of the common femoral vein and its branches and is the preferred approach in most instances. The common femoral, femoral, profunda femoris, and any other variant large tributary veins as well as the great saphenous vein at the saphenofemoral junction are all exposed and controlled with silicone rubber (Silastic) vessel loops or umbilical tapes. Graduated vascular clamps can also be used to prevent vessel injury. All venous branches must be controlled in order to prevent significant blood loss during the thrombectomy.

A transverse[6] or longitudinal[7] venotomy, centered over the appropriate venous tributary, may be chosen at the surgeon's discretion. Most often this is the common femoral vein. While a transverse incision takes less time to close and has less risk of narrowing the vessel, a longitudinal venotomy can be extended and allows for a more complete thrombectomy of all branches, especially in cases whereby the clot is subacute and more adherent to the vessel wall. Depending on the overall diameter of the common femoral vein, a longitudinal incision that has a large diameter can usually be closed primarily without critical narrowing.

Step 2: thrombus removal
Infrainguinal thrombus The initial maneuver is to squeeze the leg in order to milk the thrombus cephalad out through the common femoral venotomy. This maneuver is facilitated by forcible dorsiflexion of the foot[8] to make use of the calf muscle pump as well as vigorous compression of the leg with an Esmarch rubber bandage, wrapping tightly in a sequential manner from the foot to the high thigh. This maneuver is repeated several times to initially clear the major tributaries of the tibial, popliteal, and femoral veins and then further clear smaller venous tributaries. In many instances, particularly with fresh thrombus, most of the venous drainage of the leg is cleared with this maneuver alone.

If there is persistent infrainguinal thrombus, then balloon thrombectomy can be attempted. Depending on the vein segments being treated, small to large embolectomy balloon catheters can be passed from the groin venotomy to distal venous segments. Difficulties may arise in traversing competent venous valves in a retrograde fashion, and this maneuver may injure the valves leading to further incompetence. Other maneuvers to overcome this barrier include centering the catheter in the center of the vein, repositioning the leg, partially inflating the balloon, or using a selective catheter and guidewire followed by an over-the-wire embolectomy catheter. The last technique is the preferred method, and being in a vascular hybrid room helps facilitate wire access. Selective venography, even in the presence of thrombus, will also help visualize branches and valve structures. Of particular importance is the fact that smaller venous tributaries can be in parallel to larger axial veins. Therefore, the use of venography remains paramount to avoid injury with overinflation of a balloon catheter; direct visualization of the inflated balloon under fluoroscopy will further guide the operator to the proper inflation size. A power injection of contrast should also be avoided, as smaller and medium venous tributaries can be ruptured with higher pounds per square inch levels. A controlled hand injection should be sufficient to visualize the necessary anatomy during an open thrombectomy.

Comerota[9] describes another approach to crossing competent valves in an atraumatic fashion. The posterior tibial vein is exposed, and a small embolectomy balloon catheter is advanced antegrade into the common femoral venotomy. A 14-gauge intravenous catheter is cut from its hub, and the smaller antegrade balloon catheter is inserted into it. Next, a separate larger balloon catheter is partially inserted into the other half of the 14-gauge cut intravenous catheter. Adequate pressure is applied to fix both balloons inside the intravenous catheter. The larger embolectomy balloon catheter is then pulled retrograde from the common femoral vein to the posterior tibial vein using the smaller balloon catheter. The smaller balloon catheter and intravenous catheters are removed. The larger embolectomy balloon catheter can then be inflated and pulled back antegrade towards the groin to remove more thrombus. Additional benefits of this approach are that posterior tibial vein access allows for antegrade flushing of the vein, completion venography, instillation of thrombolytics, and placement of a percutaneous posterior tibial catheter for postoperative venous access for venography and medication delivery.[9]

Iliofemoral thrombus After completion of the infrainguinal thrombectomy, the iliofemoral thrombectomy is performed. This procedure is accomplished by using a large embolectomy balloon catheter. The catheter is filled with diluted contrast to also allow for fluoroscopic guidance during inflation and pullback. Partial thrombectomy progressing from distal to proximal is preferred, with the final pass commencing past the occlusive thrombus. By first removing all distal iliac vein thrombus and maintaining proximal occlusion, the risk of pulmonary embolism is minimized.

Other steps to avoid pulmonary embolism include permanent or retrievable inferior vena cava filter placement before thrombectomy,[6] inferior vena cava balloon occlusion via contralateral femoral vein or right internal jugular vein access,[9] and continuous positive end-expiratory pressure of 10 mm Hg during thrombectomy.[10]

Step 3: venography, intravascular ultrasound, and possible venous stenting
After the iliofemoral thrombectomy has been completed, venography and intravascular ultrasound should be performed to look for obstruction due to residual thrombus or venous compression. Intravascular ultrasound remains superior to conventional venography for the detection of iliofemoral venous obstruction and is also used to guide the accurate sizing and placement of venous stents.[11] If residual obstruction is present after adequate attempts at catheter thrombectomy, then bare-metal self-expanding venous stents should be placed as necessary.

Step 4: venous closure, arteriovenous fistula creation, and wound closure
After venous thrombectomy, the vessel is closed in the standard continuous fashion with fine monofilament permanent sutures using small bites on the vein to prevent narrowing the lumen. If a horizontal incision is used, interrupted sutures can be used to avoid a purse-string effect. Patch closure of the larger axial veins is not usually necessary.

A temporary arteriovenous shunt can be created to increase blood flow and prevent recurrent proximal thrombosis. This procedure can be done with either an autogenous[9] or prosthetic approach.[12] With the autogenous approach, the end of the proximal saphenous vein or a saphenous vein tributary are sewn to the side of the superficial femoral artery. A polytetrafluoroethylene (PTFE) or Silastic band is sewn around the fistula and a large monofilament suture is looped, clipped, and left in the subcutaneous tissue for ease of ligation if needed in the future under local anesthetic. In the prosthetic approach, a 4-mm externally supported PTFE vascular graft is sewn end to side to the common femoral artery and common femoral vein. A 6-cm redundant loop helps facilitate endovascular closure at a later date.

The wound is inspected for meticulous hemostasis, as the need for postoperative anticoagulation increases the risk for hematoma. Topical hemostatic agents may be necessary. The wound is closed in layers using an absorbable, running suture to reduce the chance of postoperative lymph leak or seroma. Routine drainage remains at the discretion of the surgeon.

Immediate Postoperative Care

Patients should be maintained on therapeutic doses of unfractionated or low-molecular-weight heparin. Warfarin therapy can be initiated as soon as patients are able to take oral medications and are titrated to an international normalized ratio of 2 to 3. The leg is wrapped with compression wraps and elevated when patients are not active. Patients should be encouraged to ambulate early and often. A postoperative baseline venous duplex should be performed before discharge, and any hypercoagulable tests that had been obtained preoperatively should be followed up with hematology consultation if necessary.

REHABILITATION AND RECOVERY

A standard course of anticoagulation for LEDVT is recommended, as prescribed by the current updated guidelines.[13] An extended course (6 months or greater) is likely to be of benefit in patients who have undergone venous stenting who are not high risk for bleeding.[14] Knee-high, 30- to 40-mm Hg graded compression stockings should be worn for 2 years postoperatively to further reduce the risk of postthrombotic syndrome.[2]

CLINICAL RESULTS IN THE LITERATURE

The history of operative thrombectomy for LEDVT can be divided into 3 different eras: operative thrombectomy alone, operative thrombectomy with surgical adjuncts, and hybrid operative thrombectomy with stenting. The complication rates for open thrombectomy in all eras was low, so this discussion mainly focuses on long-term outcomes.

Operative Thrombectomy Alone

Operative thrombectomy alone became popularized in the 1950 to 1960s,[15] particularly with the report by Haller and Abrams[5] in 1963. They showed that patients with less than 10 days of symptoms treated with thrombectomy had low rates of postphlebitic syndrome (15%) and venous obstruction on venography (16%) at an average follow-up of 18 months. Patients treated between 14 and 21 days had inferior results. Subsequent reports showed similar results (**Table 1**), with low rates of postphlebitic syndrome (13%–22%).[8,16,17] However, a follow-up of the Haller and Abrams[5] study performed by Lansing and Davis[18] suggested much higher rates of postphlebitic symptoms and venographic obstruction at least 5 years after surgery.

Operative thrombectomy alone is not commonly performed today. Davenport and Xenos[19] used the American College of Surgeons National Surgical Quality Improvement Program database to identify 91 open venous thrombectomies performed in 200 hospitals that contributed data between 2005 and 2008. Arteriovenous fistula and venous angioplasty/stent were performed in only 1 and 4 patients, respectively. There were many high-risk patients (20% American Society of Anesthesiology class 4). Thirty-day outcomes were poor, with high mortality (8.8%), morbidity (25.3%),

Table 1
Results of operative thrombectomy alone

First Author, Year	Limbs Treated	Follow-up	Postthrombotic Syndrome (%)	Venous Obstruction (%)
Haller & Abrams,[5] 1963	45	18.3 mo	22	16
Hafner et al,[8] 1965	50	3.5 y	16	NA
Harris & Brown,[16] 1968	18	≤9 mo	13	13
Edwards et al,[17] 1970	61	1–9 y	20	NA

and wound complications (11.0%). These data suggest that in contemporary practice operative thrombectomy is primarily performed in high-risk patients who are not candidates for catheter-directed therapies.

Operative Thrombectomy with Surgical Adjuncts

Surgical adjuncts were added to operative thrombectomy beginning in the 1980s (**Table 2**). Arteriovenous shunts have been used in operations for venous obstruction to increase blood flow across venous grafts and prevent occlusion.[20] They are usually considered temporary adjuncts and can be occluded by either surgical or endovascular techniques at a later date.[21] Juhan and colleagues[22] reported the outcome of 42 iliac vein thrombectomies in which 31 temporary arteriovenous fistulas were constructed with a 93% patency by venography at 4 years. In a meta-analysis of surgical thrombectomy (with or without arteriovenous shunt) versus anticoagulation alone,

Table 2
Results of operative thrombectomy with surgical adjuncts

First Author, Year	Limbs Treated	Surgical Adjunct	Follow-up	Postthrombotic Syndrome (%)	Venous Reflux (%)	Venous Obstruction (%)	Graft Patency (%)
Juhan et al,[22] 1987	42	AV shunt	4 y	NA	NA	7	NA
Plate et al,[24] 1984	31	AV shunt	6 mo	58	48	24	NA
Plate et al,[28] 1985	7	Bypass	5 y	NA	NA	NA	14
Plate et al,[25] 1990	19	AV shunt	5 y	63	43	29	NA
Comerota,[42] 1994	3	Bypass, AV shunt	11–20 mo	33	NA	NA	66
Törngren et al,[27] 1996	30	AV shunt	9 y	47	33	27	NA
Plate et al,[26] 1997	13	AV shunt	10 y	70	62	58	NA
Alimi et al,[29] 1997	4	Bypass, AV shunt	11–20 mo	0	NA	NA	100
Pillny et al,[38] 2003	97	AV shunt	6 y	44	NA	NA	NA

Abbreviation: AV, arteriovenous.

there was a significant reduction in postthrombotic syndrome and venous reflux, but not venous obstruction, in the surgical group.[23] The studies used in this meta-analysis, however, were heterogeneous and of low quality, with the most favorable study comparing 3-month surgical follow-up to 9-year anticoagulation controls.

Plate and colleagues[24] performed a prospective randomized trial comparing 31 patients who underwent operative thrombectomy plus temporary arteriovenous fistula and anticoagulation to 32 patients treated with anticoagulation alone. At the 6-month follow-up, the thrombectomy group had significantly decreased postthrombotic symptoms and improved venous outflow and valvular function compared with anticoagulation alone. However, after the 5-year[25] and 10-year[26] follow-up, the differences in outcomes between the groups decreased, suggesting that the benefits of thrombectomy diminished over time, particularly in regard to venous reflux. This observation is supported by Törngren and colleagues[27] (see later discussion).

Surgical bypasses have also been used, with or without arteriovenous shunts, to improve patency after operative venous thrombectomy. Plate and colleagues[28] reported the results of 7 patients with iliofemoral venous thrombosis with thrombectomy and bypass using PTFE (4 cross-femoral and 3 ilio-caval bypasses). There was one postoperative death and one leg amputation, and only one bypass was patent at 5 years. Alimi and colleagues[29] treated 4 patients with acute iliofemoral thrombosis and iliac vein compression with thrombectomy and bypass with arteriovenous shunt with good intermediate-term patency. The use of surgical bypass to treat outflow obstruction after acute operative thrombectomy has, in most circumstances, been replaced by venous stenting.

Hybrid Operative Thrombectomy with Stenting

The current era of operative venous thrombectomy incorporates a hybrid approach with open thrombectomy for thrombus removal and ilio-caval stenting to treat residual outflow stenosis (**Table 3**).[10,30–36] The patency rates for venous stenting are excellent, with 5-year primary patency rates between 70% and 80%.[10,34] Rodriguez and colleagues[36] compared consecutive patients with acute iliofemoral DVT treated with either percutaneous techniques (31 patients) or hybrid operative thrombectomy (40 patients). Hybrid thrombectomy and stenting resulted in significantly decreased bleeding events and length of stay with no difference in mean femoral-popliteal reflux time or postthrombotic syndrome. This finding suggests that hybrid operative thrombectomy with stenting is as effective as percutaneous therapy with the potential benefits of shorter procedural time, fewer bleeding complications, and reduced hospital length of stay. Patients at risk for bleeding with thrombolytics should be considered for such a procedure. Whether hybrid operative thrombectomy is superior to anticoagulation alone has not been evaluated.

Special Scenarios

Pregnancy
Venous thromboembolism is a common complication of pregnancy and the recommended treatment is usually anticoagulation alone. The addition of thrombus removal in this patient population remains controversial and is usually reserved for cases of phlegmasia cerulean dolens or persistent pain and significant edema after a trial of anticoagulation alone. Delin and colleagues[37] performed open thrombectomy and temporary arteriovenous fistula in 9 women with pregnancy-associated iliofemoral venous thrombosis and demonstrated an 85% short-term patency rate. This finding was confirmed by Pillny and colleagues,[38] who reported a 91% short-term patency rate, a low (1.8%) surgery-related fetal mortality, and no maternal mortality or

Table 3
Results of hybrid operative thrombectomy with stenting

First Author, Year	Limbs Treated	Follow-up	Postthrombotic Syndrome (%)	Venous Reflux (%)	Venous Obstruction (%)	Stent Patency (%)
Blättler et al,[30] 2004	21	8 y	10	0	10	NA
Schwarzbach et al,[31] 2005	20	21 mo	NA	NA	NA	Primary: 80 Secondary: 90
Husmann et al,[32] 2007	11	6 mo	9	9	9	Primary: 82 Assisted primary: 91
Hartung et al,[10] 2008	29	63 mo	NA	40	12	Primary: 79 Assisted primary: 86 Secondary: 86
Lindow et al,[33] 2010	83	59 mo	20	NA	25	NA
Hölper et al,[34] 2010	25	68 mo	16	NA	12	Primary: 74 Secondary: 84
Igari et al,[35] 2014	8	16 mo	NA	NA	NA	Primary: 75
Rodriguez et al,[36] 2017	40	2 y	15	NA	NA	NA

pulmonary embolism. A Swedish study by Törngren and colleagues[27] compared 30 pregnant women with iliofemoral DVT treated with open venous thrombectomy, temporary arteriovenous fistula, and anticoagulation to a registry population treated with anticoagulation alone. At the long-term follow-up, no difference was noted between the groups with regard to iliac vein patency, postthrombotic symptoms, venous emptying, or reflux. Thrombectomy did not improve long-term outcomes compared with anticoagulation alone. However, venous outflow stenosis was not treated in this study at the time of thrombectomy. Herrera and colleagues[39] treated 13 pregnant patients with thrombus removal, 3 with open thrombectomy, with minimal morbidity or risk of preterm delivery. In their series, radiation exposure was minimized by using pelvic lead shields, low-frame rates, collimation, and judicious use of digital subtraction angiography, suggesting that adjunctive venous stenting can be added to open venous thrombectomy without subjecting the fetus to risk for injury. There are no studies comparing anticoagulation plus thrombus removal and stenting with anticoagulation alone in this patient population.

Pediatrics
Venous thromboembolism is rare in children, and the literature for the operative treatment of iliofemoral venous thrombosis is limited to case reports.[40] Open venous thrombectomy has been reported in patients as young as 2 years old.[17] It seems that operative venous thrombectomy is feasible in children, but data supporting the practice are limited.

Phlegmasia cerulean dolens

Phlegmasia cerulean dolens due to acute iliofemoral DVT is a life-threatening condition with a risk of venous gangrene and limb loss. Operative thrombectomy may be the better option depending on the severity, time frame, and comorbidities. In a Thai study, 15 patients with phlegmasia underwent operative thrombectomy with a temporary arteriovenous fistula and inferior vena cava filter. There was no perioperative pulmonary embolism or mortality, and limb salvage was successful in all patients, with amputation limited to the transmetatarsal level in patients with venous gangrene.[41]

REFERENCES

1. Prandoni P, Villalta S, Bagatella P, et al. The clinical course of deep-vein thrombosis. Prospective long-term follow-up of 528 symptomatic patients. Haematologica 1997;82(4):423–8.
2. Meissner MH, Gloviczki P, Comerota AJ, et al. Early thrombus removal strategies for acute deep venous thrombosis: clinical practice guidelines of the Society for Vascular Surgery and the American Venous Forum. J Vasc Surg 2012;55(5): 1449–62.
3. Enden T, Haig Y, Klow NE, et al. Long-term outcome after additional catheter-directed thrombolysis versus standard treatment for acute iliofemoral deep vein thrombosis (the CaVenT study): a randomised controlled trial. Lancet 2012; 379(9810):31–8.
4. Haig Y, Enden T, Grotta O, et al. Post-thrombotic syndrome after catheter-directed thrombolysis for deep vein thrombosis (CaVenT): 5-year follow-up results of an open-label, randomised controlled trial. Lancet Haematol 2016;3(2): e64–71.
5. Haller JA, Abrams BL. Use of thrombectomy in the treatment of acute iliofemoral venous thrombosis in forty-five patients. Ann Surg 1963;158(4):561–6.
6. Olearchyk AS. Insertion of the inferior vena cava filter followed by iliofemoral venous thrombectomy for ischemic venous thrombosis. J Vasc Surg 1987;5(4): 645–7.
7. Comerota AJ, Gale SS. Technique of contemporary iliofemoral and infrainguinal venous thrombectomy. J Vasc Surg 2006;43(1):185–91.
8. Hafner CD, Cranley JJ, Krause RJ, et al. Venous thrombectomy: current status. Ann Surg 1965;161(3):411–7.
9. Comerota AJ. The current role of operative venous thrombectomy in deep vein thrombosis. Semin Vasc Surg 2012;25(1):2–12.
10. Hartung O, Benmiloud F, Barthelemy P, et al. Late results of surgical venous thrombectomy with iliocaval stenting. J Vasc Surg 2008;47(2):381–7.
11. Neglen P, Raju S. Intravascular ultrasound scan evaluation of the obstructed vein. J Vasc Surg 2002;35(4):694–700.
12. de Wolf MA, Jalaie H, van Laanen JH, et al. Endophlebectomy of the common femoral vein and arteriovenous fistula creation as adjuncts to venous stenting for post-thrombotic syndrome. Br J Surg 2017;104(6):718–25.
13. Kearon C, Akl EA, Ornelas J, et al. Antithrombotic therapy for VTE disease: CHEST guideline and expert panel report. Chest 2016;149(2):315–52.
14. Protack CD, Bakken AM, Patel N, et al. Long-term outcomes of catheter directed thrombolysis for lower extremity deep venous thrombosis without prophylactic inferior vena cava filter placement. J Vasc Surg 2007;45(5):992–7 [discussion: 997].

15. Eklof B. Surgical thrombectomy for iliofemoral venous thrombosis revisited. J Vasc Surg 2011;54(3):897–900.
16. Harris EJ, Brown WH. Patency after thrombectomy for iliofemoral thrombosis. Ann Surg 1968;167(1):91–7.
17. Edwards WH, Sawyers JL, Foster JH. Iliofemoral venous thrombosis. Reappraisal of thrombectomy. Ann Surg 1970;171(6):961–70.
18. Lansing AM, Davis WM. Five-year follow-up study of iliofemoral venous thrombectomy. Ann Surg 1968;168(4):620–8.
19. Davenport DL, Xenos ES. Early outcomes and risk factors in venous thrombectomy: an analysis of the American College of Surgeons NSQIP dataset. Vasc Endovascular Surg 2011;45(4):325–8.
20. Okadome K, Muto Y, Eguchi H, et al. Venous reconstruction for iliofemoral venous occlusion facilitated by temporary arteriovenous shunt. Long-term results in nine patients. Arch Surg 1989;124(8):957–60.
21. Endrys J, Eklof B, Neglen P, et al. Percutaneous balloon occlusion of surgical arteriovenous fistulae following venous thrombectomy. Cardiovasc Intervent Radiol 1989;12(4):226–9.
22. Juhan C, Cornillon B, Tobiana F, et al. Patency after iliofemoral and iliocaval venous thrombectomy. Ann Vasc Surg 1987;1(5):529–33.
23. Casey ET, Murad MH, Zumaeta-Garcia M, et al. Treatment of acute iliofemoral deep vein thrombosis. J Vasc Surg 2012;55(5):1463–73.
24. Plate G, Einarsson E, Ohlin P, et al. Thrombectomy with temporary arteriovenous fistula: the treatment of choice in acute iliofemoral venous thrombosis. J Vasc Surg 1984;1(6):867–76.
25. Plate G, Akesson H, Einarsson E, et al. Long-term results of venous thrombectomy combined with a temporary arterio-venous fistula. Eur J Vasc Surg 1990;4(5):483–9.
26. Plate G, Eklof B, Norgren L, et al. Venous thrombectomy for iliofemoral vein thrombosis–10-year results of a prospective randomised study. Eur J Vasc Endovasc Surg 1997;14(5):367–74.
27. Törngren S, Hjertberg R, Rosfors S, et al. The long-term outcome of proximal vein thrombosis during pregnancy is not improved by the addition of surgical thrombectomy to anticoagulant treatment. Eur J Vasc Endovasc Surg 1996;12(1):31–6.
28. Plate G, Einarsson E, Eklof B, et al. Iliac vein obstruction associated with acute iliofemoral venous thrombosis. Results of early reconstruction using polytetrafluoroethylene grafts. Acta Chir Scand 1985;151(7):607–11.
29. Alimi YS, DiMauro P, Fabre D, et al. Iliac vein reconstructions to treat acute and chronic venous occlusive disease. J Vasc Surg 1997;25(4):673–81.
30. Blättler W, Heller G, Largiader J, et al. Combined regional thrombolysis and surgical thrombectomy for treatment of iliofemoral vein thrombosis. J Vasc Surg 2004;40(4):620–5.
31. Schwarzbach MH, Schumacher H, Bockler D, et al. Surgical thrombectomy followed by intraoperative endovascular reconstruction for symptomatic iliofemoral venous thrombosis. Eur J Vasc Endovasc Surg 2005;29(1):58–66.
32. Husmann MJ, Heller G, Kalka C, et al. Stenting of common iliac vein obstructions combined with regional thrombolysis and thrombectomy in acute deep vein thrombosis. Eur J Vasc Endovasc Surg 2007;34(1):87–91.
33. Lindow C, Mumme A, Asciutto G, et al. Long-term results after transfemoral venous thrombectomy for iliofemoral deep venous thrombosis. Eur J Vasc Endovasc Surg 2010;40(1):134–8.

34. Hölper P, Kotelis D, Attigah N, et al. Long-term results after surgical thrombectomy and simultaneous stenting for symptomatic iliofemoral venous thrombosis. Eur J Vasc Endovasc Surg 2010;39(3):349–55.

35. Igari K, Kudo T, Toyofuku T, et al. Surgical thrombectomy and simultaneous stenting for deep venous thrombosis caused by iliac vein compression syndrome (May-Thurner syndrome). Ann Thorac Cardiovasc Surg 2014;20(6):995–1000.

36. Rodriguez LE, Aboukheir-Aboukheir A, Figueroa-Vicente R, et al. Hybrid operative thrombectomy is noninferior to percutaneous techniques for the treatment of acute iliofemoral deep venous thrombosis. J Vasc Surg Venous Lymphat Disord 2017;5(2):177–84.

37. Delin A, Swedenborg J, Hellgren M, et al. Thrombectomy and arteriovenous fistula for iliofemoral venous thrombosis in fertile women. Surg Gynecol Obstet 1982;154(1):69–73.

38. Pillny M, Sandmann W, Luther B, et al. Deep venous thrombosis during pregnancy and after delivery: indications for and results of thrombectomy. J Vasc Surg 2003;37(3):528–32.

39. Herrera S, Comerota AJ, Thakur S, et al. Managing iliofemoral deep venous thrombosis of pregnancy with a strategy of thrombus removal is safe and avoids post-thrombotic morbidity. J Vasc Surg 2014;59(2):456–64.

40. Clyne CA, Cudmore RE, Mansfield AO, et al. Thrombectomy for ilio-femoral venous occlusion: the youngest reported case. J Pediatr Surg 1977;12(5):703–4.

41. Laohapensang K, Hanpipat S, Aworn S, et al. Surgical venous thrombectomy for phlegmasia cerulea dolens and venous gangrene of the lower extremities. J Med Assoc Thai 2013;96(11):1463–9.

42. Comerota AJ, Aldridge SC, Cohen G, et al. A strategy of aggressive regional therapy for acute iliofemoral venous thrombosis with contemporary venous thrombectomy or catheter-directed thrombolysis. J Vasc Surg 1994;20(2):244–54.

Pulmonary Embolism
Current Role of Catheter Treatment Options and Operative Thrombectomy

Michael Jolly, MD, John Phillips, MD*

KEYWORDS

- Acute pulmonary embolism • Surgical pulmonary embolectomy
- Catheter thrombectomy • Thrombolysis • Submassive pulmonary embolism

KEY POINTS

- Acute pulmonary embolism continues to have an incredibly high mortality; more than double that seen with breast cancer.
- Anticoagulation and infrequent use of systemic thrombolysis or surgery has been the mainstay treatment options for decades.
- Less invasive techniques with more targeted therapeutic modalities have become increasingly used in the contemporary management with potentially less overall risk to the patient.
- Surgical embolectomy, although more invasive, still serves a critical and undeniable role in the effective management of this diverse patient population.

INTRODUCTION

The contemporary management of acute thrombotic pulmonary embolism (PE) has evolved significantly since the landmark clinical trial reported in *Lancet* by Barritt and Jordan[1] in 1960 established anticoagulation as the foundation of medical treatment. Even to this day, acute PE remains a devastating disease with an incredibly high prevalence, especially among hospitalized patients. It is estimated that PE accounts for at least 100,000 deaths in the United States annually[2]; however, the actual number is challenging to fully estimate, because patients with sudden death more commonly have their demise attributed to underlying cardiac disease rather than a thromboembolic cause. In Europe, of the 300,000 annual deaths attributed to PE, only 7% were diagnosed antemortem, with the remainder of victims being diagnosed at the time of death or postmortem.[3] These incredible statistics are only made more

The authors have nothing to disclose.
OhioHealth Heart and Vascular Physicians, Riverside Methodist Hospital, 3705 Olentangy River Road, Suite 100, Columbus, OH 43214, USA
* Corresponding author.
E-mail address: John.Phillips2@ohiohealth.com

impressive when it is realized that annual PE mortality rates in the United States are more than double that seen with annual breast cancer mortality,[4] the latter a highly visible disease with widespread general public awareness because of an effective media campaign.

Over the past three decades, the overall understanding of venous thromboembolic disease has grown exponentially; but the treatment paradigm has changed little compared with other disease states associated with high prevalence and mortality, such as cancer, cardiovascular disease, and stroke. Undoubtedly, the use of anticoagulation and even systemic thrombolysis for a patient with massive PE has made meaningful impact on overall mortality, but it remains a binary approach to a much more complicated disease. The understanding of the natural history of PE has been greatly informed by several prospective studies and international registries. The International Cooperative Pulmonary Embolism Registry (ICOPER) followed 2454 patients over Europe and North America with the diagnosis of acute PE and found a surprisingly high mortality rate of more than 15% for all-comers at 90 days.[5] This registry is important because it exposed the fact that not all of the mortality was driven simply from patients presenting with cardiogenic shock, the so-called "massive PE" patients. Rather, this category comprised only around 4.5% of the entire patient population with the remainder 95.5% being "nonmassive PE" patients.[6] Clearly, there was great variability in the majority group, which historically was only being treated with unfractionated heparin and eventually a vitamin K antagonist. Since the late 1990s when ICOPER was published, the clinical evaluation of PE has evolved to more fully risk-stratify patients into subsets based on a host of clinical, epidemiologic, and radiographic criteria. The overall goal is to harmonize the intensity of therapy with the prognostic risk of the disease. Not all pulmonary emboli are created equally.

PATHOPHYSIOLOGY

Notwithstanding the complex cause of venous thromboembolic disease, the sequelae of PE should be viewed as a disease of the right ventricle (RV). More specifically, the sudden strain imposed on the right side of the heart from thrombotic outflow obstruction, referred to as acute cor pulmonale, sets off a complex chain of compensatory mechanisms that eventually fail if the burden is too great. The pulmonary circulation is normally a low-pressure, high-flow circuit powered by the RV, which itself has a limited ability to increase wall tension and stress. In the normal state, the nonpreconditioned, thin-walled RV cannot generate a mean pulmonary artery (PA) pressure greater than 40 mm Hg. When 30% to 50% of the total cross-sectional pulmonary arterial bed becomes occluded by thromboemboli, the PA pressures begin to increase, setting off a chain of neurohumoral compensation pathways aimed at overcoming the pressure demands.[7] In addition to the significant RV stain, acute PE is a disease of gas exchange primarily mediated through severe oxygen supply/demand mismatch from extensive dead space ventilation. These consequences lead to an unraveling of RV and left ventricular (LV) function, with evolving RV ischemia, increased deoxygenation, decreased RV cardiac output, resultant poor total cardiac output, decreased systemic blood pressure, and ultimately ensuing cardiovascular collapse and death.[8,9] Understanding the complex pathophysiology is critical in risk-stratifying patients to an individualized treatment algorithm that appropriately addresses their real-time needs. For example, if a patient has already evolved to cardiogenic shock with severe hypoxemia, they may be considered for more urgent operative treatment or placement on extracorporeal membrane oxygenation rather than treated with catheter-based therapy that is more often reserved for patients earlier in the clinical course or with a less severe presentation.

CATHETER-BASED THERAPIES

Implicit in the need for likely an expensive, clearly invasive, and potentially dangerous treatment option, for a disease that has historically been treated with a peripheral intravenous line and anticoagulation is an acknowledgment that current treatment paradigms are lacking. The use of unfractionated heparin and oral anticoagulation is a one-size-fits-all approach for such a complex disease process. Even among intermediate-risk patients with significant RV strain, some are barely symptomatic, whereas others are at extraordinary high risk for further hemodynamic decompensation and death. The PEITHO randomized multicenter clinical trial of nearly 1000 patients sought to select these highest-risk but still normotensive, patients for either standard anticoagulation or anticoagulation in addition to full dose, systemically administered tenectaplase. Although this trial was successful in showing a significant decrease in the combined end point of death or hemodynamic deterioration in those treated with thrombolysis versus those treated with heparin alone (2.6% vs 5.6%; odds ratio, 0.44; 95% confidence interval, 0.23–0.87; $P = .02$), there was a significant trade off with significantly increased extracranial and intracranial bleeding in the tenectaplase group.[10] The recognition of sobering bleeding data further underscores a primary reason for why routine use of thrombolytics has long been cautioned against, even in this higher-risk population.

The use of catheter-based technologies seeks to mitigate some of the inherent bleeding risk associated with systemic delivery of thrombolytics in several different ways. For one, delivering drug directly into and even beyond the thrombus may allow for lower dosing and potential systemic bleeding effect. Secondly, the use of adjuvant thrombectomy may decrease the overall treatment time and dosing requirements. Importantly, the use of catheters allows for direct assessment of PA pressures, cardiac output and index measurement, and an objective hemodynamic feedback response to treatment. Finally, catheter-based thrombectomy may be the only viable option in patients with life-threatening PE who are not suitable candidates for either surgical embolectomy or thrombolysis. A rapidly evolving body of scientific evidence continues to seek better understanding as to when and where the various invasive catheter approaches will prove useful in the management of these challenging patients.

THROMBOLYTIC AGENTS AND ADMINISTRATION ROUTES

There are multiple Food and Drug Administration (FDA)-approved thrombolytic agents for the treatment of acute PE; however, the best studied ones include recombinant tissue type plasminogen activator (tPA, alteplase), streptokinase, and recombinant human urokinase.[11,12] Other thrombolytic agents include lanoteplase, tenectoplase, and reteplase, and although each agent has chemically different characteristics, they all lead to increased fibrinolysis by altering plasminogen activation. Once it has been decided to administer a specific thrombolytic agent within the venous system, the most common route is via a peripheral intravenous catheter with a continuous infusion. Although bolus routes and the use of catheter-based infusion have been described, the first of which was reported more than 40 years ago for catheter-based treatment, there is a paucity of large randomized trials demonstrating clear benefit with either of these methods.[12] In a trial of 34 patients with persistent hypotension from massive PE, catheter-directed full-dose tPA comparted to full-dose intravenous infusion, the authors demonstrated that the route of administration had no impact on the severity of PE (determined by pulmonary angiogram) or the change in mean pulmonary arterial pressure.[11] Although there are several catheter-based techniques and devices available for administration of thrombolytic regimens, only one ultrasound-assisted device has been approved by the FDA. In reality, any catheter that can reach the PA can be used to deliver the thrombolytic agent to a specific location within the pulmonary arterial tree. Common catheters used for said delivery include a standard pigtail catheter, a general multipurpose catheter, and Swan Ganz catheter. For example, in our practice we typically use a 5F pigtail catheter to administer a bolus dose of thrombolytic therapy into the pulmonary arterial tree, attempting to localize the delivery to a specific segment based on the thrombus burden from the computed tomography scan.

ULTRASOUND-ASSISTED INFUSION CATHETERS

The use of ultrasound energy to augment thrombolysis was first described in 2000 using a canine model of acute myocardial infarction.[13] This technology was ultimately refined and achieved FDA approval in 2004 for "controlled and selective infusion" of thrombolytic medication into the peripheral vasculature.[14] The ultrasound-assisted device commercially available is the EkoSonic Endovascular System (EKOS Corporation, Bothell, WA; **Fig. 1**). This catheter-based system generates ultrasound energy that is thought to facilitate catheter-directed thrombolysis, thereby thought to improve thrombolysis with lower doses of agent. The mechanism of action is thought to occur by accelerating the fibrinolytic process via the application of ultrasound energy to disrupt the fibrin strands, increasing surface area of the thrombus, and ultimately making more plasminogen activator receptor sites available to the lytic agent of choice. This technology has been applied to the treatment of PE in symptomatic patients with RV dysfunction. The rationale behind this device stems from an effort to expedite thrombus removal with a lower dose of thrombolytic agent, thus reducing the risk of major bleeding that has been reported with full-dose systemic thrombolysis.

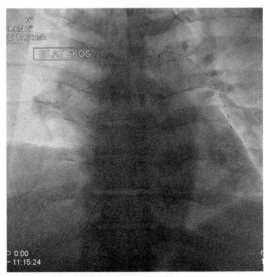

Fig. 1. Representative bilateral Ekosonic catheters placed in the pulmonary arteries via the right common femoral vein approach.

In the ULTIMA trial, 59 patients with acute intermediate-risk PE (PE of the main or low lobe PA and echocardiographic evidence of RV enlargement [RV to LV diameter ratio $\geq$1]) were randomized to ultrasound-assisted catheter-directed thrombolysis followed by intravenous heparin or intravenous heparin alone. The ultrasound-assisted group received 10 to 20 mg of tPA infused over 15 hours. At 24 hours, the ultrasound-assisted group had improved RV/LV ratio (mean difference of 0.3 vs 0.03).[15] However, at 90 days there was no difference in mortality or major bleeding between the two groups. A single-arm prospective trial (SEATTLE II) again evaluated the efficacy and safety of ultrasound-assisted, catheter-directed, low-dose fibrinolysis in 150 patients with massive and submassive PE (proximal PE, and RV/LV diameter ratio $\geq$0.9).[16] A total of 24 mg tPA was infused either at 1 mg/h for 24 hours or 1 mg/h/catheter for 12 hours with bilateral catheters. Mean RV/LV ratio decreased, as did mean PA systolic pressure, without intracranial hemorrhage.[16] The investigators concluded that this therapy decreased RV dilation, reduced pulmonary hypertension, and minimized intracranial hemorrhage in this patient population. To date the EKOS system remains the only FDA-approved device to administer thrombolytic therapy in the peripheral vasculature.

MECHANICAL THROMBECTOMY DEVICES

Unfortunately, the catheter-based removal of thrombotic pulmonary emboli is not usually as easy as advancing a catheter into the PA and applying suction. Aspirated material obtained either via catheter extraction or surgical removal commonly reveals a mixture of acute thrombus and older, more organized debris. Entrainment of the latter into a small catheter or with suction is difficult to achieve. As such, the goals of catheter-based mechanical thrombectomy are primarily aimed at removing or modifying proximal thrombus in a manner that rapidly recruits more downstream lobar and segmental arterial branches, increasing the cross-sectional area of the arterial tree, and thereby reduce the effect PA pressure and consequent RV strain pathophysiology.[17] Simple maneuvers, such as rapidly rotating a pigtail catheter within proximal thrombus or using standard percutaneous transluminal angioplasty, may be enough modification to allow for better parenchymal pulmonary perfusion, but this is more often unsuccessful as a stand-alone procedure. Thrombectomy is typically and most effectively done alongside thrombolysis but may be done without, especially in patients with contraindications to thrombolysis. Most devices in use today are adapted from their purposeful intentions elsewhere in the body and not specifically designed for the treatment of acute pulmonary embolization. The more commonly used devices in contemporary practice are reviewed next.

AngioJet

The use of hydrodynamic or rheolytic thrombectomy has emerged as a mainstay treatment option for symptomatic deep vein thrombosis but also enjoys some utility in the treatment of PE. The AngioJet (Boston Scientific, Marlborough, MA; **Fig. 2**) technology is based on the creation of high-velocity saline jets that spray backward from the catheter tip toward the catheter in a coaxial direction. The high-velocity jets create a low pressure microenvironment, creating a vacuum through the Venturi effect, ultimately entraining thrombus into the body of the catheter. In addition to its thrombectomy mechanism, it can also work as a drug delivery platform given its ability to spray thrombolytics directly into the PA. It has not been widely adopted for the treatment of acute PE, primarily because of the issues related to its secondary effects on causing bradycardia and hypotension. Other drawbacks include hemolysis and

A

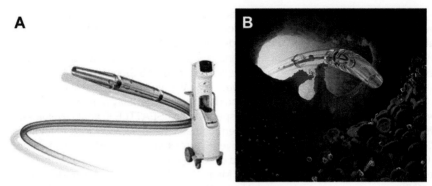

B

Fig. 2. (*A*) AngioJet catheter and console. (*B*) AngioJet rheolytic catheter. (*Courtesy of* Boston Scientific.)

hemoglobinuria that can often be significant during prolonged run times. Despite this, it continues to remain a reasonable option for this patient population and has some, primarily case series, evidence to support its continued use.[18,19]

Aspirex

The Aspirex S (Straub Medical, Wangs, Switzerland) is an up to 10F catheter device that uses a high-speed, rotational coil within the catheter body that generates a low-pressure microenvironment causing suction of thrombotic debris into the aspiration port. It then through its mechanism of action causes fragmentation, maceration, and clearing of the thrombus. Although more widely used in acute deep venous thromboembolism or dialysis access, the Aspirex catheter has some limited evidence to support its use in the treatment of high-risk PE.[20,21]

FlowTriever

The FlowTriever system (Inari Medical, Irvine, CA) uses a wide-bore, hydrophilic 20F aspiration guide catheter that can easily be delivered into the PAs over a standard supportive guidewire. Through this catheter, a series of three nitinol mesh disks are deployed and then retrieved back into the catheter with simultaneous suction (**Figs. 3** and **4**). As they are withdrawn, the often extended and flattened disks attempt to return to their baseline circular dimension. The gentle outward radial force and the porous mesh weave entrain and capture thrombus, effectively dragging often large pieces of thrombotic debris back into the 20F aspiration guide catheter. The potential advantages to this large catheter system include the ability

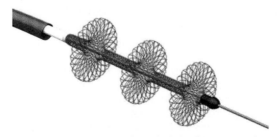

Fig. 3. FlowTriever device with three nitinol mesh disks. (*Courtesy of* Inari Medical.)

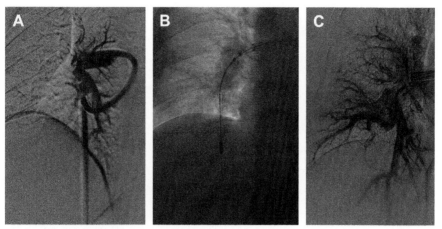

Fig. 4. (*A*) Large right main pulmonary artery embolism. (*B*) FlowTriever deployment in anterior basal right lower lobe of the pulmonary artery. (*C*) Post FlowTriever arterial flow with dramatic improvement in parenchymal perfusion.

to retrieve larger thrombi, including clot from a mixed morphology. It can be used with or without concomitant thrombolysis and is currently commercially approved for thrombectomy but undergoing a clinical trial for a specific designation to treat PE.[22]

Penumbra

The Penumbra Indigo system (Penumbra, Inc, Alameda, CA) is a general use, mechanical thrombectomy aspiration device that uses continuous suction applied through a hydrophilic, angled, up to 8F aspiration catheter (**Figs. 5** and **6**). Some mechanical disruption is achieved with the wire separator that helps assist entrainment of thrombus into the catheter, while disrupting the occasional ball-valve effect seen with completely occlusive thrombus. Like AngioJet and FlowTriever, it does not carry a specific indication for the treatment of acute PE but is often used as an adjuvant device, especially in high-risk PE when thrombolysis is contraindicated. Delivery is simple through a sheath placed into the PA. This system does not use a guidewire lumen so the forfeiture of wire access is a drawback, especially when specific arterial branch placement is sought. Like other catheter-based devices, it is often highly effective at removing fresh thrombus but struggles with chronic, more organized debris. Careful attention at controlling the suction switch is a must to avoid the unnecessary evacuation of blood.

AngioVac

An answer to many of the drawbacks of other devices listed previously is the 22F catheter AngioVac cannula and extracorporeal bypass circuit (Angiodynamics, Latham, NY). This large device overcomes the limitations of smaller devices in its ability to entrain large, even organized, debris en bloc (**Figs. 7** and **8**). Additionally, because it is recirculated through an extracorporeal membrane circuit, all blood is filtered and returned to the body with effectively no significant loss of blood. The major limitation is cannula stiffness and deliverability into the pulmonary tree with the potential for major vascular injury. Additionally, setup is more involved and typically requires perfusionists and general anesthesia. It is most commonly used in the

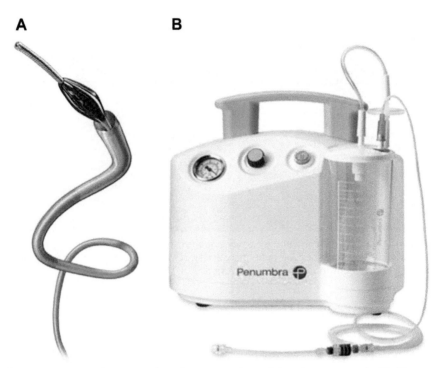

Fig. 5. Penumbra Indigo CAT-8 thrombectomy catheter (*A*) and pump console (*B*). (*Courtesy of* Penumbra, Inc.)

treatment of large vessel thrombosis, such as the inferior vena cava, or in extracting right atrial thrombi or vegetations from pacemaker leads. However, successful treatment of acute PE has been achieved in high-volume centers with appropriate expertise.[23]

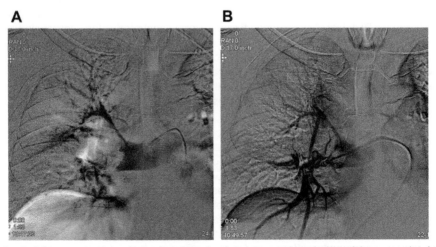

Fig. 6. (*A*) Large, nearly occlusive right distal pulmonary artery embolism. (*B*) Improved right lower pulmonary artery perfusion following suction thrombectomy using the CAT-8 Indigo catheter.

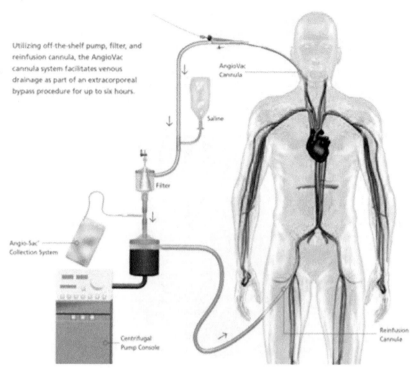

Utilizing off-the-shelf pump, filter, and
reinfusion cannula, the AngioVac
cannula system facilitates venous
drainage as part of an extracorporeal
bypass procedure for up to six hours.

AngioVac
Cannula

Saline

Filter

Angio-Sac™
Collection System

Centrifugal
Pump Console

Reinfusion
Cannula

Fig. 7. Graphical representation of the AngioVac extracorporeal circuit. (*Courtesy of* Angiodynamics.)

SURGICAL EMBOLECTOMY

Successful treatment of acute PE with surgical embolectomy was first described in the 1924 by Kirschner,[24] long before anticoagulation was recognized as a medical therapy. Today, surgical embolectomy is predominately reserved for several specific clinical scenarios. These generally include hemodynamic instability with concurrent inotropic or vasopressor support with contraindications for thrombolysis, failed thrombolysis with continued evidence of cardiopulmonary demise, and paradoxic clot-in-transit that is trapped within an atrial septal defect or patent foramen ovale. Mortality rates for patients undergoing surgery are varied across the reported literature and largely dependent on whether the patient was truly unstable, suffered from full cardiopulmonary arrest before surgery, age, and overall experience of the center. When cared for by an experienced center with a more liberal treatment paradigm that included surgery on submassive PE patients with extensive thrombus burden and RV strain, the operative mortality was 11%.[25] However, when a more representative sample of patients with true cardiogenic shock and contraindications to lysis is followed, the mortality climbs to 30% and up to 59% to 74% for those with a preoperative cardiac arrest.[26,27]

Technically, the operative procedure is straightforward. Transesophageal echocardiography should be used in all patients before incision to detect the presence of atrial septal defect, patent foramen ovale, or evidence of clot-in-transit because this may affect the choice of cannulation and myocardial protection strategy. Next, patients undergo standard median sternotomy, heparinization, and cannulation for cardiopulmonary bypass. Importantly, this is done under normothermic conditions in the absence of cardioplegic arrest unless concomitant atrial septal defect or patent

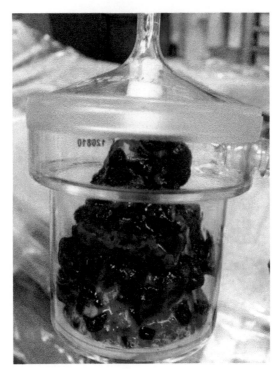

Fig. 8. Large-volume thrombus evacuated from a thrombosed inferior vena cava.

foramen ovale repair is required. A longitudinal incision is made in the main PA and in the right PA between the ascending aorta and the superior vena cava. Thrombus is manually aspirated with typical suction or forceps (**Fig. 9**). Fogarty-type embolectomy catheters are generally avoided to minimize PA injury. Variations of arteriotomy access may be required and brief reductions in cardiopulmonary bypass flow may be needed to assist with thrombus visualization.[28] The preoperative use of thrombolysis is clearly associated with increased operative bleeding but should not be considered an absolute contraindication to this procedure.[29]

Despite surgical embolectomy's important place in the overall armamentarium for treatment of severe PE, its overall use and adoption is varied across hospitals. In the two largest registries of acute PE, surgery was used in only 1% of patients presenting with cardiogenic shock and massive PE.[5,30] Review of more contemporary case series and hospital systems that have effectively reintroduced this old surgical procedure should help increase its implementation in places where it is not routinely considered. It is recognized that the location of the procedure, major referral system or smaller community hospital, did not seem to have a significant impact on inpatient mortality rates.[31] The use of multidisciplinary medical teams also seems to have a measureable benefit, likely by selecting more appropriate patients for the operating room.[32–34] The use of a PE response team should be a key consideration for any hospital that routinely takes care of this patient subset.[35]

FUTURE DIRECTIONS

In the hemodynamically unstable, or massive, PE patients, the achievement of unsupported stability and eventual hospital discharge are major clinical milestones that

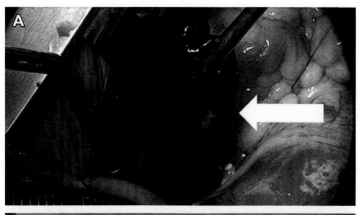

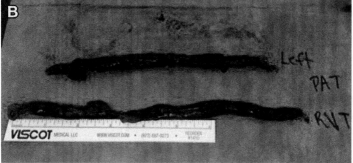

Fig. 9. (A) Operative en masse removal of a large, thrombus (arrow) via the main pulmonary artery with forceps. (B) Organized thrombus shaped as a cast of the femoral vein from where it originated. (Courtesy of Jeff Lyons, MD, Columbus, OH.)

correlate with survival. However, the full spectrum and long-term sequelae of PE is more nuanced and difficult to quantify. Several difficult clinical decisions must be made along the inpatient and outpatient journey of these patients. Should one treat with a catheter-based approach? Should thrombolysis be used? If so, for how long? What are the early or late indicators of success? How long should the patient be anticoagulated? What is his or her risk of recurrence or decompensation? Most of the answers to these questions remain clinical unknowns. Technology is maturing but still remains extremely limited for the efficient removal of acute and chronic thrombotic debris. Each device currently available has major drawbacks and limitations. A great deal has been learned about the use of surrogate markers of overall risk, such as RV strain, elevated cardiac biomarkers, and combined clinical scoring algorithms. In our opinion, keeping the patient alive, minimizing bleeding risk, and treating symptoms are excellent benchmarks to aim for. It is hoped that in the future there will be better understanding at how acute PE may lead to chronic thromboembolic pulmonary hypertension and, more importantly, how this may be prevented. Better protocols and treatment algorithms that are derived from sound, large-scale randomized clinical trials will be crucial. The advent of the PE response team will serve as a useful framework to collate data from many different centers but also to rapidly disperse the latest advancement in care.

SUMMARY

The contemporary use of catheter-based or surgical-based treatment of acute PE remains varied and often center-specific. Catheter-based treatments are evolving a niche for those patients in the intermediate-risk categories or high risk with contraindications for thrombolysis. With modern and near ubiquitous axial imaging, the recognition and diagnosis of PE is at an all-time high. The treatment of this ancient disease is finally at a precipice where it is hoped that meaningful and improved impact will begin to be made on mortality and quality of life over the upcoming generation.

REFERENCES

1. Barritt DW, Jordan SC. Anticoagulant drugs in the treatment of pulmonary embolism. Lancet 1960;275(7138):1309–12.
2. Horlander KT, Mannino DM, Leeper KV. Pulmonary embolism mortality in the United States, 1979-1998: an analysis using multiple-cause mortality data. Arch Intern Med 2003;163(14):1711–7.
3. Cohen AT, Agnelli G, Anderson FA, et al. Venous thromboembolism (VTE) in Europe. The number of VTE events and associated morbidity and mortality. Thromb Haemost 2007;98(4):756–64. Available at: http://www.ncbi.nlm.nih.gov/pubmed/17938798. Accessed July 13, 2017.
4. DeSantis CE, Fedewa SA, Goding Sauer A, et al. Breast cancer statistics, 2015: convergence of incidence rates between black and white women. CA Cancer J Clin 2016;66(1):31–42.
5. Goldhaber SZ, Visani L, De Rosa M, et al. Acute pulmonary embolism: clinical outcomes in the International Cooperative Pulmonary Embolism Registry (ICOPER). Lancet 1999;353(9162):1386–9.
6. Kucher N, Rossi E, De Rosa M, et al. Massive pulmonary embolism. Circulation 2006;113(4):577–82.
7. McIntyre KM, Sasahara AA. The hemodynamic response to pulmonary embolism in patients without prior cardiopulmonary disease. Am J Cardiol 1971;28(3):288–94. Available at: http://www.ncbi.nlm.nih.gov/pubmed/5155756. Accessed July 22, 2017.
8. Molloy WD, Lee KY, Girling L, et al. Treatment of shock in a canine model of pulmonary embolism. Am Rev Respir Dis 1984;130(5):870–4.
9. Burrowes KS, Clark AR, Tawhai MH. Blood flow redistribution and ventilation-perfusion mismatch during embolic pulmonary arterial occlusion. Pulm Circ 2011;1(3):365–76.
10. Meyer G, Vicaut E, Danays T, et al. Fibrinolysis for patients with intermediate-risk pulmonary embolism. N Engl J Med 2014;370(15):1402–11.
11. Verstraete M, Miller GA, Bounameaux H, et al. Intravenous and intrapulmonary recombinant tissue-type plasminogen activator in the treatment of acute massive pulmonary embolism. Circulation 1988;77(2):353–60. Available at: http://www.ncbi.nlm.nih.gov/pubmed/3123091. Accessed July 18, 2017.
12. Hirsh J, Hale GS, McDonald IG, et al. Streptokinase therapy in acute major pulmonary embolism: effectiveness and problems. BMJ 1968;4(5633):729–34. Available at: http://www.bmj.com/content/4/5633/729. Accessed August 28, 2017.
13. Siegel RJ, Atar S, Fishbein MC, et al. Noninvasive, transthoracic, low-frequency ultrasound augments thrombolysis in a canine model of acute myocardial infarction. Circulation 2000;101(17):2026–9. Available at: http://www.ncbi.nlm.nih.gov/pubmed/10790341. Accessed August 29, 2017.
14. Owens C. Ultrasound-enhanced thrombolysis: Ekos Endowave infusion catheter system. Semin Intervent Radiol 2008;25(1):037–41.
15. Kucher N, Boekstegers P, Müller O, et al. Randomized controlled trial of ultrasound-assisted catheter-directed thrombolysis for acute intermediate-risk

pulmonary embolism. Circulation 2014;129(4):479–86. Available at: http://circ.ahajournals.org/content/early/2013/11/13/CIRCULATIONAHA.113.005544.short. Accessed July 21, 2017.

16. Piazza G, Hohlfelder B, Jaff MR, et al. A prospective, single-arm, multicenter trial of ultrasound-facilitated, catheter-directed, low-dose fibrinolysis for acute massive and submassive pulmonary embolism. JACC Cardiovasc Interv 2015; 8(10):1382–92.

17. Engelberger RP, Kucher N. Catheter-based reperfusion treatment of pulmonary embolism. Circulation 2011;124(19):2139–44.

18. Chauhan MS, Kawamura A. Percutaneous rheolytic thrombectomy for large pulmonary embolism: a promising treatment option. Catheter Cardiovasc Interv 2007;70(1):123–30.

19. Bonvini RF, Roffi M, Bounameaux H, et al. AngioJet rheolytic thrombectomy in patients presenting with high-risk pulmonary embolism and cardiogenic shock: a feasibility pilot study. EuroIntervention 2013;8(12):1419–27.

20. Bayiz H, Dumantepe M, Teymen B, et al. Percutaneous aspiration thrombectomy in treatment of massive pulmonary embolism. Heart Lung Circ 2015;24(1):46–54.

21. Eid-Lidt G, Gaspar J, Sandoval J, et al. Combined clot fragmentation and aspiration in patients with acute pulmonary embolism. Chest 2008;134(1):54–60.

22. FlowTriever Pulmonary Embolectomy Clinical Study - Full Text View - ClinicalTrials.gov. Available at: https://clinicaltrials.gov/show/NCT02692586. Accessed July 22, 2017.

23. Donaldson CW, Baker JN, Narayan RL, et al. Thrombectomy using suction filtration and veno-venous bypass: single center experience with a novel device. Catheter Cardiovasc Interv 2015;86(2):E81–7.

24. Kirschner M. Ein durch die trendelenburgsche operation geheilter fall von bolie der arterien pulmonalis. Arch Klin Chir 1924;133:312.

25. Aklog L, Williams CS, Byrne JG, et al. Acute pulmonary embolectomy. Circulation 2002;105(12). Available at: http://circ.ahajournals.org/content/105/12/1416.long. Accessed July 6, 2017.

26. Stein PD, Alnas M, Beemath A, et al. Outcome of pulmonary embolectomy. Am J Cardiol 2007;99(3):421–3.

27. Clarke DB, Abrams LD. Pulmonary embolectomy: a 25 year experience. J Thorac Cardiovasc Surg 1986;92(3 Pt 1):442–5. Available at: http://www.ncbi.nlm.nih.gov/pubmed/3747572. Accessed July 20, 2017.

28. Leacche M, Unic D, Goldhaber SZ, et al. Modern surgical treatment of massive pulmonary embolism: results in 47 consecutive patients after rapid diagnosis and aggressive surgical approach. J Thorac Cardiovasc Surg 2005;129(5): 1018–23.

29. Aklog L, Williams CS, Byrne JG, et al. Acute pulmonary embolectomy: a contemporary approach. Circulation 2002;105(12):1416–9. Available at: http://www.ncbi.nlm.nih.gov/pubmed/11914247. Accessed July 20, 2017.

30. Kasper W, Konstantinides S, Geibel A, et al. Management strategies and determinants of outcome in acute major pulmonary embolism: results of a multicenter registry. J Am Coll Cardiol 1997;30(5):1165–71. Available at: http://www.ncbi.nlm.nih.gov/pubmed/9350909. Accessed July 23, 2017.

31. Kilic A, Shah AS, Conte JV, et al. Nationwide outcomes of surgical embolectomy for acute pulmonary embolism. J Thorac Cardiovasc Surg 2013;145(2):373–7.

32. Malekan R, Saunders PC, Yu CJ, et al. Peripheral extracorporeal membrane oxygenation: comprehensive therapy for high-risk massive pulmonary embolism. Ann Thorac Surg 2012;94(1):104–8.

33. Fukuda I, Taniguchi S, Fukui K, et al. Improved outcome of surgical pulmonary embolectomy by aggressive intervention for critically ill patients. Ann Thorac Surg 2011;91(3):728–32.

34. Aymard T, Kadner A, Widmer A, et al. Massive pulmonary embolism: surgical embolectomy versus thrombolytic therapy—should surgical indications be revisited? Eur J Cardiothoracic Surg 2013;43(1):90–4.

35. Provias T, Dudzinski DM, Jaff MR, et al. The Massachusetts General Hospital Pulmonary Embolism Response Team (MGH PERT): creation of a multidisciplinary program to improve care of patients with massive and submassive pulmonary embolism. Hosp Pract 2014;42(1):31–7.

Inferior Vena Cava Filters

Current Indications, Techniques, and Recommendations

Cindy P. Ha, MD, John E. Rectenwald, MD, MS*

KEYWORDS

- Vena cava filter • PE Prevention • DVT

KEY POINTS

- Anticoagulation is the first-line treatment of venous thromboembolic events (VTEs).
- Vena cava filters (VCFs) provide a mechanical barrier to prevent progression of lower extremity deep venous thrombosis to pulmonary embolism.
- Absolute indications for VCF are presence of VTE with contraindication or failure of anticoagulation.
- Available VCF types can be divided into permanent and retrievable filters with increasing use of the latter in recent years.
- Complications include filter tilt, migration, strut fracture, malposition, and inferior vena caval thrombosis.

INTRODUCTION

Venous thromboembolism remains the most common cause of preventable in-hospital mortality with a morality rate ranging from 5% to 10%, and the prevalence of venous thromboembolic events (VTEs) is increasing with time. In a retrospective analysis of health care claims data in the United States from 2002 to 2006, there was a 33.1% increase in prevalence of VTEs from 2002 to 2006.[1] Left untreated, VTEs can be a significant source of morbidity and mortality. Although anticoagulation remains the first-line treatment of VTEs,[2] a small percentage of patients will experience recurrence despite anticoagulation, up to 7% at 6 months.[3] In addition, there is a subset of patients that cannot tolerate anticoagulation or may have other barriers that require alternative therapies for prevention of pulmonary embolism (PE). As a

The authors have nothing to disclose.
Division of Vascular and Endovascular Surgery, University of Texas Southwestern Medical Center, Professional Office Building 1, Suite 620, 5959 Harry Hines Boulevard, Dallas, TX 75390-9157, USA
* Corresponding author.
E-mail address: john.rectenwald@utsouthwestern.edu

result, vena cava filters (VCFs) remain an important tool in the armamentarium of the treating physician.

HISTORY

Vena caval interruption to prevent the occurrence of PE in the setting of deep venous thrombosis (DVT) has been in practice for centuries. It was first suggested by Trousseau in 1868, and the first successful inferior vena caval (IVC) ligation was performed by Bottini in 1893.[4] In the 1930s, Homan[5] recognized the relationship between DVT and PE and advocated femoral vein ligation. Femoral vein ligation eventually fell out of favor due to relatively high rates of recurrent VTE, with 5% to 8% fatal PE, in particular, due to the risk of PE from the contralateral lower extremity.[6] Around the same time, other surgeons, such as Ochsner and colleagues,[7] and others, proposed IVC ligation as Bottini had performed it almost a century earlier. By the 1960s, it became the preferred treatment of the prevention of massive PE. Unfortunately, IVC ligation was also associated with significant morbidity and mortality, including recurrent PE rate of 6% and venous stasis rate of 33%.[6] The collateral venous channels that provided venous return over time became a source of recurrent emboli.[8] Mortality with IVC ligation was reported at approximately 15% and was especially high in patients with preexisting cardiac disease, with mortality up to 55% in patients with class 4 heart failure.[9] Acute ligation of the vena cava was associated with up to 47% decrease in cardiac output.[10] Later, attempts to plicate or clip the vena cava were performed[11,12] but they also were associated with poor results, with operative mortality rates of 12%, IVC patency rates of 67%, and recurrent PE rates of 4%.[6] With lackluster results from surgical ligation and plication for vena caval interruption, the stage was set for the development of intraluminal filters.

The Mobin-Uddin umbrella, the first VCF, was introduced in 1967. This filter was initially placed via venotomy and consisted of a perforated silicone filter in the shape of an inverted umbrella with 6 stainless steel struts.[13,14] Although the transvenous approach avoided the previous morbidity and mortality of laparotomy, the filter itself was associated with migration and high rates of IVC occlusion and postthrombotic syndrome.[15] In 1973, the Greenfield filter (Boston Scientific, Natick, MA, USA) was developed.[16] It consisted of multiple struts arranged in a conical shape with the apex directed cephalad and struts that imbedded it into the caval wall. It was placed via an open venotomy, such as the Mobin-Uddin umbrella, but could be placed by either a femoral or an internal jugular approach, the former unique to it. The conical shape allowed for a significant clot packing ability within the center of the IVC while preserving caval flow and pressure gradients, which in turn provided exposure of the trapped clot to endogenous fibrinolysis.[17] It was also associated with much lower rates of caval occlusion and migration.[15] The percutaneous Greenfield filter was introduced in 1984[18] and, since then, it has become the template for multiple generations of filters to follow (see later discussion of currently available filters).

The purpose of the VCF was to prevent the progression of DVT to PE and, since its advent, the absolute indications have remained relatively unchanged. Over the recent years, however, the indications for VCF placement have expanded, likely due in part to newer retrievable IVC filters and minimally invasive techniques.

INDICATIONS

In 1960, Barritt and Jordan[19] established therapeutic anticoagulation as the treatment of VTEs, which then consisted of heparin and vitamin K antagonists. Since then, anticoagulation remains the cornerstone for treatment of VTE, including in the most recent 2016 CHEST and 2012 National Institute of Health and Clinical Excellent Guidelines.[2,20] VCFs provide a mechanical barrier to prevent the progression of DVT of the lower extremities and pelvis to PE but do not treat the underlying VTE itself. With the introduction of retrieval filters, there has been an increase in the number of VCF placements. Stein and colleagues[21] found a more than 20-fold increase from 2000 in 1979 to 49,000 in 1999. Another study showed an exponential increase from 1979 to 2006, with a 3-fold increase from just 2001 to 2006, with the largest expansion for prophylactic indications.[22] Because VCFs are sometimes associated with complications, it is of utmost importance for treating physicians to know the risks and benefits of VCFs. The available literature on VCFs has been predominately nonrandomized studies with significant heterogeneity of study design, leading to difficulty in defining indications for IVC filter placement.[23]

The Prevention du Risque d'Embolie Pulmonaire par Interruption Cave (PREPIC) trial published by Decousus and colleagues[24] randomized 400 subjects with proximal DVT to receive a VCF or not, and to receive unfractionated heparin or low-molecular-weight heparin. Anticoagulation was bridged to warfarin on day 4 and continued for at least 3 months. Four types of permanent filters were placed for the IVC filter arm, including Vena Tech (B Braun, Evanston, IL, USA), titanium Greenfield, Cardial (St. Etienne, France), and Bird's Nest (Cook, Inc, Bloomington, IN, USA). All subjects underwent baseline ventilation-perfusion scan or computed tomography (CT) angiography between days 8 and 12 if any signs or symptoms developed concerning for new or recurrent PE. The subjects were evaluated at 12 days and 2 years, and additional data were published on a follow-up study at 8 years. Of note, 99% of subjects were discharged on anticoagulation, 94% were still on anticoagulation at 3 months, and 38% were on anticoagulation at 2 and 8 years. At 12 days, there was a significant reduction in PE in the VCF group (4.8% vs 1.1%) but at 2 years the reduction in symptomatic PE was no longer significant. At 8 years, the reduction in symptomatic PE was again statistically significant but there was no significant reduction in mortality at 2 or 8 years. Most importantly, the investigators found a significantly increased risk of recurrent DVT at 1, 2, and 8 years, with a cumulative incidence of 8.5%, 20.8%, and 35.7%, respectively. There was a 13% rate of IVC thrombosis at 8 years and the incidence of postthrombotic syndrome was equivalent in both groups. Overall, this study confirmed the benefits and risks of VCFs decrease and increase, respectively, with time, further highlighting the need to understand indications for VCFs.[24,25] Similarly, White and colleagues[26] published a population-based observation study using the linked California Patient Discharge Data Set. From January 1991 to 1995, 4044 patients received a VCF for VTE versus 70,687 patients who did not. Analysis showed no statistically significant difference in the rate of recurrent PE requiring readmission over 1 year of follow-up and a 2-fold increase in readmission for VTE in patients with initial presentation of PE.

Other potential complications (see later discussion) of VCFs include filter malposition, strut fracture and/or embolization, guidewire entrapment, and IVC thrombosis. With all these complications in mind, physicians must be aware of indications for VCF placement and the associated risks and benefits. The indications can be subdivided into absolute, relative, and prophylactic indications (**Box 1**), and there are multiple guidelines available for reference.

Absolute

The development of PE or DVT is associated with a relatively high risk for recurrence without treatment. Recurrence, in turn, is associated with a high risk of morbidity and mortality. Without treatment, approximately 50% of patients with symptomatic

---

Box 1
Indications for inferior vena caval filter placement

Indications for VCF Placement

Absolute
  Presence of VTE and contraindication to anticoagulation
  Failure of anticoagulation to prevent VTE

Relative
  PE with limited cardiopulmonary reserve or right heart failure
  Chronic thromboembolic pulmonary hypertension undergoing pulmonary
  thromboendarterectomy
  Massive PE undergoing embolectomy or thrombolysis
  Thrombolysis of iliocaval thrombus
  Free-floating iliocaval thrombus

Prophylactic
  High-risk trauma patients with multiple risk factors (eg, long bone fractures, immobility) and
  inability to undergo anticoagulation
  Paraplegia patients or other high-risk patients with inability to undergo anticoagulation

---

proximal DVT or PE will have recurrent thrombosis within 3 months.[26,27] Although anti-coagulation is the first-line treatment of VTEs, there is a distinct subset of patients who are not candidates for anticoagulation. All published guidelines (American College of Chest Physicians [ACCP], Society of Interventional Radiology [SIR], American College of Radiology Appropriateness Criteria, and American Heart Association [AHA]) recommend the placement of VCF in patients with VTE and a contraindication to, or a failure of, anticoagulation.[2,20–32] For patients who fail anticoagulation, it is important to confirm a true failure of treatment because often these patients are found to be subtherapeutic, representing inadequate treatment with anticoagulation rather than failure of treatment. Once failure of anticoagulation is confirmed, systemic workup to rule out hypercoagulable syndromes, malignancy, and other systemic causes of hypercoagulability must be performed before VCF placement. In addition, if the recurrent thrombotic events repeatedly occur in the same location, anatomic variants, such as May-Thurner syndrome, must be considered. A VCF in this situation would not adequately address this issue and treatment may include stenting of the left common iliac vein.[33] All guidelines recommend the initiation of anticoagulation as soon as possible, even in the presence of an IVC filter, for treatment of the underlying DVT. Providers must reassess these patients to determine if the contraindication to anticoagulation, such as recent trauma, surgery, or bleed, has passed.[34]

In addition, the SIR defines failure of anticoagulation as the development of complications of anticoagulation or the inability to achieve therapeutic anticoagulation, the latter including noncompliance, and recommends placement of a VCF in these settings.[29,30]

Relative

Relative indications differ between the 4 major guidelines. The SIR guidelines report more clinical settings in which VCF placement may be indicated. The prior ACCP guidelines in 2012 and current SIR guidelines recommend consideration of adding a VCF in addition to anticoagulation in patients, with unstable patients with PE and/or patients with limited cardiopulmonary reserve receiving anticoagulation.[29,35] Billet and colleagues[36] compared VCF and anticoagulation to anticoagulation alone. The former was mostly used for management of massive PE or VTE or anticoagulation failure. They found no difference in PE incidence at 90 days or 5 years, and a trend toward increased incidence of DVT in the VCF and anticoagulation group, although this did not reach statistical significance. Similar results were found in a more recent randomized trial comparing VCF with anticoagulation versus anticoagulation alone. At 6 months, there was no difference in recurrent PE, and 3 subjects in the former group developed filter thrombosis.[37] With results from these and other similar studies, the most recent ACCP CHEST guidelines do not recommend VCF in the setting of anticoagulation, although it remains a relative guideline for SIR guidelines. As a result, the decision must be individualized per patient.

Another relative indication includes patients with recurrent or persistent PE with subsequent chronic thromboembolic pulmonary hypertension (CTEPH) requiring pulmonary thromboendarterectomy.[38] Although data are limited, inadequate caval filtration has been associated with repeat thromboendarterectomy in patients with CTEPH.[39] Given the high risk for recurrence and limited treatments options, a VCF is often placed, along with lifelong anticoagulation.[34]

The SIR guidelines include more relative indications for VCF placement. These include large, free-floating proximal DVT, thrombolysis for iliocaval DVT, iliocaval DVT, massive PE treated with thrombolysis or embolectomy, noncompliance, and a high risk of anticoagulation complications.[29]

Large free-floating proximal iliocaval thrombus has been inconsistently reported as an increased risk for PE.[40–46] Pacouret and colleagues[43] published a prospective trial that showed no evidence of increased risk. Other studies have shown that most PEs occurred before the finding of the free-floating DVT, suggesting no significant benefit in placing a VCF on diagnosis of a free-floating iliocaval thrombus.[34,41,45] Similarly, the use of a VCF for protection during thrombolysis for proximal iliofemoral DVT has shown conflicting evidence of benefit. In a retrospective study, Kölbel and colleagues[46] evaluated catheter-directed thrombolysis with routine VCF use and found that 45% of filters had visible thrombi on venogram and no PE occurred, suggesting a protective benefit. However, other studies have shown very rare to no incidence of PE with thrombolysis in the absence of a VCF.[47,48]

Overall, given the variety of relative indications across the guidelines and conflicting data, the use of VCFs for relative indications must be individualized for each patient, weighing the risks and benefits of adding VCF placement.

Prophylactic

Prophylactic indications are applied to patients without confirmed VTE but considered high risk for VTE, with either a contraindication to anticoagulation or inadequate protection with anticoagulation. The increased use of VCFs over the past decade has been correlated with the introduction of retrieval filters and expansion of prophylactic indications. These are the least well-defined, and data are limited to predominately nonrandomized studies.[49] In various available guidelines, there is some overlap with relative indications.

The ACCP CHEST and AHA guidelines do not provide any prophylactic indication recommendations in the absence of VTE. The SIR guidelines, similar to relative indications, have delineated the most prophylactic indications, and these include high-risk trauma, oncologic, and surgical patients.[2,29–31]

Trauma patients commonly develop VTE, especially in the setting of multisystem traumas, pelvic or long bone fractures, and spinal trauma. The incidence of DVT has been reported as high as 50% to 58%, usually presenting within the first few weeks of hospitalization, and of PE as high as 32%.[50–55] Beyond the injury pattern, immobility, inflammation, and venous stasis likely contribute to the pathophysiology.[56] A prospective study by Geerts and colleagues[51] showed increased risk of DVT in lower extremity orthopedic injuries and spinal trauma with DVT rates of 69% and 62%, respectively. In addition, trauma patients not uncommonly have concurrent injuries that are contraindications to anticoagulation, such as severe intracranial hemorrhage or injury or spinal cord injury, and traditional prophylactic anticoagulation may be inadequate.[57] Consequently, the Eastern Association of Surgery of Trauma published guidelines in 2002 recommending consideration of VCF placement in high-risk patients, even in the setting of only level III evidence.[52] Multiple nonrandomized observational trials have evaluated VCF use in trauma patients, and shown a reduction in PE with a low complication rate.[53,58–60] A recent study of prophylactic and therapeutic VCFs in trauma subjects showed improved mortality in subjects with a VCF for prophylactic versus therapeutic reasons and a decrease in the recurrent PE rate of 0% versus 18%, respectively. Over the 10-year period, they reported a 50% reduction of PE risk.[60] However, an important consideration in trauma patients is the low retrieval rate. A multicenter trial by AAST (American Association for the Surgery of Trauma) showed that despite 76% of VCFs being placed for prophylactic reasons, only 22% were ultimately retrieved.[61] Currently, high-risk trauma patients, especially those with the high-risk trauma injury patterns, should be considered for VCF placement on an individualized basis.

In the past, bariatric surgery patients were considered for prophylactic a VCF due to a high risk of postoperative VTE, which is among the most common reasons for postoperative death in bariatric surgery.[62–64] The incidence of DVT is reported to be 1% to 3% and of PE to be 0.3% to 2%, and reported mortality with PE is up to 30%.[64] The use of prophylactic anticoagulation has been become commonplace in bariatric surgery patients, but there is no defined regimen. The risk is greatest in the first couple of months postoperatively and, as such, despite the relatively high incidence of VTE, no data have shown that VCFs improve outcomes. Two recent large retrospective studies showed no benefit with VCF use,[65–67] and a systemic review of available literature, including 11 observational studies, demonstrated poor evidence to support the use of VCFs in this patient population.

Patients with advanced cancer are another population historically associated with increased incidence of VTE and increased bleeding risk. Theoretically, VCFs could be beneficial in these patients. However, the hypercoagulopathy with malignancy is a systemic complication, and VCFs provide only regional protection. In addition, the risk of recurrent VTE and bleeding were directly related to cancer stage, especially metastases versus localized recurrence.[68] As such, it seems the oncologic patients who may benefit the most from a VCF may not be candidates due to a relatively short lifespan. Anticoagulation has been established as the standard prevention treatment of VTE in patients with cancer based on multiple studies.[2,69,70] A retrospective study evaluating the addition of a VCF showed improved median survival with anticoagulation alone versus a VCF alone or combined anticoagulation and a VCF.[71] Overall, the data do not support the routine use of VCFs in oncologic patients.

VENA CAVA FILTERS

The first available filters were the Mobin-Uddin and Greenfield filters,[13,16] and the latter would form the template for most filters to come. Since then, there have been ongoing developments in VCFs and, although quite fascinating, a detailed history of the various generations over the past decades is beyond the scope of this article. The currently available filters can be divided into permanent and optional filters, with the latter further subdivided into retrievable and temporary filters.

Permanent Filters

By definition, permanent filters are those that lack a mechanism for retrieving and are meant to remain in place indefinitely. Although the use of retrievable filters has surpassed permanent filters, there is still a subset of patients who benefit from permanent filters. In addition, the data and follow-up are much more robust with permanent filters (**Table 1**).

Greenfield filter

The original stainless steel Greenfield filter (see: http://www.bostonscientific.com/en-US/products/embolic-protection/greenfield-vena-cava-filter.html) is the basis of most vena caval filters to follow and has the longest follow-up data available.[16] It is conical, measures 4.6 cm from apex to base, and consists of 6 struts with hooks at the end for caval fixation. The spacing between the struts is 2 mm at the apex to 5 to 6 mm at the base, allowing effective trapping of most emboli as small as 3 mm. The conical shape allows for efficient clot trapping with preservation of caval flow so that when the thrombus fills 70% of the filter, only 49% of the cross-sectional area is blocked. Venous pressures are maintained until 80% of the filter is filled, and the preservation of flow also allows for progressive lysis of the trapped thrombus due to mechanical flow and endogenous fibrinolysis.[17,72] Greenfield and Michna[73] noted a 4% incidence of recurrent embolism and 98% filter patency rate at 12 years. At 20 years, there were similar rates of recurrent embolism, with 96% long-term patency rate and 8% rate of filter movement of no clinical significance.[74] The high rate of patency has allowed for the unconventional locations for placement, such as in the suprarenal IVC[75] and superior vena cava,[76–78] as well as for unconventional indications, such as septic thrombophlebitis. In the latter setting, preserved caval flow allows for sterilization of septic thrombus through parenteral antibiotics.[76,79]

The currently available forms of the Greenfield filter are the over-the-wire stainless steel and the titanium Greenfield filters. The over-the-wire stainless steel Greenfield

Table 1
Permanent filters

	Material	Maximum IVC Diameter	Insertion Approaches	Sheath Diameter	Magnetic Resonance (MR) Compatibility
Over-the-Wire Greenfield (1995)	Stainless steel	28 mm	Femoral, jugular	12-French	Yes, with moderate artifact
Titanium Greenfield (1989)	Beta II titanium alloy	28 mm	Femoral, jugular	12-French	Yes, minimal artifact
Simon Nitinol (1990)	Nitinol (nickel-titanium alloy)	28 mm	Femoral, jugular, antecubital	9-French	Yes, minimal artifact
Bird's Nest (1990)	Stainless steel	40 mm	Femoral, jugular	12-French	Yes, significant artifact
Vena Tech (1989)	Phynox (cobalt-chromium-nickel alloy)	28 mm	Femoral, jugular	12-French	Yes
Vena Tech LP (2001)	Phynox	28 mm	Femoral, jugular	7-French	Yes
TrapEase	Nitinol	30 mm	Femoral, jugular, antecubital	6-French	Yes, minimal artifact

filter was introduced in 1994 and approved by the US Food and Drug Administration (FDA) in 1995.[80] It maintains the conical shape with 6 stainless steel struts, but the struts fuse into an apical nose with a central hole to allow passage of a guidewire to reduce tilting and asymmetry. The anchor hooks are positioned bidirectionally and are recurved, with 4 directed superiorly and 2 inferiorly, and it measures 49 mm in length and 32 mm in base diameter. The filter is inserted via a 12-French catheter (15-French outer diameter [OD]). It is for use in IVCs measuring up to 28 mm in diameter. It is magnetic resonance (MR) safe but has significant artifact due to the stainless steel.[17,34,72,80]

The titanium Greenfield filter was introduced in 1988 and approved for use by the FDA in 1989.[81] It is similar in design to the original stainless steel Greenfield filter but is made of beta II titanium alloy to confer increased flexibility and lower profile. It retains the conical shape of the original with 6 struts. Due to frequent migration and IVC perforation, it was later modified, altering the hooks to prevent caudal migration and wall penetration. This modified hook titanium filter is inserted through a 12-French catheter, 14-French OD. Compared with the original titanium filter, the diameter and length was increased and, although the sheath is inserted over a guidewire, the filter is not. It can be used in IVCs measuring up to 28 mm in diameter and comes in femoral and jugular versions.[17,34,81]

Simon Nitinol Filter

The Simon Nitinol filter (Bard Peripheral Vascular, Covington, GA, USA) was introduced in 1989 and approved by the FDA in 1990.[82] Composed of the nickel-titanium alloy, nitinol, which has thermal properties, the filter is made of straight wires that unfold at body temperature into an umbrella filter with 7 petals. Due to the thermal expansion property, insertion requires continuous cold saline infusion through the 9-French delivery catheter until it is ready for placement, at which point the cooled filter wire is advanced by a feeder pump and discharged from the storage catheter (see: http://www.bardpv.com/portfolio/simonnitrol/). The filter itself is conical and consists of 6 struts with hooks at the base and a 28-mm dome of 8 overlapping loops. It can be placed in IVCs measuring up to 28 mm in diameter and its small delivery system allows placement from jugular, femoral, or antecubital approaches. It is MR compatible with minimal artifact.[17,34,72]

The Simon Nitinol initial multicenter study showed a 5% recurrent PE rate, a 28% insertion site thrombosis rate as confirmed on duplex ultrasound, and a 18% vena caval occlusion rate. On follow-up, 11% of patients had venous stasis and there was only 1 report of proximal migration.[82] Hann and Streiff[50] reviewed 11 available studies on the Simon Nitinol filter with a total of 975 subjects. The average recurrent PE rate was 3.3% (range 0%–5.3%) with 1.8% fatal. Recurrent DVT occurred in 8.9%, vena caval thrombosis in 5.2% (range 0%–50%), and postthrombotic syndrome in 12.9%. Insertion-site thrombosis occurred in 11.5% (range 0%–64%) with 31% in studies with routine screening for it. A later meta-analysis by Rajasekhar and Streiff[34] included 12 studies had similar findings. The Nitinol filter is associated with a relatively high rate of IVC penetration, reported at 95% to 100% in 2 recent studies, but all were asymptomatic.[83,84]

Bird's Nest Filter

The Bird's Nest Filter was introduced in 1982 and approved by the FDA in 1990.[85,86] This filter deviates from the Greenfield conical shape, consisting of 4 stainless steel wires preshaped into a crisscross and attached to 2 V-shaped struts. The 2 V-shaped struts have small barbs to fixate to the caval wall. The filter is preloaded in a 12-French catheter, and deployment is performed in a stepwise manner with, first, extrusion of the first set of hooks that are set into the caval wall; second, extrusion of the 4 wires in random distribution; and third, extrusion of the second set of hooks. It is 7 cm in length, although this varies based on overlap of the struts, and it is the only filter that can be used in mega cavas (IVCs up to 40 mm in diameter).[87] It may be placed via jugular or femoral approach with the only difference being sheath length, and this flexibility allows for advancement through tortuous anatomy and left-sided approaches.[17] It is MR safe but generates a very large artifact due to its stainless steel construction.[88]

The initial series in 1988 evaluated 440 subjects of a total of 568 subjects who had a Bird's Nest filter. These 440 subjects were followed clinically for at least 6 months. Recurrent PE occurred in 2.7% and vena caval obstruction was found in 7 of 37 subjects who underwent imaging. There were 5 instances of migration with the initial filter design but, after modification to the anchors, there were no further cases of migration seen.[89] Meta-analysis of 18 studies with 1742 subjects with the Bird's Nest filter shows a 3.4% recurrent PE rate (range 0%–7.1%), 6% recurrent DVT rate (range 0%–20%), 2.8% vena cava thrombosis rate (range 0%–15%), and 14% rate of postthrombotic syndrome (range 4%–41%). Insertion site thrombosis was seen in 7.4% in all included studies, and 23% in those studies with routine screening.[34,50] Similar to other filters, the Bird's Nest filter is associated with asymptomatic perforation in a large percentage, 85.3%, in a small series by Nicholson and colleagues.[90]

Vena Tech filter

The Vena Tech LGM filter was introduced in 1986 and approved by the FDA in 1989. It is a conical filter composed on Phynox, a cobalt-chromium-nickel alloy used in pacemaker leads. There are 6 angled radial struts arranged in a cone shape, and each strut is connected to a stabilizing side rail, which anchors the filter into the caval wall. It is inserted via a 12-French sheath (14-French OD) via a jugular or femoral approach and can be used in IVCs measuring up to 28 mm in diameter. Initial experience by Ricco and colleagues[91] included 100 subjects with most on concurrent anticoagulation. Of these, 98 filters were successfully placed with a 16% malposition incidence, which was deemed likely due to operator learning curve. There was a 2% recurrent PE rate, both in incompletely opened filters, and an 8% caval occlusion rate at 1 year. Venous insufficiency was seen in 29%. There was a 9% proximal and 4% distal migration rate. A later series by Ricco and colleagues[92] showed a 2.2% recurrent PE rate and 4.5% caval filter thrombosis with 7 of 10 cases occurring within 48 hours of placement. Of these, 3.6% of filters migrated and 4.4% had significant tilting, although none were associated with recurrent PE. Another series showed a 22% caval occlusion rate.[93] Crochet and colleagues[94,95] evaluated 142 subjects with Vena Tech filters for caval thrombosis using routine imagine surveillance and found a 22% IVC thrombosis rate at 5 years and 33% at 9 years. The occlusion rate was higher in those with anticoagulation failure, and concurrent use of anticoagulation did not significant improve IVC patency. Of subjects with caval occlusion, 50% developed lower extremity edema.

A more recent version of the Vena Tech LGM was introduced in 2001: the Vena Tech LP filter. Also made of Phynox, there are 8 wires that form a cone with attached lateral side rails, which have anchor hooks oriented superiorly and inferiorly for caval wall fixation. It is lower profile, deployed via a 7-French sheath (9-French OD) and measures 43 mm in height and 40 mm in diameter in its constrained state. It is currently approved for IVCs up to 28 mm in diameter, although it may be used in IVCs up to 35 mm. It is also MR compatible and may deployed via jugular or femoral approaches.[17] Meta-analysis of 2 studies and 91 subjects with average follow-up of 2.3 months showed no reported PE recurrence, 3.2% recurrent DVT rate, and 3.2% IVC thrombosis rate,[34] although results are limited by small subject number and short follow-up.

TrapEase filter

The TrapEase filter (Cordis Corp, Bridgewater, NJ, USA) was approved in 2000 by the FDA. It deviates from the typical conical geometry and consists of 2 conical filter baskets, 1 facing cephalad, and the other caudal, to create a double-basket filter. Six struts composed of nitinol oriented in trapezoidal configuration converge to make the filter baskets, creating 6 diamond-shaped flow corridors. The 6 struts have proximal and distal hooks as anchors to fixate to the caval wall. It is inserted with a 6-French sheath via jugular, femoral, or antecubital approaches and may be used in IVCs up to 30 mm in diameter. It is MR compatible with minimal artifact.[96]

A multicenter prospective trial in 2001 evaluated 65 subjects with 42 subjects undergoing the full 6 months follow-up, which included surveillance imaging. There was no recurrent PE at 6 months, and they also did not note any filter migration, fracture, penetration, or insertion-site thrombosis. Two subjects had early caval thrombosis, 1 symptomatic and treated with thrombolysis.[97] Hann and Streiff[50] compiled 2 studies on the TrapEase filter with a total of 254 subjects and found a recurrent PE rate of 0.4%; a recurrent DVT rate of 1.2%, an insertion-site thrombosis rate of 0.4%, and a vena caval thrombosis rate of 2%. The average follow-up was 4.2 months (range 4–6 months).

Retrievable Inferior Vena Caval Filters

In 2003, the FDA approved adaptations to 3 permanent filters that would allow retrieval. Since then, multiple versions of optional filters have emerged. Retrievable filters can be subdivided into retrieval and temporary filters.

Retrievable filters function like their permanent counterparts, maintained in place by hooks, barbs, and/or radial force. However, they differ from permanent filters owing to the inclusion of features that allow retrieval if possible but may also be left permanently. All retrievable filters currently on the market in the United States were first approved by the FDA for use as permanent IVC filters and then later approved for retrieval. Because the use of all IVC filters has increased exponentially in recent years,[21,98] it is the use of retrieval filters in particular that has exponentially expanded, estimated to be 80% of the market by 2012.[18] There are multiple retrievable filters on the market currently (see following section), which are summarized in **Table 2**.

Gunther Tulip filter

The Gunther Tulip Filter (Cook, Inc, Bloomington, IN, USA) was first available for use in the United States in 2001 and was approved for retrieval in 2003. It consists of 4 leg struts made of Conichrome, a cobalt, nickel, chromium, iron, molybdenum, and manganese alloy, which join to form a half-basket filter. The struts extend beyond the basket and anchor the filter via small barbed hooks. In addition, there are 4 secondary wire loops that extend three-quarters down the length of each leg and form tulip-shaped petals, which force a clot to the center of the filter. A hook at the apex is used for retrieval (see: https://www.cookmedical.com/products/ea845922-f1f5-4038-a4bc-f1a14e768a2d/). The filter is inserted with an 11-French OD sheath via a femoral or jugular approach and is retrieved from the jugular vein.[99]

Although the instructions for use recommend retrieval within 14 days, there are several reports of retrieval after a prolonged dwell time,[18,100–102] and the lifespan

Table 2
Retrievable filters

Filter Type (FDA Approval)	Material	Maximum IVC Diameter	Insertion Approaches	Extraction Approaches	Introducer Sheath Diameter	MR Compatibility
Gunther Tulip (2001, 2003)	Conichrome (cobalt, nickel, chromium, iron, molybdenum, manganese alloy)	30 mm	Femoral, jugular	Jugular	11-French	Yes
Celect (2008)	Conichrome	30 mm	Femoral, jugular	Jugular	7-French (jugular), 8.5-French (femoral)	Yes
ALN (2008)	Stainless Steel	32 mm	Femoral, jugular, or brachial vein	Jugular	7-French	Yes
Denali (2010)	Nitinol	28 mm	Femoral, jugular, subclavian	Jugular	8.4-French	Yes
Option (2009)	Nitinol tubing	30 mm	Femoral, jugular	Jugular	6.5-French	Yes
OptEase (2002)	Nitinol	30 mm	Femoral, jugular, antecubital	Femoral	6-French	Yes
Crux (2013)	Nitinol and PTFE (polytetrafluoroethylene)	28 mm	Femoral, jugular	Femoral, jugular	9-French	Yes
Vena Tech Convertible (2016)	Chromium-cobalt alloy	28 mm	Femoral, jugular	Jugular	6-French	Yes

may be lengthened with periodic filter repositioning.[103,104] There was a report of retrieval after 317 days and, although successful, the investigators did note an increase in difficulty with longer dwell times, recommending caution with retrieval of these filters.[105,106] A prospective study evaluated attempted retrievals in 275 subjects out of 554 subjects with implanted Gunther Tulip filters and found a 90.2% successful retrieval rate with a mean dwell time of 58.9 days. Failed retrieval was associated with a longer dwell time with a mean dwell time of 114 days in failed attempts.[107]

A retrospective study evaluating 369 subjects with a mean follow-up of 780 days found a 3.3% rate of new or recurrent PE, a 14.4% rate of new or recurrent DVT, and a 4.1% rate of IVC thrombosis. Filter migration was seen in 12.5% and strut fracture in 0.4%, all asymptomatic. Caval penetration was seen in 43.3%. Only 10 subjects had retrieval attempted.[108] Meta-analysis of 19 studies with 2215 subjects with a mean follow-up of 11.3 months showed a 0.7% rate of PE, a 0.6% rate of DVT, and a 0.8% rate of IVC thrombosis, although these may be underrepresented due to relatively short follow-up.[34]

Celect filter

The Celect filter (Cook, Inc, Bloomington, IN, USA) has been available for use since 2008 and is based on the Gunther Tulip filter. Compared with its predecessor, the secondary struts no longer form wire loops and contact the primary struts, thus it consists of 4 primary and 8 secondary independent struts. This modification was done to reduce filter tilt and improve filter retrieval. The Celect Platinum added platinum markers to increase visibility and altered the anchors. It is inserted with a 7-French or 8.5-French catheter via a jugular or a femoral approach, respectively, and can be used in IVCs up to 30 mm.[34,106]

A meta-analysis of available studies on the Celect filters shows an average rate of recurrent PE of 1.3%, of recurrent DVT of 2.1%, and of IVC thrombosis of 0.5%.[34] A commonly noted complication is filter perforation, with reported rates of up to 28.5% to 49% in retrospective reviews.[109–111] Despite this, a prospective review showed perforation was not associated with breakthrough PE or retrieval success, with successful retrieval in 96.6% of attempts and an association with dwell time.[112]

ALN filter

The ALN filter (ALN Implants Chirurgicaux, Ghisonaccia, France) is composed of nonferromagnetic stainless steel and consists of 6 short anchoring legs and 3 long legs for central positioning. It may be inserted via femoral, jugular, or brachial vein approaches via a 7-French sheath and can be used in IVCs up to 32 mm in diameter. A prospective study from Mismetti and colleagues[113] evaluating 220 subjects with 18 months of follow-up in 148 reported an 11.8% immediate complication rate, mostly filter tilt (5.7%) and access hematoma (4.2%). Review of ALN literature showed overall rates of recurrent PE of 0.7%, recurrent DVT of 4.9%, and IVC thrombosis of 1.8%.[34] There are reports of both early and late successful retrievals, and case reports of strut fracture and embolization exist, usually associated with long dwell times.[114,115]

Denali filter

The Denali filter (Bard Peripheral Vascular, Tempe, AZ, USA) was approved by the FDA in 2010 and is the newest generation from Bard, replacing the Eclipse filter and prior generations of Bard retrievable IVC filters (Recovery Nitinol, G2, and the Meridian). It is a conical filter composed of 12 nitinol struts, 6 upper and 6 lower to provide 2 filtration levels. The 6 lower arms have cranial and caudal anchors for fixation. Femoral or jugular-subclavian approaches for insertion are available via 8.4 French catheters (10-French OD) and can accommodate IVCs up to 28 mm in diameter.[116]

Stavropoulos and colleagues[117,118] reported initial and final data from a prospective study evaluating 200 subjects followed for 2 years or 30 days after retrieval. They found recurrent PE in 3% and new or worsening DVT in 13%. Prior Bard filters were associated with relatively high rates of filter fracture, embolization, and migration, and the study reported no incidence of these complications, with successful retrieval in 97.3% with mean dwell times of 200.8 days. However, a case report was also published describing embolization of fractured struts, resulting in cardiac tamponade and requiring open retrieval,[119] suggesting that, although these complications may be less common in the Denali filter, it may still be prone to them and require further evaluation.

Option filter

The Option filter (Argon Medical Devices, Inc, Athens, TX, USA) is another conical filter composed of Nitinol tubing and consists of 6 collapsible legs with anchoring struts at the ends. It is placed via a 6.5-French sheath from a jugular or a femoral approach and, similar to other retrieval filters, there is an apical hook for retrieval from a jugular approach. The maximum IVC diameter for use is 30 mm. A prospective trial with 100 subjects followed for 180 days after placement or 30 days after retrieval showed an 8% recurrent PE rate, a 3% IVC thrombosis rate, a 18% recurrent DVT rate, and a 2% filter migration rate. Retrieval was successful in 92.3% of attempts with a mean dwell time of 67.1 days.[120]

OptEase filter

The OptEase filter (Cordis Corp, Bridgewater, NJ, USA), available since 2002, is similar to its permanent counterpart, the TrapEase, in its double-basket design composed of 6 nitinol struts with superior fixation. It can be inserted in IVCs up to 30 mm in diameter and via a 6-French sheath from jugular, femoral, or antecubital approaches with differing orientations of the anchoring barbs depending on the approach. Contrary to other retrieval filters other than the Crux filter, it has a caudal hook for retrieval from a femoral approach.

The prospective multicenter PROOF trial, with 1 and 6 month follow-up, showed a 0.9% rate of migration and a 0.8% rate of symptomatic thrombus.[121,122] Meta-analysis of 7 studies with 798 subjects showed a 0.9% rate of recurrent or new PE, a 1.5% rate of recurrent DVT, and a 0.9% rate of IVC thrombosis.[34] For retrieval, a long-term retrospective study with a mean follow-up of 20 months reported retrieval success at 70.6%. Although other studies have shown better retrieval rates at 92% to 100%, retrieval failure was increased with longer dwell times, likely due to its double-basket design with the 6 vertical struts.[123,124]

Crux filter

The Crux filter (Volcano, San Diego, CA, USA) is a unique filter, deviating from the conical and basket design. It consists of 2 opposing nitinol spiral wireforms with the caudal half containing a web of expanded polytetrafluoroethylene. There are 5 anchors, and a sinusoidal retrieval tail at each end to allow retrieval from either a jugular or femoral approach. It is the only filter with the option for a femoral or jugular approach for either placement or retrieval, placed using a 9-French sheath and retrieved with a 6-French or 10-French sheath depending on the approach. It can be deployed in IVCs 17 to 28 mm in diameter. The RETRIEVE trial, a prospective multicenter trial, included 125 subjects followed for 180 days total or 30 days after retrieval.

A recurrent PE rate of 2.4% confirmed and 4% suspected or confirmed, a recurrent DVT rate of 10.4%, and a filter thrombosis rate of 7.2% were reported. Retrieval was successful in 98.1% of cases with mean dwell time of 84.6 days.[125]

Vena Tech Convertible filter

The Vena Tech Convertible filter is similar in design to the permanent Vena Tech filter. Deviating from the usual retrieval filter, this filter is not retrieved but rather converted after it is no longer used by unlocking it from a jugular approach and converting it into a stent-like configuration, which remains in place. It can be used in IVCs up to 28 mm in diameter, inserted via a 6-French sheath. There are no human studies yet on this filter, only a preclinical trial evaluating its use in sheep.[126]

Temporary filters

Temporary filters are a subclass of optional filters designed only for short-term use. They are tethered to catheters or wires that are either externalized or tunneled subcutaneously at a central venous site. These filters do not have any fixation features to anchor it to the caval wall and must be removed before they become embedded, usually within 2 to 6 weeks.[127] Although they are easy to insert and remove, there are numerous potential pitfalls, such as infection, decreased protection due to the increased potential for filter malpositioning and migration, and difficult management. With their short life spans and multiple complications, indications for temporary filters are very limited.[34,99] Although used in Europe, only 1 temporary IVC filter, the Angel catheter (Bio2 Medical, Golden [CO]), is currently approved for use in the United States and is used primarily in trauma intensive care patients. The device is a temporary filter and central venous catheter combination, consisting of a self-expanding nitinol IVC filter attached to a 9-French triple-lumen central venous catheter (**Fig. 1**). It is inserted via the femoral vein and sutured to the skin. Tapson and colleagues[128] recently published a multicenter, prospective, single-arm clinical trial evaluating the efficacy and safety of the Angel catheter. From February 2015 to December 2015, 172 subjects from 20 clinical US sites were enrolled and, of these, 163 subjects successfully had the Angel catheter placed. Eligibility criteria included age of at least 18 years old, an expected intensive care unit (ICU) stay of at least 72 hours, contraindications to standard prophylactic pharmacologic anticoagulation, and/or confirmed acute proximal lower extremity DVT or acute PE with recognized anticoagulation contraindications. Of the subjects, 93% were critically ill trauma subjects. The primary efficacy endpoint was freedom from clinically significant PE or fatal PE at discharge or up to 72 hours after device removal, and secondary endpoints were acute proximal DVT, catheter-related thrombosis, catheter-related bloodstream infections, severe bleeding events, and clinically significant thrombus in the filter (>25% filter volume).

Although not required by protocol, the placing physicians in the study used existing images to identify the renal veins in relationship to lumbar vertebrae before placement.

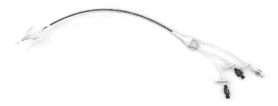

Fig. 1. Angel catheter. (*Courtesy of* Bio2 Medical.)

The filters were placed via ultrasound-guided femoral access, and a 0.035-inch J-tip 100-cm guidewire was introduced into the IVC with advancement of the catheter over the wire without fluoroscopic guidance. The filter was deployed by retracting the 9-French outer sheath over the coaxial catheter until the hubs were locked together, and the catheter was sutured to the skin with placement of a secured dressing as well. Plain films were used to confirm placement below the L1-L2 and above the L4-L5 intervertebral spaces. Placement was done in 96.3% at the bedside in the ICU, 2.5% in the operating room, 0.6% (1) in the interventional radiology suite, and another 0.6% (1) in another location. Before removal, cavogram was performed via the catheter sheath to evaluate filter thrombus and, if present, an interventional radiologist was consulted to provide the best treatment option, such as aspiration, thrombolysis, or placement of an IVC filter. The Angel catheter was retrieved by pulling the multilumen catheter into the outer sheath, allowing collapse of the filter over the former. Median time from ICU admission to device insertion was 1.7 days, and it remained in place for a mean of 7.2 plus or minus 3.8 days.

Statistical analysis was performed with a performance goal agreed on by the FDA and the sponsor company based on clinical trials and historical controls of freedom from clinically significant PE or fatal PE of greater than 96.8%. The outcomes showed no clinically significant or fatal PE in any subjects. Of the subjects, 8.6% had large filter thrombus, most of which were treated with therapeutic anticoagulation for an average of 4.1 days followed by retrieval of the filter with residual large thrombi left in the iliac and femoral veins. Major bleeding occurred in 3.1%, and unintentional catheter removal occurred in 7.4% without major venous injury or bleeding. New or worsening acute proximal DVT occurred in 7% by day 11 and 18% by day 30, reflecting importance of removing the Angel catheter and filter as soon as feasible. Although additional data are needed and there are limitations to this study, this initial clinical trial shows the Angel catheter may be a feasible treatment option.[128]

TECHNIQUE

Currently, VCF placement is a commonly performed procedures. Although in the long-term VCFs are associated with complications, their placement is a relatively safe procedure. Highlights of technique and approach are discussed in the following sections.

Preoperative Workup and Planning

Preoperative workup consists of diagnosis of VTE and establishment of indication for VCF placement. In addition, relative contraindications to VCF use include a life expectancy less than 3 months, bacteremia, and uncorrectable severe coagulopathy.[30] Subjects should have preoperative imaging with at least lower extremity venous duplex to evaluate for DVT extent. CT or MR venogram should be considered if there is evidence of proximal extension to evaluate for caval thrombosis and assist in planning for approach because many filters can be placed from either jugular, femoral, or other approaches.

Filter Placement Approach

The patient is positioned supine. Equipment to monitor for heart rate, cardiac rhythm, and blood pressure should be available, as well as pulse oximetry if sedation will be provided. VCFs are most often placed using fluoroscopy in an angiogram suite or at bedside if a portable C-arm is available. Filters may also be placed using intravascular ultrasound (IVUS) alone or in conjunction with fluoroscopy.[129–132] Ashley and colleagues[131] reported IVUS was actually more accurate the conventional venogram for VCF placement, allowing for identification of the renal veins and IVC measurements for proper filter selection. Regardless of the approach, imaging of the IVC is essential to evaluate for anatomic anomalies, such as duplicated IVCs, mega vena cava, and retro-circumaortic left renal vein.[29,30,133,134]

The right internal jugular approach is the most commonly used, and the right femoral vein is often used as well. Depending on the filter type, less common alternatives include the antecubital and subclavian veins (see previous discussion of the filter types and available approaches) (**Fig. 2**).

Postoperative Care

All patients should be in bedrest and observed initially to assess for any complications, including access site complications. In some cases, patients may be discharged home the same day but often they are critically ill and need to remain hospitalized for other

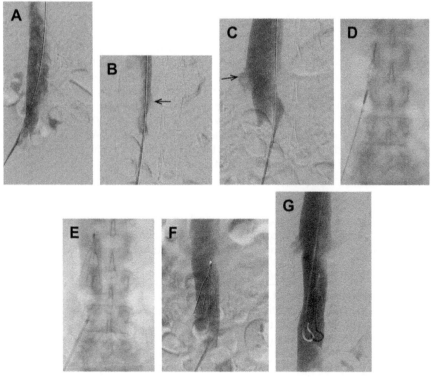

Fig. 2. Filter placement for left common femoral deep venous thrombosis in postsurgical patient with contraindication to immediate anticoagulation. (*A*) IVC access via right common femoral vein with 10-French sheath. Initial venogram demonstrates single normal caliber IVC with bifurcation at L4-L5. (*B*) Left renal vein (*black arrow*) identified on venogram. (*C*) Right renal vein (black arrow) identified on venogram. Both renal veins at L1 level. (*D*) Introduction of filter, positioned with apex at L2. (*E*) Filter fully deployed with completion venogram showing adequate positioning. (*F*) Two months later, after patient cleared for and tolerating full anticoagulation, initial venogram before VCF removal demonstrating VCF still in adequate position below renal veins. (*G*) After successful retrieval of the IVC filter, the completion venogram shows no evidence of thrombosis, contrast extravasation, or caval stenosis.

reasons. Criteria for short-term observation include ability to ambulate independently, that they are neurologically intact with full recovery from sedation if given, and the ability to follow directions and identify potential complications. Patients with high risk for contrast-induced nephropathy, medical comorbidities, electrolyte abnormalities or coagulopathies, hemodynamic changes, or impaired neurologic status should be observed at least overnight. In addition, any patients with intraoperative complications or difficulties should also be observed long-term.[31] Patients with VTE, regardless of VCF placement, should be periodically reevaluated and started on therapeutic anticoagulation as soon as possible.[29]

Filter Retrieval

If an optional filter was placed, it may be removed once its indication has resolved. For example, if the risk of bleeding has resolved and the patient can now tolerate therapeutic anticoagulation, he or she is now a candidate for removal of the VCF. The physician must periodically weigh the risks of VTE against the risks of continued VCF use to decide when retrieval is appropriate.

In general, for retrieval, there must be no indication for permanent VCF use and the risk of PE must be acceptably low. Patients must be able to tolerate and stay on anticoagulation with no foreseeable recurrence of the high risk of VTE or bleeding that required the VCF placement. SIR guidelines recommend therapeutic anticoagulation for at least 2 to 3 weeks before retrieval, which can be continued safely during the retrieval procedure. In addition, life expectancy must be greater than 6 months. For prophylactic filters, clinical examination and imaging must be performed to confirm the absence of new VTE, including lower extremity venous duplex.[29,127] Overall retrieval rates are relatively low and rates improve with creation of follow-up programs.[135]

The retrieval technique varies to some degree on the filter type, and most filters have unique retrieval systems. Characteristics suggestive of difficult or failed retrievals based on a recent retrospective review included prolonged dwell time and filter hook opposition to the caval wall. Significant filter tilt was associated with difficulty but not failure of retrieval.[135,136]

The approach for filter removal depends on the filter type. Briefly, other than the OptEase and the Crux filters, the other available retrievable filters are removed via a jugular approach. The OptEase is retrieved only via the femoral approach, and the Crux filter may be retrieved from either the jugular or femoral vein.

The retrievable filters mostly come with unique retrieval systems; however, occasionally, advanced techniques are needed. Review of the multiple advanced techniques included descriptions of various single and dual access techniques. The single access techniques include use of an angled catheter or sheath to orient the snare toward the tilted retrieval hook or use of a tip-deflecting wire to realign the filter. A stiff wire may also be used to deflect the filter and orient it centrally, after which the over-the-wire snare or retrieval cone can be advanced and used to grasp the filter. Alternatively, a coaxial loop snare can be used to grasp both the stiff wire and the reoriented filter tip. A wire can also be snared around the filter and used a sling to retrieve the filter (**Fig. 3**). Dual access techniques entail use of both jugular and femoral access and a through-and-through wire, which can be used to deflect the filter centrally itself or provide a conduit to a balloon catheter to deflect the filter centrally. Another dual access technique, called the sandwich technique, involves advancing sheaths from both the jugular and femoral approaches and with a through-and-through wire, using them to rock the filter into a central position and guide the hook into the retrieval snare. For severely embedded filters, endoscopic laser sheaths or rigid bronchoscopy snares have been used to dissect the filters free for retrieval.[137] Reported major

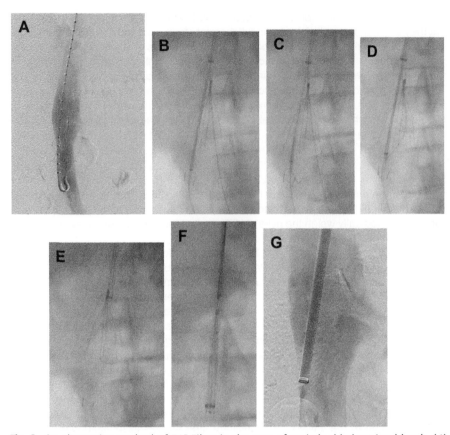

Fig. 3. An alternative method of IVC Filter in the case of an imbedded retrieval hook. (*A*) Initial venogram with filter in place. (*B*) 12-French 80-cm sheath placed from basilic vein approach under ultrasound guidance. A guidewire advanced laterally past VCF struts, over which a snare advanced past the VCF struts. (*C*) Second 260-mm guidewire introduced and advanced through VCF struts more medially. (*D*) The medial guidewire snared. (*E*) Snared guidewire retracted and used to create a sling around the VCF apex. (*F*) Snared guidewire used to retract the VCF into the 12-French sheath and remove it. (*G*) Completion venogram shows normal intact inferior vena cava with no wall defects or abnormalities.

complications of these advanced techniques are rare and they can be performed safely in the setting of anticoagulation.[138]

OUTCOMES AND COMPLICATIONS

Complications of VCF procedures include filter tilt, malposition, migration, fracture and/or embolization, and thrombosis. Overall, the complication rate is low and mostly associated with prolonged dwell times.

Based on the PREPIC results, permanent filters reduce the risk of symptomatic PE but at the cost of increased recurrent DVT. Mortality was unchanged. A systemic review by Angel and colleagues[139] compared outcomes of retrievable and permanent filters using the Manufacturer and User Facility Device Experience database and a MEDLINE literature review. Overall, retrievable filters were found to have a PE rate of 1.7% after placement, suggestive of effective protection from PE. Also, using the MAUDE database, Andreoli and colleagues found a higher rate of complications with retrievable versus permanent filters with 86.8% of reported adverse events from 2009 to 2012 involving retrievable filters. However, these findings are all limited by self-reporting and lack of large and/or randomized trials.

As stated previously, the use of VCFs is increasing exponentially. Kuy and colleagues[140] found the number of VCFs implanted over the decade from 2000 to 2009 increased by 234%. In light of these findings and the potential adverse effects, the FDA issued 2 alerts in 2010 and 2014 regarding VCF use.[141,142] In 2010, the FDA issued an initial communication to physicians responsible for the ongoing care of patients with IVC filters. The FDA noted the rapid increase in VCF use as well as the reported adverse effects with a total of 921 since 2005. Most of the adverse effects were thought to be related to long indwelling duration times with the potential for adverse outcomes to the patient. In conclusion, the FDA recommended all physicians responsible for the care of patients with retrievable VCFs to consider removal of the filter as soon as PE protection is no longer needed. In addition, the FDA initiated the development of a quantitative decision analysis model to evaluate the risk and benefits of VCF use over time, which was published by Morales and colleagues[143] in October 2013. A comprehensive literature review of VCFs and transient PE risk with emphasis on off-label prophylactic VCF use in patients with a VCF already implanted was conducted. Adverse effects were identified and assigned weights reflecting the relative severity by 3 physicians. These were later validated by 6 other physicians. They used a mathematical model to evaluate the risk in situ, the risk of removal, the relative risk without filters, and the risks and benefits of VCF use over time. The conclusion was that, once the risk of PE passed, the net risk score reached a minimum between days 29 and 54 postimplantation. The model validated the FDA recommendation, supporting the retrieval of VCFs between 1 to 2 months.

In 2014, the FDA released an updated safety communication, again recommending the retrieval of VCFs as soon as PE protection is no longer needed. In addition to citing the decision analysis model by Morales and colleagues,[143] the FDA also initiated a requirement for the collection of clinical data for all marketable filters in the United States. Manufacturers were given 2 options for data collection participation: the PREdicting the Safety and Effectiveness of InferioR VCFs (PRESERVE) study or engage in an individual FDA 522 Postmarket Surveillance Study.[142]

Since the release of the FDA alerts, there has been a decrease in overall VCF use and increase in the proportion of VCF implantation for therapeutic indications. Wadhwa and colleagues[144] reviewed the Nationwide Inpatient Sample from 2005 to 2014, preceding and following the FDA alerts of 2010 and 2014. They found VCF placements increased by a growth rate of 5.81% from 2005 to 2010, peaked in 2010, and decreased by a rate of 6.48% from 2010 to 2014. The proportion of VCFs placed for therapeutic indications also increased from 69.8% in 2005 to 80.4% in 2014, reflecting the physician response to the FDA alerts. Although there has been progress in VCF off-label use and retrieval, continued vigilance by caring physicians is needed to maintain these improvements for the sake of patient safety.

SUMMARY

Although anticoagulation has been well-established as the treatment of choice for VTE, VCFs still serve an important role as an adjunct in the management of VTE. Available VCFs can be subdivided into permanent and optional filters. With the introduction of temporary filters, there has been increasing placement of VCFs with particular expansion of the prophylactic indications. However, VCFs are associated with their own set of complications, and it is of utmost importance that physicians remain cognizant of the indications and balance the risks and benefits for placement for each patient. In addition, once inserted, physicians must continue to weigh the risks and benefits through the life of the filter and patient, and advocate for filter removal as soon as possible because filter complications tend to increase with prolonged dwell times, in particular for the retrievable filters. Given the paucity of data, there remains a very strong need for additional randomized trials to elucidate the risks and benefits of VCF use, and better follow-up programs are needed to improve retrieval rates, all of which may lead to a decrease in complications.

REFERENCES

1. Deitelzweig SB, Johnson BH, Lin J, et al. Prevalence of clinical venous thromboembolism in the USA: current trends and future projections. Am J Hematol 2011; 86(2):217–20.
2. Kearon C, Akl EA, Ornelas J, et al. Antithrombotic therapy for VTE disease: CHEST guideline and expert panel report. Chest J 2016;149(2):315–52.
3. Kinney TB. Inferior vena cava filters. In: Seminars in interventional radiology, vol. 23, No. 03. New York: Thieme Medical Publishers, Inc; 2006. p. 230–9, 333 Seventh Avenue.
4. Andrew DW. Ligation of the inferior vena cava for thromboembolism. Surgery 1958;43(1):24–44.
5. Homans J. Thrombosis of deep veins of the lower leg, causing pulmonary embolism. N Engl J Med 1934;211(22):993–7.
6. Greenfield LJ. Evolution of venous interruption for pulmonary thromboembolism. Arch Surg 1992;127(5):622–6.
7. Ochsner A, Ochsner JL, Sanders HS. Prevention of pulmonary embolism by caval ligation. Ann Surg 1970;171(6):923.
8. Gurewich V, Thomas DP, Rabinov KR. Pulmonary embolism after ligation of the inferior vena cava. N Engl J Med 1966;274(24):1350–4.
9. Amador E, Li TK, Crane C. Ligation of inferior vena cava for thromboembolism: Clinical and autopsy correlations in 119 cases. JAMA 1968;206(8):1758–60.
10. Maraan BM, Taber RE. The effects of inferior vena caval ligation on cardiac output: an experimental study. Surgery 1968;63(6):966–9.
11. Goldhaber SZ, Buring JE, Lipnick RJ, et al. Interruption of the inferior vena cava by clip or filter. Am J Med 1984;76(3):512–6. APA.
12. Moretz WH, Rhode CM, Shepherd MH. Prevention of pulmonary emboli by partial occlusion of the inferior vena cava. Am Surg 1959;25:617.
13. Mobin-Uddin K, McLean R, Bolooki H, et al. Caval interruption for prevention of pulmonary embolism: Long-term results of a new method. Arch Surg 1969; 99(6):711–5.
14. Mobin-Uddin K, McLean R, Jude JR. A new catheter technique of interruption of inferior vena cava for prevention of pulmonary embolism. Am Surg 1969;35(12): 889–94.
15. Cimochowski GE, Evans RH, Zarins CK, et al. Greenfield filter versus Mobin-Uddin umbrella. J Thorac Cardiovasc Surg 1980;79(3):358–65.
16. Greenfield LJ, McCurdy JR, Brown PP, et al. A new intracaval filter permitting continued flow and resolution of emboli. Surgery 1973;73(4):599–606.
17. Kinney TB. Update on inferior vena cava filters. J Vasc Interv Radiol 2003;14(4): 425–40.

18. Tadavarthy SM, Castaneda-Zuniga W, Salomonowitz E, et al. Kimray-Greenfield vena cava filter: percutaneous introduction. Radiology 1984;151(2):525–6.
19. Barritt DW, Jordan SC. Anticoagulant drugs in the treatment of pulmonary embolism: a controlled trial. Lancet 1960;275(7138):1309–12.
20. Chong LY, Fenu E, Stansby G, et al. Management of venous thromboembolic diseases and the role of thrombophilia testing: summary of NICE guidance. BMJ 2012;344:e3979.
21. Stein PD, Kayali F, Olson RE. Twenty-one-year trends in the use of inferior vena cava filters. Arch Intern Med 2004;164(14):1541–5.
22. Stein PD, Matta F, Hull RD. Increasing use of vena cava filters for prevention of pulmonary embolism. Am J Med 2011;124(7):655–61.
23. Girard P, Stern JB, Parent F. Medical literature and vena cava filters: so far so weak. Chest 2002;122(3):963–7.
24. Decousus H, Leizorovicz A, Parent F, et al. A clinical trial of vena caval filters in the prevention of pulmonary embolism in patients with proximal deep-vein thrombosis. N Engl J Med 1998;338(7):409–16.
25. PREPIC Study Group. Eight-year follow-up of patients with permanent vena cava filters in the prevention of pulmonary embolism. Circulation 2005;112(3):416–22.
26. White RH, Zhou H, Kim J, et al. A population-based study of the effectiveness of inferior vena cava filter use among patients with venous thromboembolism. Arch Intern Med 2000;160(13):2033–41.
27. Barker NW, Nygaard KK, Priestley JT. A statistical study of postoperative venous thrombosis and pulmonary embolism. I. Incidence in various types of operations. The Journal of the American Society of Anesthesiologists 1941;2(2):241.
28. Kearon C. Natural history of venous thromboembolism. Circulation 2003;107(23 suppl 1):I–22.
29. Kaufman JA, et al. Guidelines for the use of retrievable and convertible vena cava filters: report from the Society of Interventional Radiology multidisciplinary consensus conference. World J Surg 2007;31(2):251–64.
30. Caplin DM, Nikolic B, Kalva SP, et al. Quality improvement guidelines for the performance of inferior vena cava filter placement for the prevention of pulmonary embolism. J Vasc Interv Radiol 2011;22(11):1499–506.
31. National Guideline Clearinghouse (NGC). Guideline summary: ACR appropriateness criteria® radiologic management of inferior vena cava filters. In: National guideline clearinghouse (NGC). Rockville (MD): Agency for Healthcare Research and Quality (AHRQ); 2012. Available at: https://www.guideline.gov. Accessed September 13, 2017.
32. Jaff MR, McMurtry MS, Archer SL, et al. Management of massive and submassive pulmonary embolism, iliofemoral deep vein thrombosis, and chronic thromboembolic pulmonary hypertension. Circulation 2011;123(16):1788–830.
33. O'Sullivan GJ, Semba CP, Bittner CA, et al. Endovascular management of iliac vein compression (May-Thurner) syndrome. J Vasc Interv Radiol 2000;11(7):823–36.
34. Rajasekhar A, Streiff MB. Vena cava filters for management of venous thromboembolism: a clinical review. Blood Rev 2013;27(5):225–41.
35. Holbrook A, Schulman S, Witt DM, et al. Evidence-based management of anticoagulant therapy: antithrombotic therapy and prevention of thrombosis: American College of Chest Physicians evidence-based clinical practice guidelines. Chest 2012;141(2 Suppl):e152S–84S.

36. Billett HH, Jacobs LG, Madsen EM, et al. Efficacy of inferior vena cava filters in anticoagulated patients. J Thromb Haemost 2007;5(9):1848–53.
37. Mismetti P, Laporte S, Pellerin O, et al. Effect of a retrievable inferior vena cava filter plus anticoagulation vs anticoagulation alone on risk of recurrent pulmonary embolism: a randomized clinical trial. JAMA 2015;313(16):1627–35.
38. Jamieson SW, Kapelanski DP, Sakakibara N, et al. Pulmonary endarterectomy: experience and lessons learned in 1,500 cases. Ann Thorac Surg 2003;76(5): 1457–62.
39. Mo M, Kapelanski DP, Mitruka SN, et al. Reoperative pulmonary thromboendarterectomy. Ann Thorac Surg 1999;68(5):1770–6.
40. Radomski JS, Jarrell BE, Carabasi RA, et al. Risk of pulmonary embolus with inferior vena caval thrombosis. Am Surg 1987;53(2):97–101.
41. Baldridge ED, Martin MA, Welling RE. Clinical significance of free-floating venous thrombi. J Vasc Surg 1990;11(1):62–9.
42. Monreal M, Ruiz J, Salvador R, et al. Recurrent pulmonary embolism: a prospective study. Chest 1989;95(5):976–9.
43. Pacouret G, Alison D, Pottier JM, et al. Free-floating thrombus and embolic risk in patients with angiographically confirmed proximal deep venous thrombosis: a prospective study. Arch Intern Med 1997;157(3):305–8.
44. Berry RE, George JE, Shaver WA. Free-floating deep venous thrombosis. A retrospective analysis. Ann Surg 1990;211(6):719.
45. Voet D, Afschrift M. Floating thrombi: diagnosis and follow-up by duplex ultrasound. Br J Radiol 1991;64(767):1010–4.
46. Kölbel T, Alhadad A, Acosta S, et al. Thrombus embolization into IVC filters during catheter-directed thrombolysis for proximal deep venous thrombosis. J Endovasc Ther 2008;15(5):605–13.
47. Protack CD, Bakken AM, Patel N, et al. Long-term outcomes of catheter directed thrombolysis for lower extremity deep venous thrombosis without prophylactic inferior vena cava filter placement. J Vasc Surg 2007;45(5):992–7.
48. Mewissen MW, Seabrook GR, Meissner MH, et al. Catheter-directed thrombolysis for lower extremity deep venous thrombosis: report of a national multicenter registry. Radiology 1999;211(1):39–49.
49. Rutherford RB. Prophylactic indications for vena cava filters: critical appraisal. Semin Vasc Surg 2005;18(3):158–65.
50. Hann CL, Streiff MB. The role of vena caval filters in the management of venous thromboembolism. Blood Rev 2005;19(4):179–202.
51. Geerts WH, Code KI, Jay RM, et al. A prospective study of venous thromboembolism after major trauma. N Engl J Med 1994;331(24):1601–6.
52. Winchell RJ, Hoyt DB, Walsh JC, et al. Risk factors associated with pulmonary embolism despite routine prophylaxis: implications for improved protection. J Trauma Acute Care Surg 1994;37(4):600–6.
53. Rogers FB, Cipolle MD, Velmahos G, et al. Practice management guidelines for the prevention of venous thromboembolism in trauma patients: the EAST practice management guidelines work group. J Trauma Acute Care Surg 2002;53(1): 142–64.
54. Velmahos GC, Kern J, Chan LS, et al. Prevention of venous thromboembolism after injury: an evidence-based report—part I: analysis of risk factors and evaluation of the role of vena caval filters. J Trauma Acute Care Surg 2000;49(1): 132–9.
55. Velmahos GC, Kern J, Chan LS, et al. Prevention of venous thromboembolism after injury: an evidence-based report—part II: analysis of risk factors and

evaluation of the role of vena caval filters. J Trauma Acute Care Surg 2000;49(1): 140–4.

56. Martin MJ, Salim A. Vena cava filters in surgery and trauma. Surg Clin North Am 2007;87(5):1229–52.

57. Velmahos GC, Nigro J, Tatevossian R, et al. Inability of an aggressive policy of thromboprophylaxis to prevent deep venous thrombosis (DVT) in critically injured patients: are current methods of DVT prophylaxis insufficient? J Am Coll Surg 1998;187(5):529–33.

58. Rogers FB, Shackford SR, Ricci MA, et al. Routine prophylactic vena cava filter insertion in severely injured trauma patients decreases the incidence of pulmonary embolism. J Am Coll Surg 1995;180(6):641–7.

59. Kidane B, Madani AM, Vogt K, et al. The use of prophylactic inferior vena cava filters in trauma patients: a systematic review. Injury 2012;43(5):542–7.

60. Carlin AM, Tyburski JG, Wilson RF, et al. Prophylactic and therapeutic inferior vena cava filters to prevent pulmonary emboli in trauma patients. Arch Surg 2002;137(5):521–5.

61. Karmy-Jones R, Jurkovich GJ, Velmahos GC, et al. Practice patterns and outcomes of retrievable vena cava filters in trauma patients: an AAST multicenter study. J Trauma Acute Care Surg 2007;62(1):17–25.

62. Byrne TK. Complications of surgery for obesity. Surg Clin North Am 2001;81(5): 1181–93.

63. Sapala JA, Wood MH, Schuhknecht MP, et al. Fatal pulmonary embolism after bariatric operations for morbid obesity: a 24-year retrospective analysis. Obes Surg 2003;13(6):819–25.

64. Brolin RE. Gastric bypass. Surg Clin North Am 2001;81(5):1077–95.

65. Li W, Gorecki P, Semaan E, et al. Concurrent prophylactic placement of inferior vena cava filter in gastric bypass and adjustable banding operations in the bariatric outcomes longitudinal database. J Vasc Surg 2012;55(6):1690–5.

66. Birkmeyer NJ, Share D, Baser O, et al. Preoperative placement of inferior vena cava filters and outcomes after gastric bypass surgery. Ann Surg 2010;252(2): 313–8.

67. Rajasekhar A, Crowther M. Inferior vena caval filter insertion prior to bariatric surgery: a systematic review of the literature. J Thromb Haemost 2010;8(6):1266–70.

68. Prandoni P, Lensing AW, Piccioli A, et al. Recurrent venous thromboembolism and bleeding complications during anticoagulant treatment in patients with cancer and venous thrombosis. Blood 2002;100(10):3484–8.

69. Farge D, Debourdeau P, Beckers M, et al. International clinical practice guidelines for the treatment and prophylaxis of venous thromboembolism in patients with cancer. J Thromb Haemost 2013;11(1):56–70.

70. Akl EA, Vasireddi SR, Gunukula S, et al. Anticoagulation for the initial treatment of venous thromboembolism in patients with cancer. Cochrane Database Syst Rev 2011;6:CD006649.

71. Barginear MF, Gralla RJ, Bradley TP, et al. Investigating the benefit of adding a vena cava filter to anticoagulation with fondaparinux sodium in patients with cancer and venous thromboembolism in a prospective randomized clinical trial. Support Care Cancer 2012;20(11):2865–72.

72. Rectenwald JE. Vena cava filters: uses and abuses. Semin Vasc Surg 2005; 18(3):166–75.

73. Greenfield LJ, Michna BA. Twelve-year clinical experience with the Greenfield vena caval filter. Surgery 1988;104(4):706–12.

74. Greenfield LJ, Proctor MC. Twenty-year clinical experience with the Greenfield filter. Cardiovasc Surg 1995;3(2):199–205.

75. Greenfield LJ, Cho KJ, Proctor MC, et al. Late results of suprarenal Greenfield vena cava filter placement. Arch Surg 1992;127(8):969–73.

76. Hoffman MJ, Greenfield LJ. Central venous septic thrombosis managed by superior vena cava Greenfield filter and venous thrombectomy: a case report. J Vasc Surg 1986;4(6):606–11.

77. Ascher E, Hingorani A, Tsemekhin B, et al. Lessons learned from a 6-year clinical experience with superior vena cava Greenfield filters. J Vasc Surg 2000;32(5):881–7.

78. Owen EW, Schoettle GP, Harrington OB. Placement of a Greenfield filter in the superior vena cava. Ann Thorac Surg 1992;53(5):896–7.

79. Peyton JW, Hylemon MB, Greenfield LJ, et al. Comparison of Greenfield filter and vena caval ligation for experimental septic thromboembolism. Surgery 1983;93(4):533–7.

80. Cho KJ, Greenfield LJ, Proctor MC, et al. Evaluation of a new percutaneous stainless steel Greenfield filter. J Vasc Interv Radiol 1997;8(2):181–7.

81. Greenfield LJ, Cho KJ, Pais SO, et al. Preliminary clinical experience with the titanium Greenfield vena caval filter. Arch Surg 1989;124(6):657–9.

82. Simon M, Athanasoulis CA, Kim D, et al. Simon nitinol inferior vena cava filter: initial clinical experience. Work in progress. Radiology 1989;172(1):99–103.

83. Poletti PA, Becker CD, Prina L, et al. Long-term results of the Simon nitinol inferior vena cava filter. Eur Radiol 1998;8(2):289–94.

84. Wolf F, Thurnher S, Lammer J. Simon nitinol vena cava filters: effectiveness and complications. Rofo 2001;173(10):924–30.

85. Roehm JOF. "The bird's nest filter: a new percutaneous transcatheter inferior vena cava filter. J Vasc Surg 1984;1(3):498–501.

86. Roehm JO Jr, Gianturco C, Barth MH, et al. Percutaneous transcatheter filter for the inferior vena cava. A new device for treatment of patients with pulmonary embolism. Radiology 1984;150(1):255–7.

87. Reed RA, Teitelbaum GP, Taylor FC, et al. Use of the bird's nest filter in oversized inferior venae cavae. J Vasc Interv Radiol 1991;2(4):447–50.

88. Watanabe AT, Teitelbaum GP, Gomes AS, et al. MR imaging of the bird's nest filter. Radiology 1990;177(2):578–9.

89. Roehm JO Jr, Johnsrude IS, Barth MH, et al. The bird's nest inferior vena cava filter: progress report. Radiology 1988;168(3):745–9.

90. Nicholson AA, Ettles DF, Paddon AJ, et al. Long-term follow-up of the bird's nest IVC filter. Clin Radiol 1999;54(11):759–64.

91. Ricco JB, Crochet D, Sebilotte P, et al. Percutaneous transvenous caval interruption with the "LGM" filter: early results of a multicenter trial. Ann Vasc Surg 1988; 2(3):242–7.

92. Ricco JB, Dubreuil F, Reynaud P, et al. The LGM Vena-Tech caval filter: results of a multicenter study. Ann Vasc Surg 1995;9(Suppl):S89–100.

93. Millward SF, Peterson RA, Moher D, et al. LGM (Vena Tech) vena caval filter: experience at a single institution. J Vasc Interv Radiol 1994;5(2):351–6.

94. Crochet DP, Stora O, Ferry D, et al. Vena Tech-LGM filter: long-term results of a prospective study. Radiology 1993;188(3):857–60.

95. Crochet DP, Brunel P, Trogrlic S, et al. Long-term follow-up of Vena Tech-LGM filter: predictors and frequency of caval occlusion. J Vasc Interv Radiol 1999; 10(2 Pt 1):137–42.

96. Nutting C, Coldwell D. Use of a TrapEase device as a temporary caval filter. J Vasc Interv Radiol 2001;12(8):991–3.

97. Rousseau H, Perreault P, Otal P, et al. The 6-F nitinol TrapEase inferior vena cava filter: results of a prospective multicenter trial. J Vasc Interv Radiol 2001;12(3): 299–304.

98. Millward SF, Bormanis J, Burbridge BE, et al. Preliminary clinical experience with the Gunther temporary inferior vena cava filter. J Vasc Interv Radiol 1994;5(6): 863–8.

99. Berczi V, Bottomley JR, Thomas SM, et al. Long-term retrievability of IVC filters: should we abandon permanent devices? Cardiovasc Intervent Radiol 2007; 30(5):820–7.

100. Millward SF, Oliva VL, Bell SD, et al. Günther tulip retrievable vena cava filter: results from the registry of the Canadian Interventional Radiology Association. J Vasc Interv Radiol 2001;12(9):1053–8.

101. Millward SF, Bhargava A, Aquino J Jr, et al. Günther Tulip filter: preliminary clinical experience with retrieval. J Vasc Interv Radiol 2000;11(1):75–82.

102. Terhaar OA, Lyon SM, Given MF, et al. Extended interval for retrieval of Günther Tulip filters. J Vasc Interv Radiol 2004;15(11):1257–62.

103. Tay KH, Martin ML, Fry PD, et al. Repeated Günther Tulip inferior vena cava filter repositioning to prolong implantation time. J Vasc Interv Radiol 2002;13(5):509–12.

104. de Gregorio MA, Gamboa P, Gimeno MJ, et al. The Günther Tulip retrievable filter: prolonged temporary filtration by repositioning within the inferior vena cava. J Vasc Interv Radiol 2003;14(10):1259–65.

105. Binkert CA, Bansal A, Gates JD. Inferior vena cava filter removal after 317-day implantation. J Vasc Interv Radiol 2005;16(3):395–8.

106. Montgomery JP, Kaufman JA. A critical review of available retrievable inferior vena cava filters and future directions. Semin Intervent Radiol 2016;33(2): 79–87 [Thieme Medical Publishers].

107. Smouse HB, Rosenthal D, Thuong VH, et al. Long-term retrieval success rate profile for the Günther Tulip vena cava filter. J Vasc Interv Radiol 2009;20(7):871–7.

108. Hoffer EK, Mueller RJ, Luciano MR, et al. Safety and efficacy of the Gunther Tulip retrievable vena cava filter: midterm outcomes. Cardiovasc Intervent Radiol 2013;36(4):998–1005.

109. Sangwaiya MJ, Marentis TC, Walker TG, et al. Safety and effectiveness of the celect inferior vena cava filter: preliminary results. J Vasc Interv Radiol 2009; 20(9):1188–92.

110. Lyon SM, Riojas GE, Uberoi R, et al. Short-and long-term retrievability of the Celect vena cava filter: results from a multi-institutional registry. J Vasc Interv Radiol 2009;20(11):1441–8.

111. McLoney ED, Krishnasamy VP, Castle JC, et al. Complications of Celect, Günther tulip, and Greenfield inferior vena cava filters on CT follow-up: a single-institution experience. J Vasc Interv Radiol 2013;24(11):1723–9.

112. Bos A, Van Ha T, van Beek D, et al. Strut penetration: local complications, breakthrough pulmonary embolism, and retrieval failure in patients with Celect vena cava filters. J Vasc Interv Radiol 2015;26(1):101–6.

113. Mismetti P, Rivron-Guillot K, Quenet S, et al. A prospective long-term study of 220 patients with a retrievable vena cava filter for secondary prevention of venous thromboembolism. Chest 2007;131(1):223–9.

114. Pellerin O, Barral FG, Lions C, et al. Early and late retrieval of the ALN removable vena cava filter: results from a multicenter study. Cardiovasc Intervent Radiol 2008;31(5):889–96.

115. Pontone G, Andreini D, Bertella E, et al. Asymptomatic struts fracture and multiple embolization as a late complication of ALN removable vena cava filter implantation. Eur Heart J 2013;34(30):2353.
116. Hahn D. Retrievable filter update: the Denali vena cava filter. Semin Intervent Radiol 2015;32(4):379–83 [Thieme Medical Publishers].
117. Stavropoulos SW, Sing RF, Elmasri F, et al, DENALI Trial Investigators. The DENALI Trial: an interim analysis of a prospective, multicenter study of the Denali retrievable inferior vena cava filter. J Vasc Interv Radiol 2014;25(10):1497–505.
118. Stavropoulos SW, Chen JX, Sing RF, et al. Analysis of the final DENALI trial data: a prospective, multicenter study of the DENALI inferior vena cava filter. J Vasc Interv Radiol 2016;27(10):1531–8.e1.
119. Kuo WT, Robertson SW. Bard Denali inferior vena cava filter fracture and embolization resulting in cardiac tamponade: a device failure analysis. J Vasc Interv Radiol 2015;26(1):111–5.e1.
120. Johnson MS, Nemcek AA Jr, Benenati JF, et al. The safety and effectiveness of the retrievable option inferior vena cava filter: a United States prospective multicenter clinical study. J Vasc Interv Radiol 2010;21(8):1173–84.
121. Ziegler JW, Dietrich GJ, Cohen SA, et al. PROOF trial: protection from pulmonary embolism with the OptEase filter. J Vasc Interv Radiol 2008;19(8):1165–70.
122. Kalva SP, Marentis TC, Yeddula K, et al. Long-term safety and effectiveness of the "OptEase" vena cava filter. Cardiovasc Intervent Radiol 2011;34(2):331–7.
123. Scher D, Venbrux A, Okapal K, et al. Retrieval of TRAPEASE and OPTEASE inferior vena cava filters with extended dwell times. J Vasc Interv Radiol 2015;26(10):1519–25.
124. Rimon U, Bensaid P, Golan G, et al. Optease vena cava filter optimal indwelling time and retrievability.". Cardiovasc Intervent Radiol 2011;34(3):532–5.
125. Smouse HB, Mendes R, Bosiers M, et al. The RETRIEVE trial: safety and effectiveness of the retrievable crux vena cava filter. J Vasc Interv Radiol 2013;24(5):609–21.
126. Le Blanche AF, Ricco JB, Bonneau M, et al. The optional VenaTech™ convertible™ vena cava filter: experimental study in sheep. Cardiovasc Intervent Radiol 2012;35(5):1181–7.
127. Kaufman JA. Optional vena cava filters: what, why, and when. Vascular 2007;15(5):304–13.
128. Tapson VF, Hazelton JP, Myers J, et al. Evaluation of a device combining an inferior vena cava filter and a central venous catheter for preventing pulmonary embolism among critically ill trauma patients. J Vasc Interv Radiol 2017;28(9):1248–54.
129. Rosenthal D, Wellons ED, Levitt AB, et al. Role of prophylactic temporary inferior vena cava filters placed at the ICU bedside under intravascular ultrasound guidance in patients with multiple trauma. J Vasc Surg 2004;40(5):958–64.
130. Wellons ED, Matsuura JH, Shuler FW, et al. Bedside intravascular ultrasound-guided vena cava filter placement. J Vasc Surg 2003;38(3):455–7.
131. Chiou AC. Intravascular ultrasound-guided bedside placement of inferior vena cava filters. Semin Vasc Surg 2006;19(3):150–4. WB Saunders.
132. Ashley DW, Gamblin TC, Burch ST, et al. Accurate deployment of vena cava filters: comparison of intravascular ultrasound and contrast venography. J Trauma 2001;50(6):975–81.

133. Savin MA, Panicker HK, Sadiq S, et al. Placement of vena cava filters: factors affecting technical success and immediate complications. AJR Am J Roentgenol 2002;179(3):597–602.

134. Doe C, Ryu RK. Anatomic and technical considerations: inferior vena cava filter placement. Semin Intervent Radiol 2016;33(2):88–92. Thieme Medical Publishers.

135. Avgerinos ED, Bath J, Stevens J, et al. Technical and patient-related characteristics associated with challenging retrieval of inferior vena cava filters. Eur J Vasc Endovasc Surg 2013;46(3):353–9.

136. Al-Hakim R, Kee ST, Olinger K, et al. Inferior vena cava filter retrieval: effectiveness and complications of routine and advanced techniques. J Vasc Interv Radiol 2014;25(6):933–9.

137. Iliescu B, Haskal ZJ. Advanced techniques for removal of retrievable inferior vena cava filters. Cardiovasc Intervent Radiol 2012;35(4):741–50.

138. Schmelzer TM, Christmas AB, Taylor DA, et al. Vena cava filter retrieval in therapeutically anticoagulated patients. Am J Surg 2008;196(6):944–6 [discussion: 946–7].

139. Angel LF, Tapson V, Galgon RE, et al. Systematic review of the use of retrievable inferior vena cava filters. J Vasc Interv Radiol 2011;22(11):1522–30.e3.

140. Kuy S, Dua A, Lee CJ, et al. National trends in utilization of inferior vena cava filters in the United States, 2000-2009. J Vasc Surg Venous Lymphat Disord 2014;2(1):15–20.

141. Center for Devices and Radiological Health. Safety communications - removing retrievable inferior vena cava filters: initial communication. Internet Archive Wayback Machine, Center for Devices and Radiological Health; 2010. Available at: wayback.archive-it.org/7993/20161022180008/http://www.fda.gov/Medical-Devices/Safety/AlertsandNotices/ucm221676.htm.

142. Center for Devices and Radiological Health. Safety communications - removing retrievable inferior vena cava filters: FDA safety communication. Internet Archive Wayback Machine, Center for Devices and Radiological Health; 2014. Available at: wayback.archive-it.org/7993/20170722215731/https://www.fda.gov/Medical-Devices/Safety/AlertsandNotices/ucm396377.htm.

143. Morales JP, Li X, Irony TZ, et al. Decision analysis of retrievable inferior vena cava filters in patients without pulmonary embolism. J Vasc Surg Venous Lymphat Disord 2013;1(4):376–84.

144. Wadhwa V, Trivedi PS, Chatterjee K, et al. Decreasing utilization of inferior vena cava filters in post-FDA warning era: insights from 2005 to 2014 nationwide inpatient sample. J Am Coll Radiol 2017;14(9):1144–50.

Endovenous and Operative Treatment of Superior Vena Cava Syndrome

Manju Kalra, MBBS*, Indrani Sen, MBBS, Peter Gloviczki, MD

KEYWORDS

- Superior vena cava • Endovenous stenting • SVC bypass • Spiral saphenous
- Femoral vein

KEY POINTS

- The incidence of superior vena cava (SVC) syndrome is increasing secondary to venous thrombosis associated with the escalating use of central venous lines and cardiac pacemakers.
- Endovenous treatment, previously reserved for malignant SVC obstruction, if technically feasible, has become the first line of treatment of all causes of severely symptomatic SVC syndrome.
- Balloon and self-expanding stents have been used, depending on cause and lesion characteristics, with recent introduction of covered stents for this indication.
- Open surgical treatment, though significantly more invasive, has an important role to play in patients with benign SVC syndrome in whom endovenous treatment has either been technically unsuccessful or has eventually failed.
- Ideal conduits for surgical reconstruction of the SVC include spiral saphenous vein graft, femoral vein, and expanded polytetrafluoroethylene, which only perform well in the long-term for short reconstructions limited to within the mediastinum.

INTRODUCTION: NATURE OF THE PROBLEM

In the United States each year about 15,000 patients develop symptoms of venous congestion of the head and neck due to occlusion of the superior vena cava (SVC) or innominate veins. Metastatic lung cancer with mediastinal lymphadenopathy and primary mediastinal malignancy is the most common cause (60% of cases).[1,2] Nonmalignant causes are, however, increasing because of the more frequent use of central venous lines and cardiac pacemakers. Other causes include mediastinal fibrosis; granulomatous fungal disease, such as histoplasmosis; previous radiation to the mediastinum; retrosternal goiter; and aortic dissection. Signs and symptoms

The authors have nothing to disclose.
Mayo Clinic College of Medicine, 200 2nd Street SW, Rochester, MN 55905, USA
* Corresponding author.
E-mail address: kalra.manju@mayo.edu

of venous congestion of the head, neck, and upper extremities make up SVC syndrome and are determined by the duration, progression, and extent of the venous occlusive disease, and by the amount of collateral venous circulation that develops. Mortality is high in patients with metastatic malignant disease, and usually occurs at 6 to 12 months after the onset of symptoms. Treatment of SVC syndrome in patients with advanced malignancy is frequently palliative but a more durable mode of reconstruction needs to be considered in patients with benign disease.

CLINICAL PRESENTATION

The most frequent symptom of SVC syndrome is the feeling of fullness in the head and neck, which is more severe when the patient bends over or lies flat in bed. These patients can sleep only by elevating the head on multiple pillows. Headache, dizziness, visual symptoms, or occasional blackout spells may result from cerebral venous hypertension and can be incapacitating.[1,3,4] Additional symptoms may include mental confusion, dyspnea, orthopnea, or cough, as well as swelling of the face, eyelids, and upper extremities (**Fig. 1**). Ecchymosis and dilated jugular veins accompany cyanosis of the upper body. Extensive venous collaterals of the chest will frequently develop (**Fig. 2**). Mild to moderate upper extremity swelling may occur, but the primary symptoms are in patients with endstage renal disease. Asymptomatic SVC occlusion may be unmasked on creation of an arteriovenous fistula with rapid development of arm swelling and neck engorgement. Symptoms of malignant SVC syndrome may include hemoptysis, hoarseness, dysphagia, weight loss, lethargy, or palpable cervical tumor or lymph nodes. Patients with lymphoma may present with fever and night sweats.

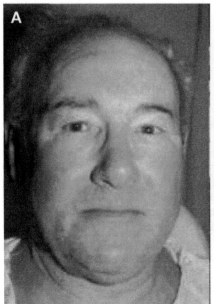 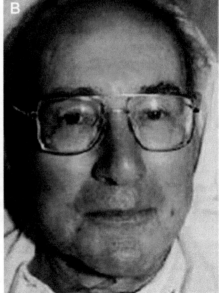

Fig. 1. (*A*) Severe symptomatic superior vena cava (SVC) syndrome in a 69 year old in man. (*B*) Photograph of the patient 5 days after right internal jugular vein–right atrial appendage spiral saphenous vein graft placement. The clinical result is excellent 8 years after the operation. (*Courtesy of* Mayo Clinic, Rochester, MN.)

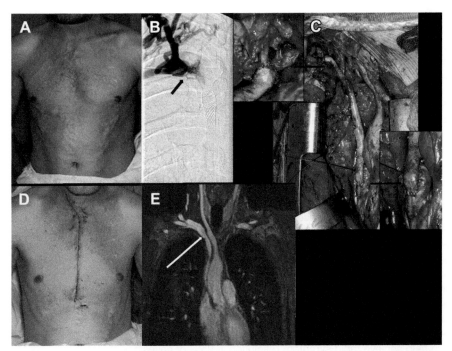

Fig. 2. (A) Symptomatic recurrent SVC obstruction following occlusion of Wallstent prominent abdominal and chest wall collaterals. (B) Venogram demonstrating occlusion until the peripheral vein. Right internal jugular vein (IJV) and subclavian veins patent with large draining collaterals (black arrow). (C) Bypass from right IJV-SCV confluence (top inset). Right atrial appendage (bottom inset) using femoral vein. (D) Postoperative symptom relief demonstrated by collapse of right chest wall and upper limb collaterals. (E) Magnetic resonance venogram 15 months after surgery confirms the graft to be widely patent (white arrow).

DIAGNOSTIC EVALUATION

A detailed clinical history with physical examination can usually establish the diagnosis of SVC syndrome. Routine laboratory tests, chest roentgenogram, and contrast-enhanced computed tomography (CT) (arterial and venous phase) of the chest is performed in all patients to exclude underlying malignant disease. The CT imaging accurately depicts the location and extent of the obstruction and also distinguishes various types of benign and malignant mediastinal disease. The extent of venous collateral formation is also well-demonstrated. These collateral pathways include the[1] azygos-hemiazygos pathway,[2] the internal mammary pathway,[3] the lateral thoracic-thoracoepigastric pathway,[4] the vertebral pathway, and small mediastinal veins. An additional advantage includes the ability to perform CT-guided biopsy to aid in the diagnosis of mediastinal masses. Magnetic resonance venography is also suitable to define anatomy, although patients with pacemakers are not candidates for this test. Bronchoscopy, mediastinoscopy, thoracoscopy, thoracotomy, or median sternotomy may be necessary in some patients to provide tissue diagnosis or, occasionally, to attempt resection of a localized tumor causing SVC occlusion.

Patency of at least 1 internal jugular vein should be confirmed with duplex scanning in those patients who are candidates for surgical reconstruction.

Evaluation of patients considered for endovascular or open surgical treatment is continued with bilateral upper extremity venography. Based on the extent of venous occlusion, as defined by bilateral upper extremity venography, Stanford and Doty[5] described 4 venographic patterns of SVC syndrome, each having a different venous collateral network depending on the site and extent of SVC obstruction. Type I is partial and type II is complete or near-complete SVC obstruction, with flow in the azygos vein remaining antegrade. Type III is 90% to 100% SVC obstruction with reversed azygos blood flow. Type IV is extensive mediastinal central venous occlusion with venous return occurring through the inferior vena cava (**Fig. 3**).

SURGICAL TECHNIQUE
Preoperative Planning

Conservative measures are used first in every patient to relieve symptoms of venous congestion and to decrease progression of venous thrombosis. These measures include elevation of the head during the night on pillows, modifications of daily activities by avoiding bending over, and avoidance of wearing constricting garments or a tight collar. Patients frequently need diuretic agents to decrease, at least temporarily, excessive edema of the neck and head. Patients with acute SVC syndrome caused by malignant disease are generally treated with intravenous unfractionated or low-molecular-weight heparin followed by warfarin to prevent recurrence and protect the venous collateral circulation. Symptoms frequently improve after irradiation, chemotherapy, or combination chemoradiation based on the tumor histology. Endovascular treatment with stenting can help achieve rapid symptom resolution in 95% of cases.[6]

Patients with severe incapacitating symptoms not responding to conservative therapy should be considered for interventional treatment, depending on the cause and anatomy of the SVC lesion. In the past 2 decades, endovascular therapy with stents has become the dominant primary therapy for SVC occlusion of both malignant and benign cause. In contemporary practice, surgical reconstruction is reserved for patients with extensive chronic venous thrombosis not anatomically suitable for endovascular treatment and for those with less extensive disease who have failed prior endovascular treatment.[3]

Endovenous Approach

The endovenous approach is an achievement that has served patients with malignant disease well with rapid symptomatic relief; however, long-term results of stents placed in young patients for benign lesions are still not well known, and rethrombosis or intimal hyperplasia can be significant. Despite this, endovascular treatment is now accepted as the first-line treatment in benign and malignant, cases. Treatment modalities include percutaneous transluminal balloon angioplasty (PTA), stenting, and thrombolysis performed alone or in combination. External compressive lesions and dense elastic fibrosis results in a high early restenosis rate with angioplasty alone.

Procedure

The technique of endovenous repair involves ultrasound-guided percutaneous venous access of the common femoral vein and placement of 6 to 10 F sheaths, followed by crossing the stenotic or occlusive lesion with hydrophilic guidewires and catheters. The right internal jugular or arm vein can be an alternate or additional venous access site in patients with short focal lesions or if the lesion cannot be crossed from the femoral approach, respectively. Access of a hemodialysis arteriovenous fistula (if present) is a viable option. Long sheaths extending to the site of a long occlusion can

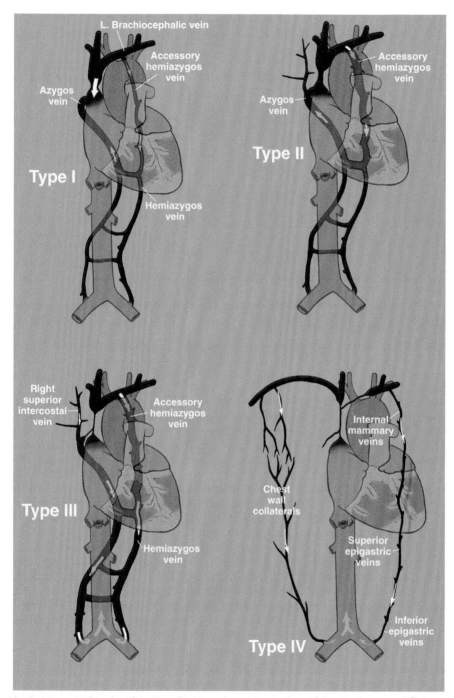

Fig. 3. Venographic classification of SVC syndrome according to Stanford and Doty.[5] Type I: high-grade SVC stenosis with normal direction of blood flow but still normal direction of blood flow through the SVC and azygos veins. Increased collateral circulation through hemiazygos and accessory hemiazygos veins. Type II: greater than 90% stenosis or occlusion of

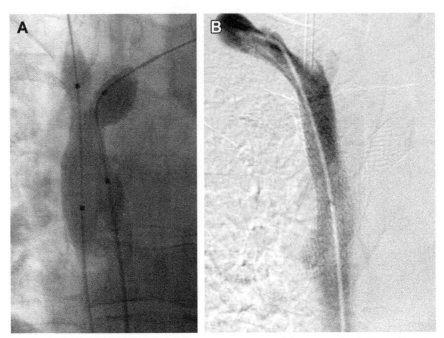

Fig. 4. (*A*) Bilateral self-expanding kissing stents placement. (*B*) Poststenting balloon dilatation.

be helpful in providing the necessary support to cross the lesion. Once wire access across the lesion is obtained, primary PTA using standard 10 to 16 mm angioplasty balloons is performed, followed by stenting. Venous stenoses can be very resistant, often requiring angioplasty with high pressure balloons (eg, Mustang [Boston Scientific, Natick, MA], Atlas [Bard, NJ]) (**Fig. 4**). The choice of stent is tailored to the cause, degree, length, and tortuosity of the SVC stenosis. The earliest stents deployed were Gianturco Z stents (Cook Medical, Bloomington, IN), available in large diameters with hooks for fixation to prevent migration. These had the advantages of ease of placement, rigidity, and lack of shortening. The large stent interstices, however, are worrisome for allowing tumor ingrowth. Palmaz (Cordis Corporation, Miami, FL, USA) balloon expandable stents are ideally suited for short, focal fibrotic or compressive lesions because of their precise deployment and good radial force but are relatively inflexible (**Fig. 5**). Disadvantages include poor flexibility and availability only in short lengths. In recent years, other self-expanding stents, such as Wallstent (Boston Scientific Corp, Natick, MA, USA), Smart stents (Cordis Endovascular, Warren, NJ, USA), Protégé stents (Plymouth, MN, USA), E*Luminexx (Bard GmbH, Angiomed, Karlsruhe, Germany), Sinus-XL (OptiMed Medizinische Instrumente GmbH, Ettlingen, Germany), and Zilver Vena (Cook Medical Inc, Bloomington, IN, USA) have been used more frequently for longer SVC stenoses because of their flexibility and availability in multiple sizes.

---

the SVC but patent azygos vein with normal direction of blood flow. Type III: occlusion of the SVC with retrograde flow in both the azygos and hemiazygos veins. Type IV: extensive occlusion of the SVC and innominate and azygos veins with chest wall and epigastric venous collaterals. (*From* Alimi YS, Gloviczki P, Vrtiska TJ, et al. Reconstruction of the superior vena cava: the benefits of postoperative surveillance and secondary endovascular interventions. J Vasc Surg 1998;27:298–99; with permission.)

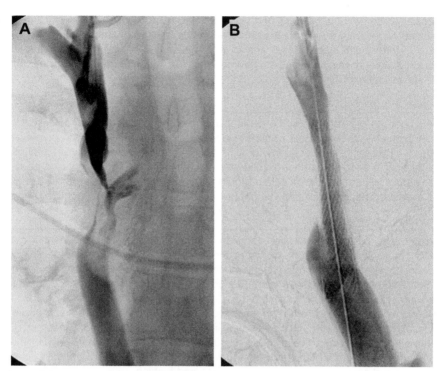

Fig. 5. (*A*) Venogram showing type II SVC obstruction due to mediastinal fibrosis in a 31-year-old man. Successful placement of a Palmaz sent resulted in immediate resolution of symptoms. (*B*) Eleven months later, the patient underwent balloon dilatation for in-stent stenosis and remains asymptomatic.

Perforation can occur during this process and, if minor, manifest as a mild peri-venous blush without hemodynamic changes. It can be managed successfully with prolonged balloon inflation. Placement of a covered stent is required to control larger, more significant perforations, especially if associated with hemodynamic instability. Rarely, SVC rupture can result in pericardial tamponade. Rapid diagnosis and immediate ultrasound-guided pericardial drainage is necessary. The authors are now electively using covered stents in selected cases to poten-tially control tumor ingrowth and provide better freedom from the need for reintervention.[6,7]

Adjunctive thrombolysis may be performed alone for acute or subacute SVC throm-bosis related to indwelling catheters, or before angioplasty or stenting to resolve the thrombosis and reveal the underlying stenotic lesion for definitive treatment. If throm-bolysis is determined to be appropriate before PTA or stenting, a suitable length cath-eter with side-holes is placed across the lesion for catheter-directed lytic therapy. Successful catheter-directed thrombolysis, as well as pharmacomechanical throm-bectomy, has been reported not only in various catheter-related thromboses but also in malignant SVC occlusions.[8]

Immediate Postprocedure Care

Care following the procedure mainly consists of care of the venous access sites. Frequently, the patient can be discharged the same day. The need for postprocedure anticoagulation is individualized based on the cause of SVC syndrome. Most patients, especially those with malignancy and catheter-related thrombosis receive oral antico-agulation for at least a few months until the stent is lined with pseudointima and the risk of rethrombosis decreases. Patients with mediastinal fibrosis are often treated with antiplatelet therapy alone. Both rethrombosis following cessation of anticoagula-tion, as well as excellent results without it, have been reported.

Surgical Approach

The procedure is performed under general anesthesia with the patient in a supine po-sition. Central venous access is obtained via the common femoral vein. The operation is performed through a median sternotomy. If the internal jugular vein is used for inflow, the midline incision is extended obliquely into the neck along the anterior border of the sternocleidomastoid muscle on the appropriate side. Dissection is carried out in the anterior mediastinum and the innominate veins, and the SVC is identified.

Surgical Procedure

Biopsy of any mediastinal mass or resection of tumor, if the cause is malignant, is car-ried out next. Once biopsy or tumor resection has been performed, the pericardial sac is opened to expose the right atrial appendage, which is the most frequent site for the central anastomosis. If not involved in the fibrosing process, a patent SVC central to the occlusion can also be used for this purpose. A side-biting Satinsky clamp is next placed on the right atrial appendage, which is opened longitudinally. Some trabecular muscle is excised to improve inflow, and an end-to-side anastomosis with the vein graft is performed with a running 5-0 monofilament suture (**Fig. 6**). The peripheral anastomosis of the graft is performed with the internal jugular or innominate vein in an end-to-side or, preferably, an end-to-end fashion.

For replacement of the SVC or the innominate vein in patients with benign disease, autogenous spiral saphenous vein graft (SSVG) has been the authors' first choice (**Fig. 7**). The great saphenous vein is harvested, opened longitudinally, the valves

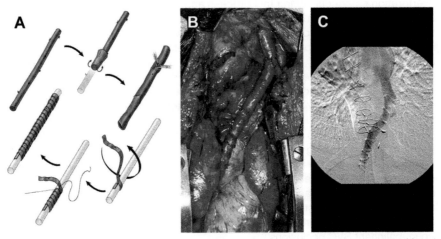

Fig. 6. (*A*) Technique for a spiral saphenous vein graft. The saphenous vein is opened longi-tudinally, valves are excised, the vein is wrapped around an argyle chest tube (*arrows*), and the vein edges are approximated with sutures. A 15-cm spiral saphenous vein graft ready for implantation. (*B*) Intraoperative image of spiral vein graft. (*C*) Postoperative venogram demonstrating the patent left internal jugular, right atrial appendage bypass graft. The graft is patent and the patient is asymptomatic 3 years later.

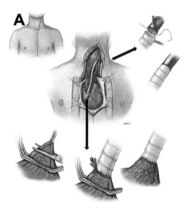 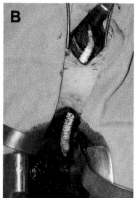 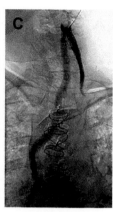

Fig. 7. (*A*) Technique of left internal jugular, right atrial spiral vein graft implantation. (*B*) Left internal jugular vein, atrial appendage externally supported ePTFE graft. (*C*) Widely patent graft at 13 months after the operation.

are excised, and the vein is wrapped around a 32 or 36 F polyethylene chest tube. The edges of the vein are then approximated with running 6-0 monofilament polypropylene sutures. The vein is continuously irrigated during this phase of preparation with heparinized papaverine solution to preserve the integrity of endothelial cells and to prevent desiccation. Spiral saphenous vein graft is a relatively nonthrombogenic autologous tissue. Disadvantages include the additional incision and the time (60–90 min) needed to prepare the graft. In addition, the length of the graft is limited by the availability of an adequate length segment of saphenous vein. The saphenous veins may also be used as a panel graft. The femoral or femoropopliteal vein been used as a conduit with success because of its excellent suitability in terms of size and length (see **Fig. 2**C; **Fig. 8**). It is an excellent graft. However, if the patient has underlying thrombotic abnormalities, removal of a deep leg vein may result in at least moderate lower extremity postthrombotic syndrome. Of the available prosthetic materials, externally supported expanded polytetrafluoroethylene (ePTFE) is used for large vein reconstruction almost exclusively because of low thrombogenicity. Short, large-diameter (10–14 mm) grafts have excellent long-term patency because flow through the innominate vein usually exceeds 1000 mL/min. If the peripheral anastomosis is performed with the subclavian vein, venous inflow is significantly less and the addition of an arteriovenous fistula is usually required in the arm to ensure graft patency. An arteriovenous fistula with direct flow into the graft has not been performed for jugular grafts. An externally supported prosthetic graft is a good choice in patients with a tight mediastinum, and usually for all patients with malignancy, because recurrent tumor is more likely to compress and occlude a vein graft. Iliocaval allograft can be considered in those patients who are treated for receive immunosuppressive treatment to protect a transplanted organ. Cryopreserved femoral vein grafts are potential alternatives, as are grafts prepared from autogenous or bovine pericardium.

The authors have performed bifurcated SSVGs grafts in a few patients but, because of a high incidence of early postoperative occlusion of 1 limb of the graft, our current operative choice is a single straight graft from the internal jugular or innominate vein. Collateral circulation in the head and neck is almost always adequate, thus unilateral reconstruction is sufficient to relieve symptoms in most patients. When only part of the

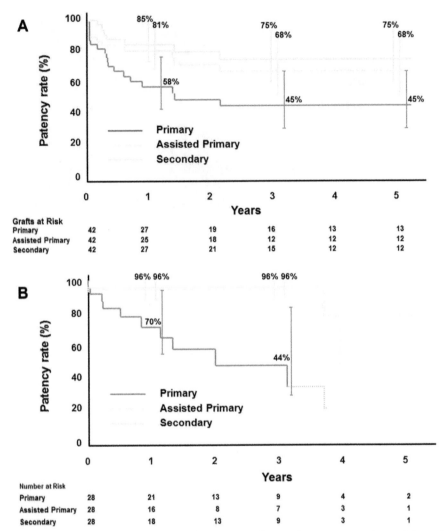

Fig. 8. (*A*) Cumulative primary, assisted primary, and secondary patency rates at 1, 3, and 5 years of open surgical reconstruction (n = 42). Solid bars represent SEM (standard error of the mean) less than 10%. (*B*) Cumulative primary, assisted primary, and secondary patency rates at 1 and 3 years of endovascular repair (n = 28). Solid bars represent SEM less than 10%. (*From* Rizvi AZ, Kalra M, Bjarnason H, et al. Benign superior vena cava syndrome: stenting is now the first line of treatment. J Vasc Surg 2008;47(2):372–80; with permission.)

circumference of the SVC is invaded by the tumor, resection and caval patch angioplasty using prosthetic patch; bovine pericardium; or autogenous material, such as saphenous vein or pericardium, are viable options.

IMMEDIATE POSTPROCEDURE CARE AND RECOVERY

Postoperative anticoagulation is started 24 hours later with heparin, and the patient is discharged on an oral anticoagulation regimen. Patients with SSVGs or femoral

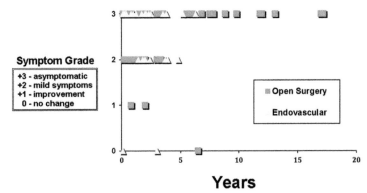

Fig. 9. Grading of symptom relief at last clinical follow-up in patients undergoing open surgical reconstruction (n = 42) or endovascular repair (n = 28). (*From* Rizvi AZ, Kalra M, Bjarnason H, et al. Benign superior vena cava syndrome: stenting is now the first line of treatment. J Vasc Surg 2008;47(2):372–80; with permission.)

vein grafts who have no underlying coagulation abnormality are maintained on warfarin (Coumadin) for 3 months only. Those with underlying coagulation disorders and most patients with ePTFE grafts continue lifelong anticoagulation therapy.

Relief of symptoms is instantaneous following successful endovenous or surgical reconstruction (**Fig. 9**). Surveillance with duplex ultrasound, computed tomography venogram, or magnetic resonance venography is done at 6-month intervals during the first 2 years, followed by annually thereafter. Reintervention for stenosis is mostly endovenous with surgical reintervention reserved for refractory cases (**Fig. 10**). In the long-term, the interval of imaging surveillance can be lengthened because restenosis is invariably associated with recurrent symptoms. Clinical results are presented in **Table 1**.

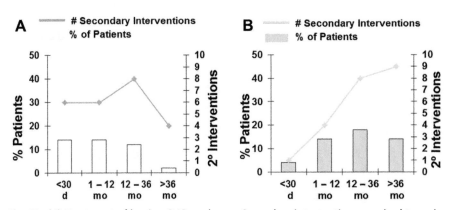

Fig. 10. (A) Treatment of benign SVC syndrome. Secondary interventions required to maintain patency in (A) the open surgical group (n = 42) and (B) the endovascular group (n = 28). The bars represent the percentage of patients in each group and the line graphs represent the total number of interventions. (*From* Rizvi AZ, Kalra M, Bjarnason H, et al. Benign superior vena cava syndrome: stenting is now the first line of treatment. J Vasc Surg 2008;47(2):372–80; with permission.)

Table 1
Clinical results in the literature

Study	Number of Subjects	Cause	Details of Intervention	Technical Success	Mean Follow-up	Patency	Mortality or Morbidity
Kee et al,[8] 1998	59	Benign[16] Malignant (43)	Catheter-directed thrombolysis 27 Stent placement 51 (Wallstent or Palmaz)	95%	Clinical 17 mo (1–27 mo)	Malignancy: primary patency 33 (79%) Secondary patency 39 (93%) Benign: primary patency 10 (77%) Secondary patency 11 (85%)	Mortality 3% Morbidity 10%
Qanaldi et al,[9] 1999	12	Benign	Stent placement (Wallstent)	100%	Clinical 11 mo (1–36 mo) Radiologic 7 mo (0–32 mo)	Primary patency 10 (85%) Secondary patency 11 (91%)	—
Barshes et al,[10] 2007	56	Malignant (40) Benign[16]	Stent placement (Wallstent or Palmaz)	100%	Malignant 8.3 mo (1–21 mo) Benign 28 mo (4–57 mo)	Primary patency 64% (malignant) 76% (benign) Secondary reintervention in 4 with benign disease: all successful	Nil
Breault et al,[11] 2017	44	Benign	Venoplasty 4 Stent placement 40	100%	41 mo (1–16 y)	Assisted patency 100%	Morbidity 13%

Study	N	Etiology	Intervention	Technical success	Follow-up	Outcome	Morbidity/Mortality
Dinkel et al,[12] 2003	44	Malignant	Stent placement (Wallstent)	99%	13.9 mo (2–55 mo)	Primary patency 90%, 81%, 76%, and 69% (1, 3, 6, and 12 mo, respectively) Secondary intervention in 7: all successful	Morbidity 28% (bilateral stents) 9% (unilateral)
Maleux et al,[13] 2013	78	Malignant	Stent placement (large-bore nitinol Zilver, Cook Medical)	100%	—	Primary patency 89% at 12 mo	Morbidity (4/78)5.2%
Fagedet et al,[14] 2013	164	Malignant	Stent placement Wallstent, Mesotherm (CR Bard, Inc, Billerica, MA, USA)	95%	—	Relapse in 36 patients (21.9%), restenting in 75%: all successful	Mortality 2.4% Morbidity 12.8%
Mokry et al,[15] 2015	23	Malignant	Stent placement Sinus-XL stent	100%	2 mo (1–25 mo)	Primary patency 95.7% Secondary patency 100%	Morbidity 17%
Gwon et al,[6] 2013	37	Malignant	Stent placement Covered ePTFE vs uncovered	100%	5 mo (0–2 y)	Covered stents cumulative patency (97%, 94%, 94%, and 94% at 1, 3, 6, and 12 mo, respectively) Uncovered stents cumulative patency (97%, 79%, 67%, and 48% at 1, 3, 6, and 12 mo, respectively)	Nil
Doty et al,[16] 1999	16	Benign	Composite spiral vein graft	100%	10.9 y (1 mo to 24 y)	Graft thrombosis in 3: patency restored in 1	Nil

(continued on next page)

Table 1
(continued)

Study	Number of Subjects	Cause	Details of Intervention	Technical Success	Mean Follow-up	Patency	Mortality or Morbidity
Dartevelle et al,[17] 1991	22	Malignant	ePTFE	100%	23 mo (1–98 mo)	Continued patency in 20 of 22	Mortality 4.5% Morbidity 4.5%
Picquet et al,[18] 2009	24	Malignant[18] Benign[6]	ePTFE (23) autologous spiral saphenous vein graft (1)	100%	28 mo	Continued patency 100%	Mortality 12% (malignant)
Rizvi et al,[3] 2008	70	Benign	Open reconstruction: spiral saphenous vein 22, ePTFE 13, femoral vein 6, human allograft 1 Endovascular reconstruction: 32; stent placement 19 PTA 14 Thrombolysis with PTA or stent placement 5	Endovascular 88% Open 100%	Open: 4.1 y (0.1–17.5 y) Endovascular: 2.2 y (0.2–6.4 y)	Primary, assisted primary, secondary patency (at 3 and 5 y) Open reconstruction: 45%, 68%, 75% Endovascular reconstruction: 44%, 96%, and 96%	Mortality: nil Morbidity Open reconstruction: 19% Endovascular reconstruction: 4%

REFERENCES

1. Wilson LD, Detterbeck FC, Yahalom J. Superior vena cava syndrome with malignant causes. N Engl J Med 2007;356(18):1862–9.
2. Rice TW, Rodriguez RM, Light RW. The superior vena cava syndrome: clinical characteristics and evolving etiology. Medicine (Baltimore) 2006;85(1):37–42.
3. Rizvi AZ, Kalra M, Bjarnason H, et al. Benign superior vena cava syndrome: stenting is now the first line of treatment. J Vasc Surg 2008;47(2):372–80.
4. Laguna Del Estal P, Gazapo Navarro T, Murillas Angoitti J, et al. Superior vena cava syndrome: a study based on 81 cases. An Med Interna 1998;15(9):470–5 [in Spanish].
5. Stanford W, Doty DB. The role of venography and surgery in the management of patients with superior vena cava obstruction. Ann Thorac Surg 1986;41(2):158–63.
6. Gwon DI, Ko GY, Kim JH, et al. Malignant superior vena cava syndrome: a comparative cohort study of treatment with covered stents versus uncovered stents. Radiology 2013;266(3):979–87.
7. Anaya-Ayala JE, Smolock CJ, Colvard BD, et al. Efficacy of covered stent placement for central venous occlusive disease in hemodialysis patients. J Vasc Surg 2011;54(3):754–9.
8. Kee ST, Kinoshita L, Razavi MK, et al. Superior vena cava syndrome: treatment with catheter-directed thrombolysis and endovascular stent placement. Radiology 1998;206(1):187–93.
9. Qanadli SD, El Hajjam M, Mignon F, et al. Subacute and chronic benign superior vena cava obstructions: endovascular treatment with self-expanding metallic stents. AJR Am J Roentgenol 1999;173(1):159–64.
10. Barshes NR, Annambhotla S, El Sayed HF, et al. Percutaneous stenting of superior vena cava syndrome: treatment outcome in patients with benign and malignant etiology. Vascular 2007;15(5):314–21.
11. Breault S, Doenz F, Jouannic AM, et al. Percutaneous endovascular management of chronic superior vena cava syndrome of benign causes: long-term follow-up. Eur Radiol 2017;27(1):97–104.
12. Dinkel HP, Mettke B, Schmid F, et al. Endovascular treatment of malignant superior vena cava syndrome: is bilateral wallstent placement superior to unilateral placement? J Endovasc Ther 2003;10(4):788–97.
13. Maleux G, Gillardin P, Fieuws S, et al. Large-bore nitinol stents for malignant superior vena cava syndrome: factors influencing outcome. AJR Am J Roentgenol 2013;201(3):667–74.
14. Fagedet D, Thony F, Timsit JF, et al. Endovascular treatment of malignant superior vena cava syndrome: results and predictive factors of clinical efficacy. Cardiovascu Intervent Radiol 2013;36(1):140–9.
15. Mokry T, Bellemann N, Sommer CM, et al. Retrospective study in 23 patients of the self-expanding sinus-XL stent for treatment of malignant superior vena cava obstruction caused by non-small cell lung cancer. J Vasc Interv Radiol 2015;26(3):357–65.
16. Doty JR, Flores JH, Doty DB. Superior vena cava obstruction: bypass using spiral vein graft. Ann Thorac Surg 1999;67(4):1111–6.
17. Dartevelle PG, Chapelier AR, Pastorino U, et al. Long-term follow-up after prosthetic replacement of the superior vena cava combined with resection of mediastinal-pulmonary malignant tumors. J Thorac Cardiovasc Surg 1991;102(2):259–65.
18. Picquet J, Blin V, Dussaussoy C, et al. Surgical reconstruction of the superior vena cava system: indications and results. Surgery 2009;145(1):93–9.

Pathophysiology of Chronic Venous Disease and Venous Ulcers

Joseph D. Raffetto, MD[a,b,*]

KEYWORDS

- Chronic venous disease • Venous leg ulcers • Inflammation • Adhesion molecules
- Endothelial dysfunction • Glycocalyx • Cytokines • Matrix metalloproteinases

KEY POINTS

- Venous reflux and obstruction leads to venous hypertension.
- Genetic predisposition and various candidate genes and their polymorphisms and environmental factors are important in the development of chronic venous disease.
- Inflammatory cells have a central role in the pathophysiology of chronic venous disease and venous leg ulcers.
- Changes in the glycocalyx and shear stress lead to dysfunctional endothelium and expression of adhesion molecules that attract leukocytes initiating events of inflammatory response.
- Cytokines and matrix metalloproteinases are expressed in chronic venous disease, particularly in venous leg ulcers, and are responsible for persistent impaired wound healing but also are necessary for wound closure.

INTRODUCTION

Chronic venous disease (CVD) is a debilitating condition that affects millions of individuals worldwide. The condition can result in varicose veins, or advance to severe skin changes and venous ulceration. Both reflux and obstruction account for the pathophysiology of CVD; however, reflux has a much higher prevalence in patients presenting with the different stages of CVD including venous leg ulcers (VLU), but obstruction has a higher rate of patients developing venous ulceration, and has a much more rapid progression of disease.[1–5] Whether reflux or obstruction is the cause for the patient's clinical presentation and symptomatology, both conditions lead to increased ambulatory venous pressure. Genetic and environmental factors influence predisposition to

The author has nothing to disclose.
[a] Harvard Medical School, VA Boston Healthcare System, Brigham and Women's Hospital, Boston, MA, USA; [b] VA Boston HCS, Surg 112, 1400 VFW Parkway, West Roxbury, MA 02132, USA
* VA Boston HCS, Surg 112, 1400 VFW Parkway, West Roxbury, MA 02132.
E-mail address: joseph.raffetto@med.va.gov

Surg Clin N Am 98 (2018) 337–347
https://doi.org/10.1016/j.suc.2017.11.002
0039-6109/18/Published by Elsevier Inc.

CVD and VLU. Inflammatory cells are activated on changes in shear stress and endothelial cell disruption. Matrix metalloproteinases (MMPs) are activated and changes in the structural components of the vein wall collagen and elastin occur, and extracellular matrix degradation resulting in CVD as seen in varicose veins, skin changes, and VLU. The fundamental basis for CVD and venous ulceration is inflammation within the venous circulation that is subjected to increased hydrostatic pressure, resulting in increased ambulatory venous pressure, increased inflammation within the vein wall and valve leaflet, and extravasation of inflammatory cells and molecules into the interstitium.[6–8] The inflammatory response involves leukocytes, in particular macrophages and monocytes, and T lymphocytes and mast cells, inflammatory modulators and chemokines, cytokine expression, growth factors, metalloproteinase activity, and many regulatory pathways that perpetuate inflammation and the resultant changes seen with CVD (**Fig. 1**).[9–14]

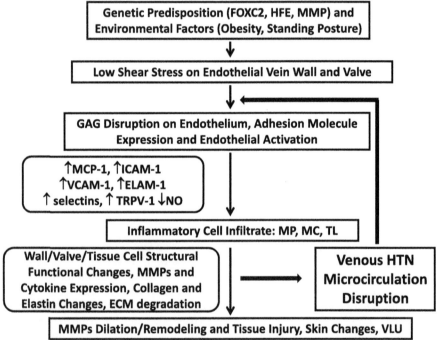

Fig. 1. Schematic flow diagram of chronic venous disease pathophysiology. Genetic and environmental factors predispose individuals to venous disease, changes in shear stress and endothelial integrity lead to adhesion molecule expression and leukocyte-endothelial activation, initiating an inflammatory response with expression of cytokines, chemokines, and matrix metalloproteinases. Changes in venous wall structure and valve function lead to venous dilation and insufficiency, venous hypertension, and disruption in the microcirculation. Persistent inflammatory state with matrix metalloproteinase and cytokine expression causes tissue damage and degradation resulting in skin changes and venous leg ulcer. ECM, extracellular matrix; ELAM-1, endothelial leukocyte adhesion molecule-1; FOXC2, forkhead box protein C2 gene; GAG, glycosaminoglycan; HFE, hemochromatosis gene; HTN, hypertension; ICAM-1, intercellular adhesion molecule-1; MC, mast cells; MCP-1, monocyte chemotactic protein-1; MP, macrophages; NO, nitric oxide; TL, T lymphocytes; TRPV-1, transient receptor potential vanilloid channels; VCAM-1, vascular cell adhesion molecule-1.

CONTENT

The pathophysiology of primary venous disease is a complex entity with genetic and environmental factors, changes in venous endothelium, inflammatory biomolecules, and structural wall changes that lead to the dilated tortuous veins, dysfunctional valves with insufficiency, venous hypertension, and the associated clinical manifestations seen with CVD.[13] Several epidemiologic studies have assessed the associated risk factors. Certainly genetic and environmental factors influence the predisposition and perpetuation of developing primary venous disease. Some important observations are a family history, female gender, pregnancy, estrogen (the latter three associated with varicose veins clinically), prolonged standing and sitting postures, and obesity.[9] Genetic conditions, such as Klippel-Trénaunay syndrome, CADASIL, FOXC2 gene mutation, desmulin dysregulation, and Ehlers-Danlos syndrome, display early onset of varicose veins.[9,15] However, most individuals with primary venous disease do not have the aforementioned genetic conditions because these are rare conditions, and a specific gene leading to primary venous disease and varicose veins has not been identified, but it seems that the trait is autosomal-dominant with variable penetrance.[15,16] In a study of 2701 patients with CVD, inherited genetic disorders leading to CVD accounted for an estimated 17%.[17] Importantly, this study did not find much difference in genetic susceptibility across the different clinical classes of CEAP (Clinical Etiology Anatomy Pathophysiology). This represents a significant proportion of individuals that may have a genetic link to venous disease. A recent genome-wide association study was performed in 2296 patients with CVD and 7765 control subjects without CVD. The study determined genetic variants in the genes EFEMP1, KCNH8, and SKAP2 in CVD susceptibility. These genes are important in regulation of extracellular matrix protein, potassium channels, and cellular signaling, and possibly implicated in the pathophysiology of CVD.[18] A review of candidate genes and their polymorphic variants that are important in the development of CVD determined that genes of significance include FOXC2, HFE, and the MMPs, all of which demonstrated strong associations with varicose veins, chronic venous insufficiency, and venous ulceration.[19]

Further studies have focused on genetic polymorphism in populations with CVD in the development and healing potential of VLU.[20] Hemochromatosis C282Y (HFE) gene mutation and certain factor XIII V34L gene variants have been demonstrated in patients with CVD and varicose veins, and may have long-term implications for increased risk of more severe forms of CVD, and the size of venous ulcers.[21,22] Factor XIII is an important cross-linking protein that plays a key role during ulcer healing.[23] HFE and FXIII genes were also evaluated in predicting venous ulcer healing following superficial venous surgery in patients with CVD. Specific FXIII genotypes had favorable ulcer healing rates, whereas the HFE gene mutation, despite its importance in venous ulcer risk, had no influence on healing time.[24] Identification of genetic susceptibility factors for CVD requires further work to establish mechanisms of disease and translation therapies for effective treatments.

It is clear from biochemical, immunohistochemical, and functional studies that the vein wall and the valve are involved in the primary events leading to venous disease. Whether it is the vein wall changes preceding valve insufficiency or the valve insufficiency causing wall distention and wall changes, is a moot point.[9] Importantly, evidence demonstrates that vein wall and vein valve are pathologically altered to cause primary venous disease. The perturbation in the microcirculation is a critical component in the pathophysiology of CVD. The endothelium is a key regulator of vascular tone, hemostasis, and coagulation. Injury, infection, immune diseases, diabetes, genetic predisposition, environmental factors, smoking, and atherosclerosis all have an adverse effect on the endothelium, which in turn must compensate to prevent further injury and maintain integrity of the vascular wall. In CVD, the sine qua non is persistent elevated ambulatory venous pressure leading to sustained venous hypertension and the effects associated with the microcirculation. The effect on the microcirculation begins with altered shear stress on the endothelial cells, causing endothelial cells to release vasoactive agents, express selectins, inflammatory molecules, chemokines, and prothrombotic precursors.[25,26] Mechanical forces, low shear stress, and stretch are sensed by the endothelial cells via intercellular adhesion molecule-1 (ICAM-1, CD54), vascular cell adhesion molecule-1 (VCAM-1, CD-106), endothelial leukocyte adhesion molecule-1 (CD-62, E-selectin), and the mechanosensitive transient receptor potential vanilloid channels that are present in the endothelium.[26,27] It is well known that patients with CVD have increased expression of ICAM-1, and likely VCAM-1 and endothelial leukocyte adhesion molecule-1, which is expressed on endothelial cells, and activate the recruitment of leukocytes and initiate endothelial transmigration, setting up an inflammatory cascade.[12,28–30] Initiating events likely involve altered shear stress and mechanical stress forces on the endothelium and its glycocalyx (a glycosaminoglycan on the surface of endothelial cells), with perturbations on nitric oxide production, vasoactive substance release, expression of macrophage chemoattractant protein-1 and VCAM-1, expression of L-selectin and E-selectin, ICAM-1, with recruitment of leukocytes leading to leukocyte transmigration into the vein wall and valve, setting up an inflammatory cascade and production of several cytokines (transforming growth factor [TGF]-β1, tumor necrosis factor-α, interleukin-1) and increased expression of MMPs.[11,26,30] In addition, the endothelial glycocalyx is an important structure that prevents leukocyte adhesion, inflammation, and thrombosis. However, altered shear stress, mechanical forces on the vein wall causing leukocyte adhesion, and inflammation lead to injury and loss of the glycocalyx.[31,32] Alterations of glycosaminoglycans by degrading enzymes have been described in varicose veins. Endothelial glycocalyx disruption has been observed in patients with CVD, and in the vein wall of varicose veins there is increased levels of degraded sulfated glycosaminoglycans, indicating the crucial role of glycosaminoglycans and CVD.[33] A key component of inflammation and in VLU is the overexpression of MMPs and cytokines, which have significant effects on the vein wall and venous valve, endothelium, and likely the glycocalyx, and surrounding tissues including destruction of the dermis with eventual skin changes and ulcer formation (**Fig. 2**).[11,34,35] A variety of MMPs have been observed in vein specimens taken from patients with CVD. Their functions may not only include degradation of adventitial extracellular matrix and collagen bundles and elastin in the medial layer, but may also have significant early effects on venous dilation.[9,30,35] MMPs can be released as a result of mechanical stretch (and hence during conditions of venous hypertension) and have significant effects on the endothelium, venous smooth muscle, and adventitia.[36] MMPs have been demonstrated in rat venous tissue to cause venous dilation via several mechanisms including hyperpolarization and inhibition of extracellular calcium mobilization, which are tightly regulated by hypoxia inducible factor (HIF).[37–39] In a study evaluating varicose veins in CVD patients, it was determined that HIF-1α and HIF-2α transcriptional factors were overexpressed compared with control nonvaricose veins, suggesting that the HIF pathway may be associated with several pathophysiologic changes in the venous wall leading to venous hypertension, and that hypoxia may be a feature contributing to the pathogenesis of varicose veins.[40]

MMPs have been found to be present in high quantities in VLU and in the wound fluid, and correlation of increased expression of proteinase activity is associated with poor healing. The regulation of MMP production and function, although not fully

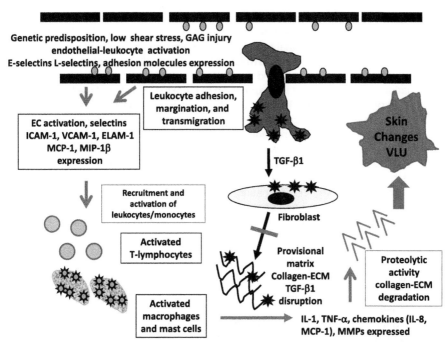

Fig. 2. Representation of the cellular events that lead to the inflammatory state in chronic venous disease, and resulting skin changes and venous leg ulcer formation. EC, endothelial cell; ECM, extracellular matrix; ELAM-1, endothelial leukocyte adhesion molecule-1; GAG, glycosaminoglycan; IL-1, interleukin-1; MCP-1, monocyte chemotactic protein-1; MIP-1β, macrophage inflammatory protein-1β; MP, macrophages; TNF-α, tumor necrosis factor-α.

understood, is likely linked to cytokines, uPA, EMMPRIN (extracellular MMP inducer CD147), PDGF-AA, and MAPK pathways.[41–52] Cytokines have important roles at different stages of CVD beginning with inflammation and expression in the interstitial space and in the venous ulcer wound bed.[11,33] In a nonrandomized trial evaluation of various cytokine levels and venous ulcer healing in patients undergoing compression therapy, a study determined that untreated ulcers typically display high levels of proinflammatory cytokines including several interleukins, tumor necrosis factor-α, and interferon-γ. After 4 weeks of compression therapy, the levels of proinflammatory cytokines decreased significantly and the wounds began to heal. After compression, levels of TGF-β1 increased significantly as the ulcers improved. When specific cytokine levels were related to the percentage of healing, those with higher levels of proinflammatory cytokines including interleukin-1 and interferon-γ healed significantly better than those with lower levels of these cytokines before compression.[53] The same authors evaluated in a similar fashion the MMP profile in 29 VLU. There was significant elevation in MMP-1, -2, -3, -8, -9, -12, and -13 (collagenases, stromelysins, gelatinases, metalloelastase) compared with healthy tissue. Following compression treatment there was significant reduction in MMP-3, -8, and -9; and reduction of MMP-1, -2, and -3 was associated with higher healing rates at 4 weeks.[54]

A recent study of patients with inflammatory and granulating VLU demonstrated that significant differences exist in the wound fluid collected with respect to cytokines, chemokines, granulocyte-monocyte colony–stimulating factor, and growth factors depending on the wound environment. The same authors also demonstrated that there were significant differences in MMPs and tissue inhibitor of metalloproteinase based again on the status of the VLU wound (inflammatory vs granulating).[55,56] These studies identify important differences that exist in healing versus nonhealing VLU wounds, provide important information of possible mechanisms of wound progression, and may offer biomarkers for targeted therapy and prognosis. As a result of venous hypertension, inflammation, remodeling, and the expression of cytokines and MMPs, a key feature is found in the postcapillary venule called the fibrin cuff, which consists of a complex process involving fibrin and collagen deposition. The result is a major abnormality in dermal microcirculation with many components forming the postcapillary cuff including collagen I and III, fibronectin, vitronectin, laminin, tenascin, fibrin, TGF-β1, and α2-macroglobulin.[11,57] In addition, macrophages and mast cells have been identified in the fibrin cuff, and their presence is a source of cytokines and MMPs, which are certainly involved in CVD, skin changes, and VLU formation.

Structural proteins have been analyzed in varicose veins from patients with CVD, and an important finding determined that overall collagen is increased, and elastin and laminin are decreased.[58] When the collagen was examined in the smooth muscle from varicose veins compared with control, the consistent finding was that there was a significant decrease of collagen type III and increased type I in varicose veins, and this finding was also observed in the dermal fibroblasts from patients with varicose vein.[58,59] These findings indicate a systemic condition with strong genetic influences, and because collagen I confers rigidity, whereas collagen III is involved in the extensibility of a tissue, modification of the collagen I/III ratio might contribute to the weakness and the decreased elasticity of varicose veins. The transcription of collagen III is normal in smooth muscle cells from varicose veins, and the activity of MMP-3 is increased leading to post-translational modification of collagen type III; these events are reversible when MMP-3 is inhibited in vitro.[60] MMPs are an important step in the development of primary venous disease; their implications are early events affecting endothelium-smooth muscle interactions and venodilation, and late with extracellular matrix degradation, structural vein wall changes and fibrosis, and tissue damage leading to venous ulceration.[9]

Venous microvalves have been identified in control specimens and in patients with CVD.[61] The interesting aspect of that study is a system of sequentially smaller generations of tributaries leading to a small venous network, with competent and incompetent microvalves. The regions are divided into six generations before reaching the small venous network. In regions where incompetence existed in microvalves out to the third-generation tributary (the boundary), resin applied in the microvasculature was able to penetrate deeper into the microvenous networks of the dermis. In limbs with varicose veins and venous ulcers, reflux into the small venous networks and capillary loops was more extensive with more dense networks and greater tortuosity. In addition to superficial axial saphenous vein insufficiency, microvalve insufficiency also exists, and once it compromises the third-generation set of microvalves, there is a greater risk for the development of dermal venous ulceration. These finding may help explain why some patients with long-standing varicose veins do not develop venous ulcers, because the microvalves may be intact at the third-generation network preventing clinical deterioration.[61] In addition, these findings may explain why skin changes consistent with venous disease (hyperpigmentation and even small skin ulceration) are seen clinically in patients with normal duplex ultrasound of the superficial, deep, and perforator venous systems. Further research on the factors responsible for initiating the altered shear stress and stretch on vein walls will make it possible to have specific pharmaceutical targets to restore the integrity of the microcirculation and treat the spectrum of CVD.

Other potential mechanisms for the development of venous insufficiency and CVD are hypoxia and apoptosis of the vein wall; however, studies evaluating these pathophysiologic alterations are more likely associations, with significant variability in results, and are inconclusive.[62,63]

Metabolic abnormalities may be critical to venous dysfunction and lead to pathology. Metabonomics is the study of metabolism in biologic systems in response to pathophysiologic stimuli and genetic modifications, and in patients with varicose veins there are significant differences in three important metabolic products involving creatine, lactate, and myoinositol metabolites that are increased and lower amounts of lipid metabolites when compared with nonvaricose control veins.[64] In an animal study of venous tissue, inferior vena cava that was stretched at high tension for 18 hours over nonstretched tissue was found to have significantly increased concentrations of valine and choline metabolites, and triglyceride moieties. The interpretation and importance to CVD of this study is that the branched chain amino acid valine and cell membrane constituent choline indicate increased muscle breakdown. The increased levels of triglyceride moieties in stretched vein segments suggest that high pressure may induce an inflammatory response. Both findings are consistent with pathology seen with varicose veins and CVD and provide insight into the mechanism and potential areas of therapy.

A recent comprehensive study assessing metabolites of varicose veins determined higher concentrations of glutamate, taurine, *myo*-inositol, creatine, and inosine were present in aqueous extracts and phosphatidylcholine, phosphatidylethanolamine, and sphingomyelin in lipid extracts in the varicose vein group compared with the control group. Pathway analysis revealed an association of phosphatidylcholine and sphingomyelin with inflammation and *myo*-inositol with cellular proliferation, providing insights into important cellular pathways that may be implicated in the pathophysiology of CVD.[65] Analyzing the cellular metabolism in varicose veins, with signature end products, reflect the metabolism of the tissue and holds key information to the disease processes. Further research in this exiting field is necessary to have a better understanding of the processes leading to CVD, and to determine if patients with VLU have certain characteristic metabolic profiles that will allow for improved targeted therapy in the prevention and active treatment of CVD and VLU.

Finally, another interesting area of research and applications to pathophysiology and therapy in CVD is in gap junctions. Gap junctions are proteins that have critical roles in the pathogenesis of chronic wounds, especially involved in inflammation, edema formation, and fibrosis. Connexins (eg, connexin43 is abnormally elevated in the wound margin of VLU) are the channel-forming components of gap junctions, and provide a channel between cells cytoplasm, allowing for small molecules to pass, and facilitating electrical propagation between excitable cells.[66] ACT1 is a peptide that inhibits connexin43, and in animal models accelerates fibroblast proliferation and epithelialization. In a study of VLU patients (46 in each group) randomized to ACT1 gel application with compression versus compression alone, VLU treated with ACT1 gel and compression had significantly greater mean percent re-epithelialization at 12 weeks, and a reduced median time to 100% ulcer healing.[66] Connexin seemed to have an important role in CVD especially in the inflammatory response and in VLU healing. Further studies in the different types of connexins and their relationship to the entire spectrum of CVD are important in understanding the pathophysiology of CVD and directed targeting of the connexin cellular pathway for treatment and possibly altering disease progression.

REFERENCES

1. Labropoulos N, Leon M, Nicolaides AN, et al. Superficial venous insufficiency: correlation of anatomic extent of reflux with clinical symptoms and signs. J Vasc Surg 1994;20:953–8.
2. Meissner MH, Moneta G, Burnand K, et al. The hemodynamics and diagnosis of venous disease. J Vasc Surg 2007;46(Suppl S):4S–24S.
3. Labropoulos N, Leon M, Nicolaides AN, et al. Venous reflux in patients with previous deep venous thrombosis: correlation with ulceration and other symptoms. J Vasc Surg 1994;20:20–6.
4. Labropoulos N, Gasparis AP, Tassiopoulos AK. Prospective evaluation of the clinical deterioration in post-thrombotic limbs. J Vasc Surg 2009;50:826–30.
5. Labropoulos N, Gasparis AP, Pefanis D, et al. Secondary chronic venous disease progresses faster than primary. J Vasc Surg 2009;49:704–10.
6. Eberhardt RT, Raffetto JD. Chronic venous insufficiency. Circulation 2014;130: 333–46.
7. Raffetto JD. Pathophysiology of wound healing and alterations in venous leg ulcers-review. Phlebology 2016;31(1 Suppl):56–62.
8. Chi YW, Raffetto JD. Venous leg ulceration pathophysiology and evidence based treatment. Vasc Med 2015;20:168–81.
9. Raffetto JD, Khalil RA. Mechanisms of varicose vein formation: valve dysfunction and wall dilation. Phlebology 2008;23:85–98.
10. Deroo S, Deatrick KB, Henke PK. The vessel wall: a forgotten player in post thrombotic syndrome. Thromb Haemost 2010;104:681–92.
11. Raffetto JD. Inflammation in chronic venous ulcers. Phlebology 2013;28(Suppl 1): 61–7.
12. Ono T, Bergan JJ, Schmid-Schönbein GW, et al. Monocyte infiltration into venous valves. J Vasc Surg 1998;27:158–66.
13. Raffetto JD, Mannello F. Pathophysiology of chronic venous disease. Int Angiol 2014;33:212–21.
14. Mannello F, Ligi D, Raffetto JD. Glycosaminoglycan sulodexide modulates inflammatory pathways in chronic venous disease. Int Angiol 2014;33:236–42.
15. Anwar MA, Georgiadis KA, Shalhoub J, et al. A review of familial, genetic, and congenital aspects of primary varicose vein disease. Circ Cardiovasc Genet 2012;5:460–6.
16. Cornu-Thenard A, Boivin P, Baud JM, et al. Importance of the familial factor in varicose disease. Clinical study of 134 families. J Dermatol Surg Oncol 1994; 20:318–26.
17. Fiebig A, Krusche P, Wolf A, et al. Heritability of chronic venous disease. Hum Genet 2010;127:669–74.
18. Ellinghaus E, Ellinghaus D, Krusche P, et al. Genome-wide association analysis for chronic venous disease identifies EFEMP1 and KCNH8 as susceptibility loci. Sci Rep 2017;7:45652.
19. Bharath V, Kahn SR, Lazo-Langner A. Genetic polymorphisms of vein wall remodeling in chronic venous disease: a narrative and systematic review. Blood 2014; 124:1242–50.
20. Zamboni P, Gemmati D. Clinical implications of gene polymorphisms in venous leg ulcer: a model in tissue injury and reparative process. Thromb Haemost 2007;98:131–7.
21. Zamboni P, Tognazzo S, Izzo M, et al. Hemochromatosis C282Y gene mutation increases the risk of venous leg ulceration. J Vasc Surg 2005;42:309–14.

22. Tognazzo S, Gemmati D, Pallazzo A, et al. Prognostic role of factor XIII gene variants in nonhealing venous leg ulcers. J Vasc Surg 2006;44:815–9.
23. Zamboni P, De Mattei M, Ongaro A, et al. Factor XIII contrasts the effects of metalloproteinases in human dermal fibroblast cultured cells. Vasc Endovascular Surg 2004;38:431–8.
24. Gemmati D, Tognazzo S, Catozzi L, et al. Influence of gene polymorphisms in ulcer healing process after superficial venous surgery. J Vasc Surg 2006;44: 554–62.
25. Schmid-Shonbein GW, Takase S, Bergan JJ. New advances in the understanding of the pathophysiology of chronic venous insufficiency. Angiology 2001;52(Suppl 1):S27–34.
26. Bergan JJ, Schmid-Shonbein GW, Coleridge Smith PD, et al. Chronic venous disease. N Engl J Med 2006;355:488–98.
27. Chen YS, Lu MJ, Huang HS, et al. Mechanosensitive transient receptor potential vanilloid type 1 channels contribute to vascular remodeling of rat fistula veins. J Vasc Surg 2010;52:1310–20.
28. Takase S, Pascarella L, Lerond L, et al. Venous hypertension, inflammation and valve remodeling. Eur J Vasc Endovasc Surg 2004;28:484–93.
29. Takase S, Bergan JJ, Schmid-Schönbein G. Expression of adhesion molecules and cytokines on saphenous veins in chronic venous insufficiency. Ann Vasc Surg 2000;14:427–35.
30. Castro-Ferreira R, Cardoso R, Leite-Moreira A, et al. The role of endothelial dysfunction and inflammation in chronic venous disease. Ann Vasc Surg 2017. [Epub ahead of print].
31. Mannello F, Raffetto JD. Matrix metalloproteinase activity and glycosaminoglycans in chronic venous disease: the linkage among cell biology, pathology and translational research. Am J Transl Res 2011;3:149–58.
32. Mannello F, Medda V, Ligi D, et al. Glycosaminoglycan sulodexide inhibition of mmp-9 gelatinase secretion and activity: possible pharmacological role against collagen degradation in vascular chronic diseases. Curr Vasc Pharmacol 2013; 11:354–65.
33. Mannello F, Ligi D, Canale M, et al. Omics profiles in chronic venous ulcer wound fluid: innovative applications for translational medicine. Expert Rev Mol Diagn 2014;14:737–62.
34. Serra R, Grande R, Butrico L, et al. Effects of a new nutraceutical substance on clinical and molecular parameters in patients with chronic venous ulceration. Int Wound J 2016;13:88–96.
35. Chen Y, Peng W, Raffetto JD, et al. Matrix metalloproteinases in remodeling of lower extremity veins and chronic venous disease. Prog Mol Biol Transl Sci 2017;147:267–99.
36. Raffetto JD, Qiao X, Koledova VV, et al. Prolonged increases in vein wall tension increase matrix metalloproteinases and decrease constriction in rat vena cava: potential implications in varicose veins. J Vasc Surg 2008;48:447–56.
37. Raffetto JD, Ross RL, Khalil RA. Matrix metalloproteinase 2-induced venous dilation via hyperpolarization and activation of K+ channels: relevance to varicose vein formation. J Vasc Surg 2007;45:373–80.
38. Raffetto JD, Barros YV, Wells AK, et al. MMP-2 induced vein relaxation via inhibition of [Ca2+]e-dependent mechanisms of venous smooth muscle contraction. Role of RGD peptides. J Surg Res 2010;159:755–64.

39. Lim CS, Qiao X, Reslan OM, et al. Prolonged mechanical stretch is associated with upregulation of hypoxia-inducible factors and reduced contraction in rat inferior vena cava. J Vasc Surg 2011;53:764–73.
40. Lim CS, Kiriakidis S, Paleolog EM, et al. Increased activation of the hypoxia-inducible factor pathway in varicose veins. J Vasc Surg 2012;55:1427–39.
41. Trengove NJ, Bielefeldt-Ohmann H, Stacey MC. Mitogenic activity and cytokine levels in non-healing and healing chronic leg ulcers. Wound Repair Regen 2000;8:13–25.
42. Tian YW, Stacey MC. Cytokines and growth factors in keratinocytes and sweat glands in chronic venous leg ulcers. An immunohistochemical study. Wound Repair Regen 2003;11:316–25.
43. Gohel MS, Windhaber RA, Tarlton JF, et al. The relationship between cytokine concentrations and wound healing in chronic venous ulceration. J Vasc Surg 2008;48:1272–7.
44. Wysocki AB, Staiano-Coico L, Grinnell F. Wound fluid from chronic leg ulcers contains elevated levels of metalloproteinases MMP-2 and MMP-9. J Invest Dermatol 1993;101:64–8.
45. Weckroth M, Vaheri A, Lauharanta J, et al. Matrix metalloproteinases, gelatinase and collagenase in chronic leg ulcers. J Invest Dermatol 1996;106:1119–24.
46. Herouy Y, May AE, Pornschlegel G, et al. Lipodermatosclerosis is characterized by elevated expression and activation of matrix metalloproteinases: implications for venous ulcer formation. J Invest Dermatol 1998;111:822–7.
47. Herouy Y, Trefzer D, Hellstern MO, et al. Plasminogen activation in venous leg ulcers. Br J Dermatol 2000;143:930–6.
48. Norgauer J, Hildenbrand T, Idzko M, et al. Elevated expression of extracellular matrix metalloproteinase inducer (CD147) and membrane-type matrix metalloproteinases in venous leg ulcers. Br J Dermatol 2002;147:1180–6.
49. Mwaura B, Mahendran B, Hynes N, et al. The impact of differential expression of extracellular matrix metalloproteinase inducer, matrix metalloproteinase-2, tissue inhibitor of matrix metalloproteinase-2 and PDGF-AA on the chronicity of venous leg ulcers. Eur J Vasc Endovasc Surg 2006;31:306–10.
50. Meyer FJ, Burnand KG, Abisi S, et al. Effect of collagen turnover and matrix metalloproteinase activity on healing of venous leg ulcers. Br J Surg 2008;95:319–25.
51. Raffetto JD, Vasquez R, Goodwin DG, et al. Mitogen-activated protein kinase pathway regulates cell proliferation in venous ulcer fibroblasts. Vasc Endovascular Surg 2006;40:59–66.
52. Raffetto JD, Gram CH, Overman KC, et al. Mitogen-activated protein kinase p38 pathway in venous ulcer fibroblasts. Vasc Endovascular Surg 2008;42:367–74.
53. Beidler SK, Douillet CD, Berndt DF, et al. Inflammatory cytokine levels in chronic venous insufficiency ulcer tissue before and after compression therapy. J Vasc Surg 2009;49:1013–20.
54. Beidler SK, Douillet CD, Berndt DF, et al. Multiplexed analysis of matrix metalloproteinases in leg ulcer tissue of patients with chronic venous insufficiency before and after compression therapy. Wound Repair Regen 2008;16:642–8.
55. Ligi D, Mosti G, Croce L, et al. Chronic venous disease - Part I: inflammatory biomarkers in wound healing. Biochim Biophys Acta 2016;1862:1964–74.
56. Ligi D, Mosti G, Croce L, et al. Chronic venous disease - Part II: proteolytic biomarkers in wound healing. Biochim Biophys Acta 2016;1862:1900–8.
57. Pappas PJ, DeFouw DO, Venezio LM, et al. Morphometric assessment of the dermal microcirculation in patients with chronic venous insufficiency. J Vasc Surg 1997;26:784–95.

58. Sansilvestri-Morel P, Rupin A, Badier-Commander C, et al. Imbalance in the syn-
    thesis of collagen type I and collagen type III in smooth muscle cells derived from
    human varicose veins. J Vasc Res 2001;38:560–8.
59. Sansilvestri-Morel P, Rupin A, Jaisson S, et al. Synthesis of collagen is dysregu-
    lated in cultured fibroblasts derived from skin of subjects with varicose veins as it
    is in venous smooth muscle cells. Circulation 2002;106:479–83.
60. Sansilvestri-Morel P, Rupin A, Jullien ND, et al. Decreased production of collagen
    type III in cultured smooth muscle cells from varicose vein patients is due to a
    degradation by MMPs: possible implication of MMP-3. J Vasc Res 2005;42:
    388–98.
61. Vincent JR, Jones GT, Hill GB, et al. Failure of microvenous valves in small super-
    ficial veins is a key to the skin changes of venous insufficiency. J Vasc Surg 2011;
    54(6 Suppl):62S–9S.
62. Lim CS, Davies AH. Pathogenesis of primary varicose veins. Br J Surg 2009;96:
    1231–42.
63. Lim CS, Gohel MS, Shepherd AC, et al. Venous hypoxia: a poorly studied etiolog-
    ical factor of varicose veins. J Vasc Res 2011;48:185–94.
64. Anwar MA, Shalhoub J, Vorkas PA, et al. In-vitro identification of distinctive meta-
    bolic signatures of intact varicose vein tissue via magic angle spinning nuclear
    magnetic resonance spectroscopy. Eur J Vasc Endovasc Surg 2012;44:442–50.
65. Anwar MA, Adesina-Georgiadis KN, Spagou K, et al. A comprehensive charac-
    terisation of the metabolic profile of varicose veins; implications in elaborating
    plausible cellular pathways for disease pathogenesis. Sci Rep 2017;7:2989.
66. Ghatnekar GS, Grek CL, Armstrong DG, et al. The effect of a connexin43-based
    Peptide on the healing of chronic venous leg ulcers: a multicenter, randomized
    trial. J Invest Dermatol 2015;135:289–98.

Optimal Compression Therapy and Wound Care for Venous Ulcers

Fedor Lurie, PhD, MD[a,b,*], Samir Bittar, MD[a], Gregory Kasper, MD[a]

KEYWORDS

- Compression therapy • Venous ulcers • Wound care

KEY POINTS

- Compression therapy is an essential component of care for patients with venous leg ulcers.
- Achieving and maintaining the appropriate level of interface pressure is the goal of compression therapy. The type of device used to achieve this goal depends on the specific patient's condition and circumstances. Whenever possible, multicomponent compression bandages should be used as the first choice.
- Coexisting peripheral arterial disease is not a contraindication to compression therapy, unless the ankle-brachial index is 0.5 or less or absolute ankle pressure is less than 60 mm Hg.
- Sufficient wound bed preparation, wound infection and bacterial control, and maintenance of moist conditions for each stage of the wound-healing process are key aspects of appropriate wound care.

INTRODUCTION

Chronic ulceration of the lower legs is a relatively common condition affecting 1% of the adult population, 3.6% of people older than 65, and more than 5% for those older than 80. It is defined as a defect in the skin below the knee that persists for more than 6 weeks, showing no tendency to heal after 3 or more months. The common causes are venous disease, arterial disease, and neuropathy.[1-4] Leg ulcers greatly reduce patients' quality of life, are a common cause of morbidity,[5] and carry a wound-related mortality rate of 2.5%.[4-6] Every year, 2 to 3 million more Americans are diagnosed with various types of chronic wounds.[7] Estimates of the annual incidence of leg

Disclosures: The authors do not have any financial disclosures.
Development of this article was funded in part by the Conrad and Caroline Jobst Foundation.
[a] ProMedica Jobst Vascular Institute, 2109 Hughes Drive, Toledo, OH 43606, USA; [b] University of Michigan, Ann Arbor, MI, USA
* Corresponding author. ProMedica Jobst Vascular Institute, 2109 Hughes Drive, Toledo, OH 43606.
E-mail address: Fedor.Lurie@ProMedica.org

ulceration in the United Kingdom and Switzerland are 3.5 and 0.2 per 1000 individuals, respectively. The prevalence of vascular-related ulcers in the United States is estimated at 500,000 to 600,000 and increases with age.[8,9]

Venous disease accounted for 81% and arterial disease for 16.3% of ulcers. Leg ulcers are an important source of morbidity in the aging population.[10] The cost of treating a venous leg ulcer (VLU) has been estimated at $15,732 per year, or $86 per day of treatment to heal an ulcer.[10–13] Because of their high prevalence, VLUs represents an economic burden on the health care system that ranges from $1.5 billion to $3 billion annually.[14,15]

Studies report that the average VLU could require as long as 6 to 12 months to heal completely and as many as 70% will recur within 5 years of closure.[12] These ulcers cause a loss of an estimated 2 million workdays due to disability. The cost for treating patients with chronic VLUs per year in the United States is estimated to exceed $3 billion per year.[13] The primary goal after an ulcer has healed should be avoidance of recurrence. Patients with chronic venous disease are prone to develop new sites of involvement over time. The ongoing venous dysfunction tends to become more destructive to the lower leg tissues as aging occurs. Progression from asymptomatic varicose veins to severe lipodermatosclerosis is estimated to occur in about 20% of cases. The aim of treatment in all patients should focus on preventing the progression of venous hypertension, which leads to lower leg tissue scarring with advanced skin and ulcer effects.

GENERAL PRINCIPLES OF COMPRESSION THERAPY

Compression therapy, one of the oldest treatment modalities, enjoys a consensus-based justification for use, with limited evidence support and even more limited scientific basis. Attempts have only recently been made to introduce quantitative parameters of compression and to develop standards for compression devices. The "dose" of compression refers to the amount of pressure that a compression device applies to the skin (interface pressure). Only graduated compression stockings are currently standardized using the interface pressure. Although these standards differ between countries, the differences are sufficiently small, allowing uniform clinical use and research studies.

To develop the standard for compression stockings, a consensus was reached to use a specific point for interface pressure measurement. The B1 point is located about 8 cm above the ankle, where the tendinous part changes into the gastrocnemius muscle. All graduated compression stockings are labeled with reference to the pressure measured ex vivo at the B1 point. This pressure is not always the same when compression stockings are used by the patients,[16,17] and what pressure is applied to the remaining surface of the leg outside the B1 point is unknown. Such points include the area of ulceration. Even when the ulcer is located at the B1 point, the actual pressure applied to the surface of the ulcer may differ significantly from the label on the stockings.

Defining the dose of compression for bandages is even more challenging. For most of the bandages and bandage systems, the only way to know what pressure is applied to the limb is to measure it. Several devices for measuring interface pressure exist, but are rarely used in clinical settings. Several bandages have printed marks that allow for the control of the degree of stretch during application, providing an estimate of the pressure applied to the limb.

The second quantitative parameter relates to the mechanical properties of the bandage or stocking material. The bandages are usually applied with a patient in the supine position; when a patient stands up, the pressure increases. The difference between the value of interface pressure in standing and supine positions is the static stiffness index. During walking, the interface pressure changes with each step, and the difference between the maximal pressure while walking (working pressure) and the pressure when a patient is standing (resting pressure) is the dynamic stiffness index. Although stiffness indexes are rarely mentioned in the literature and not used in clinical practice, they quantify the difference between different types of bandages, such as inelastic, short stretch, and long stretch bandages, terms that are important and commonly used in practice.

The interface pressure does not remain the same during the time of wear for any compression device. Changes in the leg volume, especially when edema is present, and the stretch of the bandage over time lead to a decrease in interface pressure, slippage, and change in the pressure profile. Depending on the type of the compression device, the reapplication or a change to a new bandage needs to be done with a sufficient frequency to maintain desirable range of the interface pressure.

It is a general consensus that the interface pressure should be distributed in a graduated fashion decreasing from ankle to more proximal limb. Medical compression stockings are designed to provide graduated pressure, although the specific pressure profile is different for each of the stocking models and for each individual limb. Compression bandages should be applied with the same tension along the entire limb. Because the limb circumference increases from ankle to calf, the resulting interface pressure will decrease in the proximal direction following Laplace's law, which states that the pressure is proportional to the radius of the cylinder.

Compression Devices

A large number of devices that can be used for compression therapy for VLUs can be broadly divided into 3 groups: static compression, dynamic compression, and sustained compression.

Static compression devices are applied to the limb with an initial pressure that is usually assumed to remain constant during use, because they do not change their initial tension over time. This assumption is obviously false, and most of these devices decrease interface pressure during the time of use. Potentially more dangerous is the increase in interface pressure during times of increased swelling of the limb, which in some cases leads to pressure damage of the skin and soft tissues.

Dynamic compression is provided by pneumatic compression devices. These devices are not designed specifically for VLUs and vary significantly in delivered interface pressure, time of compression cycle, and the distribution of pressure over the limb. Although dynamic compression is effective in edema reduction, which may facilitate healing, the evidence of its benefit for VLUs is inconsistent and inconclusive. This type of compression therapy is generally recommended for patients who cannot use any other type of compression devices.[14]

The sustained compression device is a new class, with only one device currently commercially available. It is also a pneumatic compression device; however, it has a built-in pressure sensor that automatically adjusts the pressure in the garment, maintaining a constant pressure level during the time of wear. The sustained compression device shows good patient acceptance and compliance, but its clinical effectiveness for VLU patients remains to be studied.[18]

Static compression is the most widely used and the most diverse class of compression device. It includes different types of bandages, bandage systems, adjustable Velcro devices, and ready-to-use and custom-made stockings. The mechanical behavior of these devices is mainly determined by their elastic properties.

The most commonly used example of inelastic material is the Unna boot, or any bandage with zinc paste. After zinc paste dries, the bandage becomes rigid and keeps its size and shape unchanged, so the interface pressure is determined by the degree of swelling and the changes in muscle volume during walking. The pressure produced by an inelastic bandage can be high enough to affect arterial flow, especially during walking. This significantly limits the use of such bandages in patients with mixed arterial and venous ulcers and in diabetic patients.

Inelastic materials are also used in Velcro devices. The major difference is that these devices allow for tension adjustment and therefore provide an easy way to maintain a desirable level of the interface pressure during the time of wear to compensate for variable edema.

Short stretch bandages have very low elasticity. They can be extended to less than 100% (usually <70%) of their initial length. The difference in the interface pressure under short stretch bandages between standing and supine positions (static stiffness index) exceeds 10 mm Hg. They are similar in their usage, advantages, and limitations to inelastic bandages. Application of a short stretch bandage requires a substantial level of skill and should be done by trained medical staff. Both inelastic and short stretch bandages start losing pressure immediately after application, as much as 25% within the first hour. Although this is due to their therapeutic effect of decreasing limb edema, it makes dosing the pressure difficult.

Long stretched materials accommodate the shape of the leg and, because of their elastic recoil, sustain desirable pressures during ambulation and at rest. Because the interface pressure is generated by the stretch of an elastic textile, the working pressure is almost the same as the resting pressure, and the static and dynamic stiffness indices have very low values, usually in the 3-mm Hg to 5-mm Hg range. Application of long stretch bandages is easier compared with short stretch materials and can be done by minimally trained personnel or self-applied by patients. Any bandage, including elastic, should be applied with at least 50% overlap, which means that even a single bandage when applied correctly has 2 layers. The friction between the layers decreases their tendency to slip down and also makes the bandage behave as less stretchable material.

Elastic textile is also used in compression stockings, and its behavior is similar to a long stretch bandage. Most stockings that are used for patients with VLUs are 2-component systems of a liner with absorbing properties and the compression stockings themselves. Similar to multicomponent bandage systems, the friction between the 2 layers decreases the elasticity of the stockings, making them behave as an intermediate or even short stretch bandage when applied to a limb.

The main advantage of stockings compared with bandages is that their pressure does not depend on the expertise of the medical personnel; moreover, they can easily be removed by the patient when needed. However, the latter is also a disadvantage because it gives patients control over usage, which can result in noncompliance. Without additional educational efforts, compliance with compression stockings is as low as 40%.[19] Reasons for noncompliance are the absence of perceived benefits, unpleasant sensation caused by stockings (heat, itching, numbness, or discomfort), poor cosmetic appearance, and difficulties in donning and doffing. When patients are educated regarding the benefits of compression, and are provided with a choice of stockings (material, color, and so forth), compliance improves. In a clinical trial setting, 70% of previously noncompliant patients became compliant with compression stockings.[4]

Multicomponent bandage systems use a combination of materials with different elastic properties. This makes the application process less operator dependent compared with short stretch bandages, decreases the slippage of the bandage, and makes the interface pressure more stable. These systems, though, are more expensive and require a certain level of expertise for appropriate application.

Mechanism of Action and Clinical Effects

The precise mechanisms of action for compression therapy remain to be defined. Some information is available regarding physiologic effects observed during application of compression devices. These effects include reduction in venous volume,[20] improvement of muscle pump function and venous blood flow,[21] and shift of blood volume from superficial into deep veins.[22] Some changes in biomarkers have been documented mainly for intermittent pneumatic compression.[23]

Compression alone can heal about 60% of VLUs within 24 weeks.[24] The remaining 40%, however, may not heal despite adequate compression and wound care. Identifying these refractory ulcers early allows the care provider to better differentiate between venous and mixed cause ulcers, use advanced wound care options, or treat underlying venous abnormality more aggressively. Clinical predictors of delayed ulcer healing include history of previous ulceration in the same extremity, large ulcer area, decreased ankle mobility, and obesity.[25–29] A slow initial healing rate with less than 25% of area reduction during the first 2 weeks also suggests delayed healing.[30]

Clinical evidence is consistent and convincing that compression therapy increases ulcer healing rates, time to healing, and the percent of ulcers healed. This evidence includes several randomized trials and systematic reviews and serves as the basis for the only grade 1 level of evidence, a recommendation in the most comprehensive clinical practice guidelines for management of VLUs.[14] The following 5 guidelines related to compression are the most current:

1. In a patient with a VLU, the authors recommend compression therapy over no compression therapy to increase VLU healing rate (Grade 1; Level of evidence A).
2. In a patient with a healed VLU, the authors suggest compression therapy to decrease the risk of ulcer recurrence (Grade 2; Level of evidence B).
3. The authors suggest the use of multicomponent compression bandage over single-component bandages for the treatment of VLUs (Grade 2; Level of evidence B).
4. In a patient with a VLU and underlying arterial disease, the authors do not suggest compression bandages or stockings if the ankle-brachial index is 0.5 or less or if absolute ankle pressure is less than 60 mm Hg (Grade 2; Level of evidence C).
5. The authors suggest use of intermittent pneumatic compression when other compression options are not available, cannot be used, or have failed to aid in VLU healing after prolonged compression therapy (Grade 2; Level of evidence C).

It is important to mention that although multiple consensus documents exist justifying different compression pressures as an optimal treatment of different venous and lymphatic disorders, including VLUs, no scientific evidence supporting levels of compression is currently available.[31]

OPTIMAL WOUND CARE
Wound Bed Preparation

Debridement, the removal of nonvital tissue, foreign material, abnormal and dysfunctional cells, and bacteria and their byproducts, including biofilms debris on the wound surface, is vital to successful wound care based on the available evidence.[32,33] One study documented faster healing of a variety of chronic wounds with weekly debridement compared with every 2 weeks.[33]

Necrotic tissue is not usually found in VLUs unless they are complicated by arterial disease or infection. Debridement of necrotic tissue in chronic wounds can be achieved using several methods: surgical removal of slough or sharp debridement to bleeding tissue; autolytic dressings, including calcium alginates, hydrogels, hydrocolloids, or biologics (eg, maggots); and enzymatic methods (eg, collagenase).[34]

Methods of debridement may be used as a single therapeutic modality or may be combined to optimize the debridement process. Selecting the optimal combination of debridement techniques will depend on the patient's individual needs and the available clinical resources.[33]

Low-frequency ultrasound (20–60 kHz) debridement is a promising technology that functions to disperse bacterial biofilms and stimulates wound healing. Ultrasound debridement appears to be most effective when used 3 times a week and has the potential to decrease exudate and slough, decrease patient pain, disperse biofilms, and increase healing in wounds of various causes.[35]

The MIST therapy in conjunction with standardized care was also reported to decrease exudate and fibrin slough.[36,37] Another study noted significant decrease in erythematous and edematous skin, undermining, tunneling, and odor and a decrease in clinical evidence of infection.[38]

Cleansing is also a vital component of wound management. At this time, there is limited research to inform the development of protocols.[39] Research has primarily focused on types of dressings with little attention given to the solutions needed for cleansing purposes. Various solutions have been applied for their supposed therapeutic value; however, in practice, the decisions have been based on experience, service policy, and personal preference.

The use of antiseptic solutions may compromise the healing process,[40,41] and, as a result, the use of normal saline as a cleansing solution is widely recommended.[40,42,43] However, there is no agreement among wound care authorities on the advantages of using sterile solutions over nonsterile solutions. Tap water has been recommended as an effective solution for wound cleansing and has the advantages of being cost-effective and easily accessible.[44,45]

Generally, antiseptics are used when the clinician perceives the need to reduce the level of bioburden as the number one priority or visualizes signs of infection.[46] Cytotoxic effects can be seen with many approved topicals, including silver, but detrimental effects are generally a result of exposure time and overall concentration.

Wound Progress

It is generally accepted that a reasonable goal is healing by 12 weeks. Healing by 12 weeks can often be achieved with diabetic ulcers. Venous ulcers can take longer; if they demonstrate less than 40% healing after 4 weeks of good therapy, they are unlikely to heal at 24 weeks, the anticipated time for healing of most VLUs.[47] Healing rates at 4 weeks predict overall healing rates, and a 10% to 15% area reduction weekly suggests an excellent prognosis.[47–49]

In the case of venous ulcers, healing rates of less than 40% after 1 month of "good" wound care should serve as a clue for the practitioner to at least consider some of the technical advances available.[49,50]

Wound Infection and Bacterial Control

Infection in chronic wounds continues to be a challenging problem, representing a considerable health care burden and leading to delays in wound healing. Wounds will be stuck in either the inflammatory or proliferative phases of healing. Antimicrobial therapy, in conjunction with debridement, is crucial for wound healing.

It is well known that control of bioburden is an important aspect of wound management.[51] Chronic wounds can become colonized with bacteria and/or fungi. However, when the microorganisms become invasive, critical colonization can result and, if left untreated, wound infection may develop. Several mnemonics are helpful in differentiating critical colonization and infection by way of wound characteristics. They can assist in the decision on whether to use topical or systemic antimicrobials. NERDS (Nonhealing, Exudate, Red friable tissue, Debris, and Smell) would suggest the wound has reached a critical colonization point and initiating antimicrobial treatment with topical agents along with debridement would be appropriate. On the other hand, STONES (Size enlargement, Temperature increase, Os/bone exposed, New breakdown, Exudate, Erythema, Edema, and Smell) suggests infection and requires systemic antimicrobial treatment.[52–54] Wound sepsis has been associated with deep tissue quantitative microbial counts of greater than 100,000 colony-forming units per gram of tissue.

In practice, quantitative wound biopsies are not routinely performed because semiquantitative surface wound swabs tend to correlate well with deep tissue quantitative counts using the Levine technique.[55] The Levine technique involves rotating the swab over a small area (1 cm^2) of the wound to extract fluid, ensuring that no contact is made with the wound edges. Topical antibacterial therapy such as silver dressings, honey, mupirocin, and iodine compounds can be used to treat colonized wounds, but systemic antibiotics are usually also necessary if the wound is infected.[52–54]

Microbes often reside in a biofilm community firmly attached to the wound and protected by an extracellular polymeric substance (EPS).[56,57] All chronic wound infections share these characteristics, and it has been suggested that biofilms play a role in the prevention of wound healing.[55] The EPS provides capsulelike protection for the community of microorganisms, thus conferring resistance to antimicrobials and host-immune responses. Chronic wounds tend to have more anaerobes than acute wounds, and these may not be identified on routine swabs unless specific culture techniques are used. The importance of adequate and repetitive debridement of necrotic tissue in chronic wounds cannot be overemphasized. This material provides an efficient growth medium for microorganisms and contributes to the development and maintenance of the biofilm. Continuous and aggressive maintenance debridement reduces the necrotic burden, microbial bioburden, excessive exudate, and biofilm.[58] Antimicrobial resistance has become a problem, not only in the hospital setting but also in the community, because of the overuse and misuse of community-provided antimicrobials.[59] Judicious antimicrobial use is critical, and all open wounds do not require antimicrobials unless they are infected.

The treatment of chronic wounds and acute or chronic infections can be challenging. Consider the possibility of anaerobic and fungal organisms when culturing; use systemic antibiotics judiciously to reduce microbial resistance and perform maintenance debridement to control necrosis and biofilm.

Leg cellulitis can often complicate VLUs and present with increasing swelling, erythema, and pain. Differential diagnosis should include venous stasis dermatitis, which often occurs in the setting of venous hypertension/insufficiency of the lower extremity. It will require topical or systemic steroid therapy instead of antimicrobial therapy (**Fig. 1**).

Primary Wound Dressings

A moist wound environment is essential to all phases of wound healing. It accelerates the reepithelialization process and collagen synthesis. It also facilitates the action of growth factors and keratinocyte and fibroblast proliferation and promotes

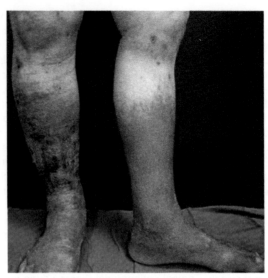

Fig. 1. Leg cellulitis (inflammation and infection of the skin and subcutaneous tissue most commonly due to streptococci or staphylococci) surrounding the venous ulcer should be treated with systemic gram-positive bactericidal antibiotics. (*Data from* Madaras-Kelly KJ, Remington RE, Oliphant CM, et al. Efficacy of oral beta-lactam versus non-beta-lactam treatment of uncomplicated cellulitis. Am J Med 2008;121:419–25.)

angiogenesis. Venous ulcers are typically heavily exudative, and the exudate contains inflammatory proteases and cytokines capable of attacking surrounding healthy skin if the exudate is not removed efficiently from the wound surface.

In VLUs, the management consideration typically is not how to maintain a moist wound environment but how to avoid an overly wet wound environment in the presence of toxic mediators. The frequency of dressing changes should be chosen based on the absorptive capacity of the dressing applied. Once a dressing becomes saturated, it should be replaced.

Many dressings have been developed to maintain moisture balance. The major categories of moisture-retentive dressings include foams, alginates, hydrofibers, hydrogels, and hydrocolloids.[49,60,61] Dressing selection is based on the wound characteristics, control of seeping, odor, and protection of periwound skin.

Antimicrobial dressings contain agents such as silver, iodine, and polyhexamethylene biguanide (PHMB). They can be used to combat bioburden and superficial infection. Silver dressings are effective against a broad spectrum of pathogens, including bacteria and fungi. PHMB is neither a primary skin irritant nor a hypersensitizing agent, which makes it well suited to chronic wound care.

Patients with VLUs often have lipodermatosclerosis, atrophie blanche, hyperpigmentation, dry, scaling, and atrophic skin, and venous stasis dermatitis. This results in vulnerable periwound skin that is thin and easily damaged by adhesives, for example. The skin condition can be further complicated by allergic or irritant reactions.

Raised intracapillary pressure as a result of damage to the venous system leads to edema, which may cause maceration. The skin directly below the wound is at greatest risk of maceration owing to the gravitational effect of wound drainage.

Stasis dermatitis, edema, and swelling are often improved with compression therapy, pneumatic pumps, and lower extremity elevation. Stasis dermatitis may occasionally require topical or systemic steroid therapy. Adequate hydration of a peri-wound dry skin is crucial to prevent potential VLUs, promote healthy epithelium, and facilitate wound healing.

FUTURE DIRECTIONS

Venous ulcers continue to be an important public health problem with a high economic burden. Two fundamental challenges are hampering the progress in addressing this issue: (1) the significant gaps in knowledge related to venous disease and to wound healing, and (2) the absence of effective prevention of VLUs. The current variability in all aspects of care for VLU patients, including the diagnosis, key therapeutic options, and outcome measures, is beyond reasonable. Standardization should be the first step leading to generation of reliable clinical data. Identification and early treatment of patients with high risk of ulceration should also become a priority. Even a moderate decrease in incidence of VLUs resulting from earlier treatment of underlying venous disease will have a significant public health and economic impact.

REFERENCES

1. Chatterjee SS. Venous ulcers of the lower limb: where do we stand? Indian J Plast Surg 2012;45:266–74.
2. Pannier F, Rabe E. Differential diagnosis of leg ulcers. Phlebology 2013;28(Suppl 1): 55–60.
3. Rayner R, Carville K, Keaton J, et al. Leg ulcers: atypical presentations and associated co-morbidities. Wound Pract Res 2009;17:168–85.
4. Rahman GA, Adigun IA, Fadeyi A. Epidemiology, etiology, and treatment of chronic leg ulcer: experience with sixty patients. Ann Afr Med 2010;9:1–4.
5. O'Brien JF, Grace PA, Perry IJ, et al. Prevalence and aetiology of leg ulcers in Ireland. Ir J Med Sci 2000;169:110–2.
6. Mekkes JR, Loots MAM, Van Der Wal AC, et al. Causes, investigation and treatment of leg ulceration. Br J Dermatol 2003;148:388–401.
7. Faria E, Blanes L, Hochman B, et al. Health-related quality of life, self-esteem, and functional status of patients with leg ulcer. Wounds 2011;23:4–10.
8. Sen CK, Gordillo GM, Roy S, et al. Human skin wounds: a major and snowballing threat to public health and the economy. Wound Repair Regen 2009;17:763–71.
9. Baker SR, Stacey MC. Epidemiology of chronic leg ulcers in Australia. Aust N Z J Surg 1994;64:258–61.
10. Ma H, Rosen NA, Iafrati MD, et al. The real costs of treating venous ulcers in a contemporary vascular practice. J Vasc Surg Venous Lymphat Disord 2013; 1(1):105.
11. O'Donnell TF Jr, Browse NL, Burnand KG, et al. The socioeconomic effects of an iliofemoral venous thrombosis. J Surg Res 1977;22:483–8.
12. Ruckley CV. Socioeconomic impact of chronic venous insufficiency and leg ulcers. Angiology 1997;48:67–9.
13. Van den Oever R, Hepp B, Debbaut B, et al. Socio-economic impact of chronic venous insufficiency. An underestimated public health problem. Int Angiol 1998; 17:161–7.
14. O'Donnell TF Jr, Passman MA, Marston WA, et al. Management of venous leg ulcers: clinical practice guidelines of the Society for Vascular Surgery ® and the American Venous Forum. J Vasc Surg 2014;60:3S–59S.
15. Browse NL, Burnand KG. The cause of venous ulceration. Lancet 1982;2:243–5.

16. Lurie F, Kistner R. Variability of interface pressure produced by ready-to-wear compression stockings. Phlebology 2014;29:105–8.

17. Ma H, Blebea J, Malgor RD, et al. Variability in leg compression provided by gradient commercial stockings. J Vasc Surg Venous Lymphat Disord 2015;3: 431–7.

18. Lurie F, Schwartz M. Patient-centered outcomes of a dual action pneumatic compression device in comparison to compression stockings for patients with chronic venous disease. J Vasc Surg Venous Lymphat Disord 2017 Sep;5(5): 699–706.

19. Raju S, Hollis K, Neglen P. Use of compression stockings in chronic venous disease: patient compliance and efficacy. Ann Vasc Surg 2007;21:790–5.

20. Partsch B, Partsch H. Calf compression pressure required to achieve venous closure from supine to standing positions. J Vasc Surg 2005;42:734–8.

21. Riebe H, Konschake W, Haase H, et al. Interface pressure and venous drainage of two compression stocking types in healthy volunteers and in patients with hemodynamic disturbances of the legs. Clin Hemorheol Microcirc 2015;61:175–83.

22. Lurie F, Scott V, Yoon HC, et al. On the mechanism of action of pneumatic compression devices: combined magnetic resonance imaging and duplex ultrasound investigation. J Vasc Surg 2008;48:1000–6.

23. Comerota AJ, Chouhan V, Harada RN, et al. The fibrinolytic effects of intermittent pneumatic compression: mechanism of enhanced fibrinolysis. Ann Surg 1997; 226(3):306–13.

24. Margolis DJ, Berlin JA, Strom BL. Which venous leg ulcers will heal with limb compression bandages? Am J Med 2000;109:15–9.

25. Abbade LPF, Lastória S, Rollo Hde A. Venous ulcer: clinical characteristics and risk factors. Int J Dermatol 2011;50:405–11.

26. Gohel MS, Taylor M, Earnshaw JJ, et al. Risk factors for delayed healing and recurrence of chronic venous leg ulcers–an analysis of 1324 legs. Eur J Vasc Endovasc Surg 2005;29:74–7.

27. Guest M, Smith JJ, Sira MS, et al. Venous ulcer healing by four-layer compression bandaging is not influenced by the pattern of venous incompetence. Br J Surg 1999;86:1437–40.

28. Milic DJ, Zivic SS, Bogdanovic DC, et al. Risk factors related to the failure of venous leg ulcers to heal with compression treatment. J Vasc Surg 2009;49: 1242–7.

29. Phillips TJ, Machado F, Trout R, et al. Prognostic indicators in venous ulcers. J Am Acad Dermatol 2000;43:627–30.

30. Parker CN, Finlayson KJ, Edwards HE. Ulcer area reduction at 2 weeks predicts failure to heal by 24 weeks in the venous leg ulcers of patients living alone. J Wound Care 2016;25:626–34.

31. O'Meara S, Cullum N, Nelson EA, et al. Compression for venous leg ulcers. Cochrane Database Syst Rev 2012;(11):CD001177.

32. Lebrun E, Kirsner RS. Frequent debridement for healing of chronic wounds. JAMA Dermatol 2013;149:1059.

33. Wilcox JR, Carter MJ, Covington S. Frequency of debridements and time to heal: a retrospective cohort study of 312 744 wounds. JAMA Dermatol 2013;149: 1050–8.

34. Sibbald RG, Goodman L, Woo KY, et al. Special considerations in wound bed preparation 2011: an update©. Adv Skin Wound Care 2011;24(9):415–36.

35. Maher SF, Halverson J, Misiewicz R, et al. Low-frequency ultrasound for patients with lower leg ulcers due to chronic venous insufficiency: a report of two cases. Ostomy Wound Manage 2014;60:52–61.
36. Bell AL, Cavorsi J. Noncontact ultrasound therapy for adjunctive treatment of nonhealing wounds: retrospective analysis. Phys Ther 2008;88:1517–24.
37. Ennis WJ, Valdes W, Gainer M, et al. Evaluation of clinical effectiveness of MIST ultrasound therapy for the healing of chronic wounds. Adv Skin Wound Care 2006;19:437–46.
38. Cole PS, Quisberg J, Melin MM. Adjuvant use of acoustic pressure wound therapy for treatment of chronic wounds: a retrospective analysis. J Wound Ostomy Continence Nurs 2009;36:171–7.
39. Lindholm C, Bergsten A, Berglund E. Chronic wounds and nursing care. J Wound Care 1999;8:5–10.
40. Bergstorm N, Bennett M, Carlson C. Pressure ulcer treatment. Clinical practice guideline. Rockville (MD): Department of Health and Human Services, Public Health Service, Agency for Health Care Policy and Research; 1994. p. 15.
41. Brennan SS, Leaper DJ. The effect of antiseptics on the healing wound: a study using the rabbit ear chamber. Br J Surg 1985;72:780–2.
42. Glide S. Cleaning choices. Nurs Times 1992;88:74, 76, 78.
43. Lawrence JC. Wound irrigation. J Wound Care 1997;6:23–6.
44. Moscati R, Mayrose J, Fincher L, et al. Comparison of normal saline with tap water for wound irrigation. Am J Emerg Med 1998;16:379–81.
45. Thompson S. Towards evidence based emergency medicine: best BETs from the Manchester Royal Infirmary. Wound cleaning methods. Arch Emerg Med 1999;16:63.
46. Fife CE, Carter MJ, Walker D, et al. A retrospective data analysis of antimicrobial dressing usage in 3,084 patients. Ostomy Wound Manage 2010;56:28–42.
47. Gelfand JM, Hoffstad O, Margolis DJ. Surrogate endpoints for the treatment of venous leg ulcers. J Invest Dermatol 2002;119:1420–5.
48. Sheehan P, Jones P, Caselli A, et al. Percent change in wound area of diabetic foot ulcers over a 4-week period is a robust predictor of complete healing in a 12-week prospective trial. Diabetes Care 2003;26:1879–82.
49. Gale SS. DOMINATE wounds. Wounds 2014;26:1–12.
50. Bittar S. Skin substitutes in the diabetic and venous stasis ulcer. Presentation at Wound Care/HBO Symposium; Perrysburg (OH), May 18, 2012.
51. Robson MC. Wound infection. Surg Clin North Am 1997;77:637–50.
52. Livingston M, Wolvos T. Scottsdale wound management guide. 2nd edition. Malvern (PA): HMP Communications; 2009.
53. Sibbald RG, Woo K, Ayello EA. Increased bacterial burden and infection: the story of NERDS and STONES. Adv Skin Wound Care 2006;19:447–61.
54. Stotts N. Infection: diagnosis and management. In: Morison M, Ovington L, Wilkie K, editors. Chronic wound care: a problem-based learning approach. Edinburgh (United Kingdom): Mosby; 2004. p. 101–16.
55. Angel DE, Lloyd P, Carville K, et al. The clinical efficacy of two semi-quantitative wound-swabbing techniques in identifying the causative organism(s) in infected cutaneous wounds. Int Wound J 2011;8:176–85.
56. James GA, Swogger E, Wolcott R, et al. Biofilms in chronic wounds. Wound Repair Regen 2008;16:37–44.
57. Wolcott RD, Ehrlich GD. Biofilms and chronic infections. JAMA 2008;299:2682–4.
58. Percival SL, Hill KE, Williams DW, et al. A review of the scientific evidence for biofilms in wounds. Wound Repair Regen 2012;20:647–57.

59. Cosgrove SE. The relationship between antimicrobial resistance and patient out-comes: mortality, length of hospital stay, and health care costs. Clin Infect Dis 2006;42:S82–9.
60. Vaneau M, Chaby G, Guillot B. Consensus panel recommendations for chronic and acute wound dressings. Arch Dermatol 2007;143:1291–4.
61. Chaby G, Senet P, Vaneau M. Dressings for acute and chronic wounds: a system-atic review. Arch Dermatol 2007;143:1297–304.

Role of Venous Stenting for Iliofemoral and Vena Cava Venous Obstruction

Adham N. Abou Ali, MD, Efthymios D. Avgerinos, MD,
Rabih A. Chaer, MD*

KEYWORDS

- Chronic venous disease • Venous stenting • Intravascular ultrasound scan
- Postthrombotic syndrome • Iliofemoral deep vein thrombosis
- Vena cava thrombosis

KEY POINTS

- Venous stenting for chronic venous disease is being increasingly used as more evidence accumulates supporting the open vein hypothesis and supporting the safety, efficacy, and durability of these interventions.
- As such, they can be offered to patients with advanced age and complex comorbidities.
- Future studies should focus on reporting outcomes specific to the underlying venous pathology (thrombotic vs nonthrombotic and acute vs chronic) to provide better evidence for stenting in chronic venous disease and the outcomes of new stent design with dedicated venous indications.

INTRODUCTION

Chronic venous disease (CVD) is a functional or morphologic abnormality of the lower extremity venous system manifesting itself as pain, swelling, skin changes, venous claudication, or ulceration.[1] Depending on the duration and severity of the venous abnormality, the presenting sign or symptom can range along a spectrum starting with painless telangiectasias and reticular veins up to painful ulcerations, tissue edema, and pigmentation. The prevalence of CVD complications fluctuates between 1% and 2% for venous ulcer disease and up to 60% for telangiectasias and reticular veins.[2,3] The postthrombotic syndrome (PTS) represents the constellation of symptoms seen with CVD and is regarded as the single most common complication of deep vein thrombosis (DVT) occurring in 20% to 50% of cases.[4]

The authors have nothing to disclose.
Division of Vascular Surgery, University of Pittsburgh Medical Center, 200 Lothrop Street, Suite A1011, Pittsburgh, PA 15213, USA
* Corresponding author.
E-mail address: chaerra@upmc.edu

Surg Clin N Am 98 (2018) 361–371
https://doi.org/10.1016/j.suc.2017.11.015
0039-6109/18/© 2017 Elsevier Inc. All rights reserved.

The diagnosis of PTS is predominantly supported by clinical signs (pain on calf compression, skin edema, induration, pigmentation, erythema, venous ectasia, and ulcers) and clinical symptoms (leg pain, cramps, heaviness, paresthesia, and itching). Initial conservative management of CVD includes lifestyle modifications (moderate physical activity and leg elevation), compression therapy, and pharmacologic therapy.

Venous reflux but not obstruction, has been the "central theme in CVD" for the last half century.[5] Venous reflux has been traditionally managed first. However, the advances in diagnosis and imaging techniques, mainly the intravascular ultrasound scan (IVUS), have allowed us to better understand the obstructive pathophysiology of venous disease. In fact, venous outflow obstruction involving the iliocaval segment has been identified in 10% to 30% of patients with severe chronic venous insufficiency.[5]

Although the combination of obstruction and reflux is present in most CVD, a recent study found that attending to the obstructive pathologic condition alone (through stenting) among patients with deep venous system reflux offered complete or partial pain relief (78% at 5 years).[6] As such, some investigators suggest stent treatment to most patients with CEAP score (clinical, etiology, anatomic, pathophysiology) ≥ 3 before addressing deep reflux.[5,6]

During the last decade, the endovascular management of iliofemoral and iliocaval obstruction has superseded open venous reconstruction for CVD. The safety, efficacy and durability of endovascular interventions for iliocaval obstruction have been extensively demonstrated.[7] This article reviews the role of venous stenting for iliofemoral and vena cava obstruction in patients with acute or chronic venous outflow obstruction.

ACUTE ILIOFEMORAL DEEP VEIN THROMBOSIS

Acute iliofemoral DVT (IFDVT) is associated with increased rates of DVT recurrence, PTS, and pulmonary embolism compared with infrainguinal DVT.[8] The benefits from restoring patency and relieving venous outflow obstruction early on with catheter-directed interventions (CDI) have been extensively studied (open vein theory) to prevent the onset of PTS.[9,10] Currently, catheter-directed thrombolysis and pharmacomechanical thrombolysis are increasingly being used for the treatment of acute IFDVT targeting thrombus clearance, restoration of patency, maintenance of valvular function, and potential reduction of PTS severity.[11–13] CDI utilization rates for patients with proximal DVT have increased from 2.3% in 2005 to 6.4% in 2011.[14] This increase is particularly true for caval thrombosis in which the CDI rates are even higher, increasing from 16% to 34.7% in that same period.[14] This may be in part attributable to the increased incidence or higher diagnosis rates of VTE in the last decade.[15,16]

Thrombolysis for acute symptomatic iliofemoral DVT can achieve relatively high rates of immediate thrombus clearance and reduce long-term PTS morbidity. Clinical success with CDI for iliofemoral DVT, defined as $\geq 50\%$ lysis without 30-day recurrence, ranges between 80% to 95% across the literature.[10,17] Iliac vein stenting with self-expanding stents is required after thrombolysis of acute IFDVT to treat venous outflow obstruction identified on venography or IVUS (traditionally defined as >50% area reduction by IVUS) to prevent recurrence. The correction of venous outflow obstruction after thrombolysis of acute IFDVT has been recommended by several guidelines, including the American College of Chest Physicians, the Society for Interventional Radiology, the Society of Vascular Surgery, and the American Heart Association.[18–21]

PATHOPHYSIOLOGY OF CHRONIC VENOUS DISEASE

Chronic iliofemoral venous obstruction can be secondary to DVT manifesting clinically as PTS or secondary to a nonthrombotic iliac vein lesion from an extrinsic compression such as arterial crossovers over the iliac vein (May-Thurner syndrome). PTS is the most frequent chronic complication of DVT, which confers a negative impact on a patient's quality of life and on the economy.[8] PTS is predominantly a clinical diagnosis supported by clinical signs (pain on calf compression, skin edema, induration, pigmentation, erythema, venous ectasia, and ulcers) and symptoms (pain, cramps, heaviness, paresthesia, and itching). Patient symptoms are variable and largely depend on the cause, extent of venous obstruction, and disease duration. Symptom production with PTS has been tied to iliac vein obstruction (vs femoral and tibial) caused by the absence of adequate collateralization at the iliac segment. These signs and symptoms constitute the Villalta scale, which is a clinically validated measure for identifying, assessing, and treating PTS.[22] A Villalta score between 0 to 4 indicates the absence of PTS, whereas a score between 5 and 9, 10 and 14, and greater than 15 indicates mild, moderate, or severe PTS, respectively.[22]

ENDOVASCULAR MANAGEMENT OF CHRONIC VENOUS OBSTRUCTION

Recanalization of chronic iliocaval obstruction has been advocated recently to treat patients with severe PTS or nonhealing venous stasis ulcers. The main goal of treating chronic venous disease is improving quality of life, and, currently, endovascular management has replaced open surgical technique as the go-to modality for chronic venous obstruction.

INDICATIONS

Current European and American guidelines recommend endovenous stenting for severe CVD even though the supporting evidence is weak.[23,24] The indications for stenting in patients with CVD are patients with a CEAP score of 3 and higher and in patients who have not responded to conservative therapy with compression.[5] Iliac vein stenting and obstruction relief has provided symptomatic improvement to patients with a combined reflux and obstruction condition.[25] However, up until recent years, there has been no dedicated venous stent, but a few stent designs have been recently tested in clinical trials in the United States and are awaiting approval from the US Food and Drug Administration (FDA) for venous indications.[26]

TECHNIQUE
Access

Ultrasound-guided access to the deep venous system is commonly performed through the ipsilateral femoral or deep femoral vein in the upper thigh or midthigh. This grants a direct route to a stenosis or obstruction with the ability of infrainguinal extensions of the stent. Other approaches include popliteal and jugular vein access. Both are viable options and can be useful in certain anatomic situations. However, popliteal access requires the patient to be in a prone position, which can increase risk of respiratory compromise, and jugular access confers less ease of instrument manipulation because of the longer distance between access and target lesion. Interventions can be done under local anesthesia and intravenous sedation or under general anesthesia.

Traversing the Lesion

Traversing nonobstructive venous lesions is usually straightforward. Using a 0.035 hydrophilic guide wire, threading the wire into the inferior vena cava (IVC) is done with ease. For delivering the appropriate-sized balloons or stents, 9 to 11F sheaths are typically required; serial dilators may be used to facilitate sheath placement. IVUS is recommended for delineating the extent of disease and stent sizing; if unavailable, venography using anteroposterior, 45° and 60° oblique projections are recommended to better delineate the stenosis.

Chronic total occlusions of the iliocaval system are traversed with relative ease despite their daunting appearance on venography using a hydrophilic guide wire because of the trabeculations within the thrombus. Stiff and soft wires with straight or angled tips along with supporting catheters are needed to cross the lesion, including the use of crossing sets and re-entry devices. The TriForce kit (Cook, Bloomington, IN) includes a crossing set of catheters and supporting sheath to achieve recanalization. Anecdotally, in our practice, we have observed that this setup has allowed crossing of venous occlusions that previously we were unable to cross or has significantly reduced crossing time. However, it is still difficult to predict which patients will be long cases versus short cases.

The most difficult cases are those in which an extravascular plane is generated and re-entry is required. Re-attempting entry after an initial failed attempt is common, as these lesions are challenging and require patience and persistence. Crossing the IVC is achieved whenever the wire easily advances into the right atrium, which is usually at the level of the tenth rib. Whenever perforation is suspected, the wire is withdrawn and re-advanced without the need for aborting the procedure because of the low venous pressures and the perivenous fibrosis.

Stenting of Iliofemoral Vein

Several points about the differences between venous and arterial stenting need to be addressed.[27] Venous balloon angioplasty alone is a suboptimal intervention, and the lesion almost always recurs. Large-caliber stents are instead required in most cases. And although venography is used to confirm deep venous occlusion, IVUS is frequently being implemented to determine the extent of the lesion and the proximal and distal stent landing zones. Cephalad landing zones include the IVC up to the level but not including the right atrium. Caudad landing zones include crossing the inguinal ligament down to the common femoral vein without jailing the profunda. IVC filters, if present, are stented across whenever encountered to optimize inflow (**Fig. 1**).

After traversing the lesion, appropriate predilation of the stenosed segment may be required. Predilation of the track over the wire is performed using 4- to 6-mm balloons. The entire track is subsequently dilated using 14- to 18-mm balloons depending on the involved vein segment. The common femoral vein can accept up to a 14-mm, the external iliac vein a 16-mm, and the IVC an 18- to 24-mm balloon. Subsequent stenting usually corresponds to the size of the balloon. IVUS is recommended for adequate placement of the stent and for stent sizing and determining the extent of disease. The extent of disease is frequently more severe than what is indicated by venography alone. In general, self-expanding stents (braided stainless) are used, although this is an off-label use, as current stents do not have a venous indication by the FDA. It is essential to postdilate the stents to allow full expansion. Re-assessing with IVUS is also advisable to ensure stent apposition.

Vein rupture secondary to balloon dilation is rare given the restrictive perivenous fibrosis. Consequently, overdilation and the use of large balloons and stents is

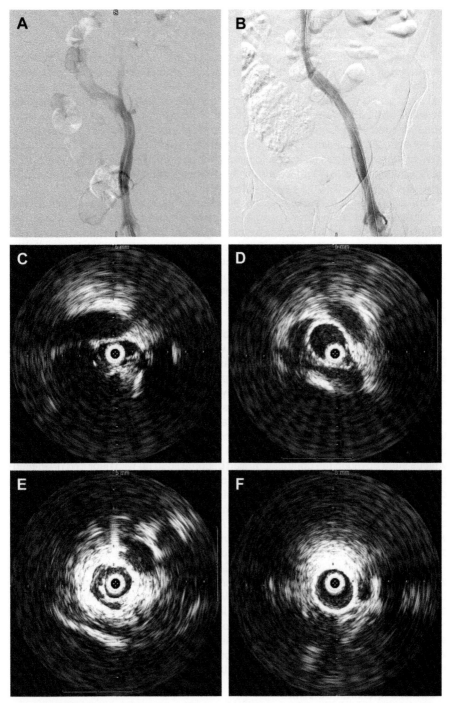

Fig. 1. Postthrombotic lesions in a 43-year-old woman with multiple prior deep venous thrombosis. (*A*) Venogram shows inconclusive findings of stenosis in the left common femoral, external iliac, and common iliac vein. (*B*) Wallstents (16 mm in diameter) extending from the caval junction crossing the inguinal ligament and down to the common femoral vein (off-label use). (*C*) IVUS examination shows stenosis in the common iliac vein before stenting. (*D*) Widely patent common iliac vein as shown by IVUS after stenting. (*E*) IVUS examination shows significant stenosis in the external iliac vein before stenting. (*F*) Widely patent external iliac vein as shown by IVUS after stenting.

acceptable and safe. The low venous pressure acts as a safety feature, particularly with perforations, which are not uncommon with venous interventions. Stent sizing is different in venous practice compared with arterial stents. Although it is agreed that stent sizing with arterial lesions is in accordance with normal adjacent vessels, the same approach would lead to significant undersizing with venous lesions. Raju[5] recommended venous stent sizing by 2 mm over standard anatomic sizes. Undersizing venous stents can lead to iatrogenic stenosis, which becomes more pronounced when in-stent restenosis (ISR) develops and possible migration. This finding is particularly important, as 61% of stents in the iliocaval outflow tract experienced ISR between 20% and 50% at 5-year of follow-up.[28]

With regard to the extent of stenting, all lesions should be stented without leaving skip areas behind, as these may cause symptom recurrence and interstent stenosis. It is acceptable to stent below the inguinal ligament into the common femoral vein (ideally avoiding to jail the origin of the deep femoral vein), as stent fracture in the venous system is infrequently encountered.[29] Contrary to arterial stenting, venous stenting across the inguinal ligament has not been associated with increased risk of stent fracture, narrowing, or ISR. Patency is rather related to whether the thrombotic obstruction is occlusive.[29] Extensive metal loading seems to be well tolerated in the iliofemoral-caval system.

The iliocaval junction is a critical and common failure point that needs to be traversed; otherwise, distal stent compression with recurrent stenosis is to be expected.[30] Extension of the self-expanding stent such as the Wallstent (Boston Scientific, Marlborough, MA) into the vena cava to avoid this problem may render subsequent contralateral stenting technically difficult and possibly contribute to partial jailing of contralateral flow. Acute jailing of the contralateral iliac is less of a concern compared with chronic subclinical jailing.[31] In addition, contralateral stenting is required in up to 20% of patients.[32] IVC stent extension has raised concerns about contralateral limb outflow obstruction, particularly in a subacute and chronic fashion.[7,31] The interstices of the venous stent covering the contralateral iliac become lined up with neointima that eventually occlude the outflow.[31] Techniques to circumvent this occurrence have been proposed including using the Gianturco Z stent (Cook Medical) that has wider interstices. One study found a higher rate of freedom from contralateral DVT with the Z stent compared with the Wallstent (99% vs 90%, P<.001).[31] The contralateral DVT incidence was around 2% with the Wallstent, which is much lower than the rate of restenosis if the stainless steel stent is not extended beyond the confluence (around 40%).[31,33]

The addition of the Gianturco Z stent (Cook Medical) to the upper portion of the Wallstent may ameliorate the above concerns. This technical modification, which requires oversizing the Z stent relative to the Wallstent, seems to facilitate simultaneous or subsequent stenting of the contralateral limb.[30] The double-barrel technique works for simultaneous bilateral stenting and is optimal whenever bilateral disease is present.[32] However, this technique does not seem to be suitable for sequential stenting. With sequential stenting, the new stent is prone to be compressed by the older stent that has already been incorporated within the surrounding tissue.

Technical and Clinical Outcomes

Technical success was 94% and 96% for thrombotic and nonthrombotic conditions, respectively. Primary patency at 1 year was 96% (95% confidence interval [CI], 93%–98%) for nonthrombotic and 79% (95% CI, 76%–83%) for thrombotic disease. Secondary patency at 1 year was 99% (95% CI, 88%–100%) for nonthrombotic and 94% (95% CI, 90%–96%) for thrombotic etiologies. Primary and secondary patency remained higher in nonthrombotic patients versus thrombotic patients through 5 years.[34] In the same meta-analysis assessing the effectiveness of stenting for iliofemoral venous obstruction, complete symptom relief at the final follow-up visit was reported in 69% to 82% of patients for pain, 64% to 68% of patients for edema, and 71% to 81% of patients for ulcer healing (**Fig. 2**).[34]

In a large series analysis between 1997 and 2005, 982 chronic nonmalignant obstructive lesions of the femoroiliocaval vein were stented. Patency was verified at a mean follow-up of 30 months after stent placement in 610 (62%) limbs. Overall primary, primary-assisted, and secondary patency rates were 67%, 89%, and 93%, respectively, at 72 months. Ipsilateral early or late stent occlusion occurred in 31 limbs and was successfully lysed in 7; 24 stents remained occluded. The stented limbs with nonthrombotic iliac vein lesions fared significantly better (P<.0001) than did those with thrombotic disease, with primary, assisted-primary, and secondary cumulative patency rates of 79%, 100%, and 100%, and 57%, 80%, and 86% at 72 months, respectively.[7]

Predictors of stent failure included a thrombotic etiology for the obstruction (vs nonthrombotic iliac vein lesion), occlusive obstruction (vs nonocclusive obstruction), and stenting extended to the common femoral vein. Those same factors were associated with increased odds of severe ISR (>50%).[7] Younger age seemed to increase the risk of occlusion but not ISR. Gender was not associated with increased odds for either occlusion or ISR. Severe ISR was around 5% at 6 years. The incidence was higher in patients with a thrombotic etiology (10%) compared with patients with a nonthrombotic etiology (1%).[7]

A subsequent analysis to examine the effect of infrainguinal stenting found that even though secondary patency rates were lower in patients with caudad versus cephalad stent termination relative to the inguinal ligament (86% vs 95%; P<.001), there was no difference in secondary patency rates when the limbs were stratified by nature of thrombotic obstruction (occlusive vs nonocclusive). The investigators concluded that stent patency depended on the etiology of the iliac obstruction rather than caudad stent extension (above or below the inguinal ligament).[29]

Primary and secondary patency rates were mainly related to the presence and severity of thrombotic disease. Further analysis of possible contributing factors confirmed that tight, long lesions of thrombotic etiology requiring multiple stents

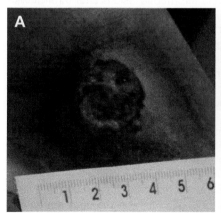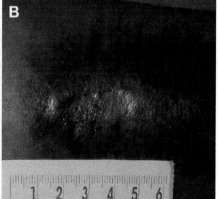

Fig. 2. Venous ulcers from the same patient in **Fig. 1** show advanced stages of postthrombotic syndrome. (*A*) Shallow 3- × 3-cm venous ulcer along the left anteromedial shin area. (*B*) Healed venous ulcer 6 months later after stenting of the common femoral, external iliac, and common iliac veins up to and including the iliocaval junction.

reaching caudad into the common femoral vein were of greatest risk to occlude. Even though the thrombotic state was such a high-risk factor, the presence of thrombophilia was not significantly associated with occlusion. The operation side and gender did not influence stent outcome, but younger age seemed to do so.

Complications

Approximately 25% of patients with iliac vein stenting will require reintervention. The incidence of poststent DVT is 1.5% within 30 days. Complication rates ranged from 0.3% to 1.1% among groups for major bleeding, defined as hematomas requiring evacuation and access site bleeding requiring transfusion. Other adverse events included pulmonary embolism (0.2%–0.9%), periprocedural mortality (0.1%–0.7%), and early thrombosis (1.0%–6.8%).[34]

Anticoagulation and Stent Surveillance

Stenting itself does not require chronic anticoagulation beyond the first 3 months after implantation unless otherwise indicated. Antiplatelets such as aspirin have been adequate for stent maintenance particularly in nonthrombotic cases. Chronic anticoagulation has been suggested in certain patients such as those with thrombophilia, recurrent venous thrombosis, unprovoked DVT, and IVC stenting procedures.[5]

Venous stent surveillance aims at detecting stent thrombosis, ISR, or stent compression. Detecting stent compression necessitates measurement of the stent diameter as a routine part of stent assessment. Duplex surveillance after the procedure, at 4 weeks, 3 months, and yearly thereafter has been proposed as a surveillance program.[5] In patients at high risk of thrombosis (recanalization of postthrombotic occlusion), anticoagulation is suggested in this patient subset. It has been reported that around 20% of stents will require re-intervention for an ISR.[35] If an ISR of greater than 50% is identified on surveillance imaging, balloon angioplasty is recommended to maintain patency regardless of symptoms.

Pregnancy

Stenting of nonthrombotic iliocaval lesions and thrombotic lesions after thrombolysis is often done to treat symptomatic lesions in women of reproductive age. However, there is a theoretic and observed concern with iliac vein stenting given the young age and the anatomic and physiologic changes of pregnancy.

The pressure of the gravid uterus on the iliac veins and the known relative venous stasis that occurs during pregnancy are considerations for potential stent complications in this anatomic region. In addition, changes in coagulation factors during pregnancy are well established and mechanistically can contribute to stent complications.

In a recent multicenter series of 12 female patients within the reproductive age group, all patients remained asymptomatic with patent stents at a median follow-up of 63 months after initial stenting.[36] Only 1 patient experienced asymptomatic stent compression 1 year after her second delivery, which was managed with balloon dilation with subsequent 3-month follow-up showing resolved stent stenosis. All the stents were self-expanding with limited radial strength. Although they may be compromised, given the inward force on the veins during pregnancy by the gravid uterus, they are expected to re-expand after delivery with resolution of the extrinsic compression. The authors concluded that iliocaval stenting is safe in this patient population given the low rate of reported stent complications.

New and Future Stent Designs

Until recently, there have been no venous dedicated stents, but 2 stent designs have completed clinical trial enrollment in the United States and are awaiting data analysis and subsequent FDA approval.

The Zilver Vena (Cook Medical) is the first stent designed specifically for treating ilio-femoral venous outflow obstruction and was recently tested as part of the VIVO clinical trial in the United States.[37] Experience with the Zilver Vena venous stent in Europe found a favorable efficacy profile even in challenging anatomy (50% of cases were malignant iliofemoral obstructions).[26] Other novel stent designs are also in the process of being approved in the United States. A prospective multicenter nonrandomized study (VIRTUS) has completed enrollment and aims to evaluate the safety and efficacy of the Veniti Vici venous stent in patients with chronic nonmalignant iliofemoral venous outflow obstruction.[38]

SUMMARY

Venous stenting for CVD is being increasingly used as more evidence accumulates supporting the open vein hypothesis and supporting the safety, efficacy, and durability of these interventions. As such, they can be offered to patients with advanced age and complex comorbidities. Future studies should focus on reporting outcomes specific to the underlying venous pathologic condition (thrombotic vs nonthrombotic and acute vs chronic) to provide better evidence for stenting in CVD, and the outcomes of new stent design with dedicated venous indications.

REFERENCES

1. Seager MJ, Busuttil A, Dharmarajah B, et al. Editor's choice– a systematic review of endovenous stenting in chronic venous disease secondary to iliac vein obstruction. Eur J Vasc Endovasc Surg 2016;51(1):100–20.

2. Rabe E, Guex JJ, Puskas A, et al. Epidemiology of chronic venous disorders in geographically diverse populations: results from the vein consult program. Int Angiol 2012;31(2):105–15.

3. Beebe-Dimmer JL, Pfeifer JR, Engle JS, et al. The epidemiology of chronic venous insufficiency and varicose veins. Ann Epidemiol 2005;15(3):175–84.

4. Kahn SR. The post-thrombotic syndrome: the forgotten morbidity of deep venous thrombosis. J Thromb Thrombolysis 2006;21(1):41–8.

5. Raju S. Treatment of iliac-caval outflow obstruction. Semin Vasc Surg 2015;28(1): 47–53.

6. Raju S, Darcey R, Neglén P, et al. Unexpected major role for venous stenting in deep reflux disease. J Vasc Surg 2010;51(2):401–8.

7. Neglen P, Hollis KC, Olivier J, et al. Stenting of the venous outflow in chronic venous disease: long-term stent-related outcome, clinical, and hemodynamic result. J Vasc Surg 2007;46(5):979–90.

8. Kahn SR, Shbaklo H, Lamping DL, et al. Determinants of health-related quality of life during the 2 years following deep vein thrombosis. J Thromb Haemost 2008; 6(7):1105–12.

9. Comerota AJ, Gale SS. Technique of contemporary iliofemoral and infrainguinal venous thrombectomy. J Vasc Surg 2006;43(1):185–91.

10. Enden T, Haig Y, Kløw NE, et al. Long-term outcome after additional catheter-directed thrombolysis versus standard treatment for acute iliofemoral deep vein

thrombosis (the CaVenT study): a randomised controlled trial. Lancet 2012; 379(9810):31–8.

11. Bashir R, Zack CJ, Zhao H, et al. Comparative outcomes of catheter-directed thrombolysis plus anticoagulation vs anticoagulation alone to treat lower-extremity proximal deep vein thrombosis. JAMA Intern Med 2014;174(9):1494–501.

12. Comerota AJ. Thrombolysis for deep venous thrombosis. J Vasc Surg 2012;55(2): 607–11.

13. Watson L, Broderick C, Armon MP. Thrombolysis for acute deep vein thrombosis. Cochrane Database Syst Rev 2014;(1):CD002783.

14. Alkhouli M, Zack CJ, Zhao H, et al. Comparative outcomes of catheter-directed thrombolysis plus anticoagulation versus anticoagulation alone in the treatment of inferior vena caval thrombosis. Circ Cardiovasc Interv 2015;8(2):e001882.

15. Huang W, Goldberg RJ, Anderson FA, et al. Secular trends in occurrence of acute venous thromboembolism: the Worcester VTE study (1985-2009). Am J Med 2014;127(9):829–39.e5.

16. Heit JA, Spencer FA, White RH. The epidemiology of venous thromboembolism. J Thromb Thrombolysis 2016;41(1):3–14.

17. Avgerinos ED, Hager ES, Naddaf A, et al. Outcomes and predictors of failure of thrombolysis for iliofemoral deep venous thrombosis. J Vasc Surg Venous Lymphat Disord 2015;3(1):35–41.

18. Meissner MH, Gloviczki P, Comerota AJ, et al. Early thrombus removal strategies for acute deep venous thrombosis: clinical practice guidelines of the society for vascular surgery and the american venous forum. J Vasc Surg 2012;55(5): 1449–62.

19. Vedantham S, Millward SF, Cardella JF, et al. Society of Interventional Radiology position statement: treatment of acute iliofemoral deep vein thrombosis with use of adjunctive catheter-directed intrathrombus thrombolysis. J Vasc Interv Radiol 2009;20(7 Suppl):S332–5.

20. Kearon C, Akl EA, Ornelas J, et al. Antithrombotic therapy for VTE disease: CHEST guideline and expert panel report. Chest 2016;149(2):315–52.

21. Jaff MR, McMurtry MS, Archer SL, et al. Management of massive and submassive pulmonary embolism, iliofemoral deep vein thrombosis, and chronic thromboembolic pulmonary hypertension: a scientific statement from the American Heart Association. Circulation 2011;123(16):1788–830.

22. Wik HS, Ghanima W, Sandset PM, et al. Scoring systems for postthrombotic syndrome. Semin Thromb Hemost 2017;43(5):500–4.

23. O'Donnell TFJ, Passman MA, Marston WA, et al. Management of venous leg ulcers: clinical practice guidelines of the Society for Vascular Surgery (R) and the American Venous Forum. J Vasc Surg 2014;60(2 Suppl):3S–59S.

24. Mahnken AH, Thomson K, de Haan M, et al. CIRSE standards of practice guidelines on iliocaval stenting. Cardiovasc Intervent Radiol 2014;37(4):889–97.

25. Raju S, Darcey R, Neglén P. Unexpected major role for venous stenting in deep reflux disease. J Vasc Surg 2010;51(2):401–8.

26. O'Sullivan GJ, Sheehan J, Lohan D, et al. Iliofemoral venous stenting extending into the femoral region: initial clinical experience with the purpose-designed zilver vena stent. J Cardiovasc Surg (Torino) 2013;54(2):255–61.

27. Raju S. Endovascular repair of chronic venous obstruction. In: Moore WS, editor. Vascular and endovascular surgery: a comprehensive review. 8th edition. Philadelphia: Elsevier; 2013.

28. Neglen P, Raju S. In-stent recurrent stenosis in stents placed in the lower extremity venous outflow tract. J Vasc Surg 2004;39(1):181–7.

29. Neglen P, Tackett TPJ, Raju S. Venous stenting across the inguinal ligament. J Vasc Surg 2008;48(5):1255–61.
30. Raju S, Ward MJ, Kirk O. A modification of iliac vein stent technique. Ann Vasc Surg 2014;28(6):1485–92.
31. Murphy EH, Johns B, Varney E, et al. Deep venous thrombosis associated with caval extension of iliac stents. J Vasc Surgery Venous Lymphat Disord 2017;5(1):8–17.
32. Neglen P, Darcey R, Olivier J, et al. Bilateral stenting at the iliocaval confluence. J Vasc Surg 2010;51(6):1457–66.
33. Neglen P, Raju S. Balloon dilation and stenting of chronic iliac vein obstruction: technical aspects and early clinical outcome. J Endovasc Ther 2000;7(2):79–91.
34. Razavi MK, Jaff MR, Miller LE. Safety and effectiveness of stent placement for iliofemoral venous outflow obstruction: systematic review and meta-analysis. Circ Cardiovasc Interv 2015;8(10):e002772.
35. Raju S, Tackett PJ, Neglen P. Reinterventions for nonocclusive iliofemoral venous stent malfunctions. J Vasc Surg 2009;49(2):511–8.
36. Dasari M, Avgerinos E, Raju S, et al. Outcomes of iliac vein stents after pregnancy. J Vasc Surgery Venous Lymphat Disord 2017;5(3):353–7.
37. Comerota AJ, Hoffman L. Obstruction, evaluation of the zilver Venatm venous stent in the treatment of symptomatic iliofemoral venous outflow. ClinicalTrials.gov [Internet]. Identifier NCT01970007. 2017.
38. Marston WA, Razavi MK. VIRTUS: an evaluation of the veniti Vicitm venous stent system in patients with chronic iliofemoral venous outflow obstruction (VIRTUS). ClinicalTrials.gov [Internet]. Identifier NCT02112877. 2017.

Open Surgical Reconstruction for Deep Venous Occlusion and Valvular Incompetence

Katherin E. Leckie, MD*, Michael C. Dalsing, MD

KEYWORDS

- Deep venous insufficiency • Deep venous obstruction • Venous bypass
- Venous valve repair • Venous valve replacement • Venous valvuloplasty
- Venous transplantation • Venous transposition

KEY POINTS

- First-line therapy for patients with deep venous obstruction is compression therapy and treatment of pathologic superficial or perforator disease. In patients who fail conservative management and have failed or have no endovascular options, open venous bypass can be considered.
- Of venous bypasses, the Palma procedure has the best patency and clinical outcomes. Hybrid procedures for femoral occlusive disease and complex reconstructions for iliocaval disease have a more guarded outcome.
- First-line therapy for patients with deep venous valvular insufficiency is compression therapy and treatment of any concomitant superficial or perforator reflux or obstructive disease amenable to endovascular techniques. In patients who have persistent significant clinical disease, open surgical repair can be considered.
- Valvuloplasty is first choice in patients with significant clinical symptoms who have intact and incompetent valves.
- In patients without intact valves, the options are vein transposition, valve transplant, and autologous neovalve creation, which are generally selected in that order and based on available anatomic conditions.

INTRODUCTION

Venous insufficiency and/or venous occlusive disease affecting the superficial, perforator, or deep veins of the lower extremity are common problems affecting a significant proportion of the United States population. These conditions are

Disclosure Statement: The authors have nothing to disclose.
Division of Vascular Surgery, Department of Surgery, Indiana University School of Medicine, 1801 North Senate Boulevard, Suite 3500, Indianapolis, IN 46202, USA
* Corresponding author.
E-mail address: kleckie@iu.edu

frequently comorbid in patients[1,2] and, either alone or in combination, manifest as lower extremity venous hypertension with resultant signs and symptoms (the venous stasis syndrome). The underlying pathologic complication, regardless of the anatomic location, can manifest itself on a spectrum ranging from no physical findings, telangiectasias, or reticular or varicose veins, to swelling, chronic skin changes, or ulcerations (clinical, etiologic, anatomic, and pathologic [CEAP] classification).[3] Patients may have no or mild or moderate associated discomfort (eg, pain, itching), venous claudication, or constant pain. It is estimated that 150,000 new cases of venous stasis syndrome and more than 20,000 new venous ulcers are diagnosed annually.[4] In a population study, 7% to 20% of adults older than age 50 years were noted to have venous stasis skin changes. Another study reported trophic changes in 6.2% of adults studied with incidence increasing with age; 22% of legs with trophic changes had deep functional disease defined as either reflux or obstruction (9% of individuals and 5.6% of legs). In this study, superficial disease alone was almost 3 times more common that deep disease with or without commitment superficial disease (14.9% vs 5.6%). Superficial disease was present in 48% of legs with deep disease.[5] So, although a significant component of venous disease is located in the superficial (great saphenous vein [GSV] or small saphenous vein) or perforator systems, and is treated conservatively and/or with endovascular options, there remains a subset of patients afflicted with deep venous disease who require treatment to alleviate persistent symptoms. Some deep venous occlusive disease is amenable to endovascular options, which is generally the first option chosen by the patient and their physician due to its minimally invasive nature. However, a smaller number of patients with deep venous disease will ultimately require an open surgical repair to provide some relief. The goal of this article is to outline general indications for intervention and options for reconstruction for deep venous occlusive disease and deep venous valvular incompetence.

DEEP VENOUS OCCLUSIVE DISEASE

With limited data available, recommendations for surgical intervention in venous obstructive disease are based on a mixture of observational studies, case series, and expert opinion (grade 2C recommendations).[6] Similar to endovascular interventions, patients should have failed conservative management, which generally includes at least 3 months of compression therapy, as well as elevation of the extremity, especially at night, with or without wound care as needed. Because of the increased risks and potentially modest benefit associated with an open operative approach, surgical interventions are often considered in patients with more advanced venous disease. Based on the CEAP classification of venous disease, these patients generally have significant skin changes and are at risk of (C4b) or have had (C5) or have (C6) lower leg ulcers. According to the most recent Society for Vascular Surgery and American Venous Forum guidelines, patients with infrainguinal obstruction and CEAP score of C4b or greater might be considered for surgical reconstruction. However, in patients with iliac vein or inferior vena cava (IVC) occlusive disease, surgical reconstruction is currently recommended only in patients with recalcitrant venous ulcers who have failed endovascular reconstruction.[6] It should be noted, however, that the level of evidence is 2C at best. Symptomatic patients without ulcerations and a CEAP score of C3 and higher have been offered surgery by experienced practitioners with acceptable outcomes.[1,7–9]

Approaches for open surgical reconstruction for deep venous occlusion are based on the anatomic location, the extent of the obstruction, and the availability of autogenous venous conduit. These options include the saphenopopliteal bypass,[10] cross-femoral venous (Palma procedure), or synthetic graft (often polytetrafluoroethylene [PTFE] bypass),[8] femorocaval or iliocaval bypass using various conduits, hybrid approaches,[1] and spiral vein grafts.[11] Regardless of choice of conduit or anatomic location, the principle remains to bypass from a nondiseased distal vein segment to a nondiseased proximal vein segment. Considerations for conduit selection include the availability of adequate vein as well as size matching. Proximal occlusions are often bypassed with synthetic conduits (often PTFE) due to the availability of large diameter grafts in sufficient lengths.[1,8] The various surgical options for deep venous obstruction are considered as a progression from distal to proximal disease.

Saphenopopliteal vein bypass is used for patients with chronic symptomatic occlusion of the femoral or proximal popliteal vein. This operation is a relatively rare procedure due to the often successful ability to conservatively control the patients' symptoms, the anatomic need for patent proximal common femoral and iliocaval systems, and a competent GSV. The procedure involves transection of the GSV at a length sufficient for the bypass and creation of an end-to-side anastomosis with the popliteal vein distal to the occlusion. This effectively drains the deep system of the lower leg via the proximal GSV. In a series of 17 subjects, 82% had resolution of venous claudication and 3 of 5 subjects healed chronic ulcerations. Secondary patency was 75% at a median follow-up of 103 months.[10]

For patients with common femoral vein occlusion and proximal iliac disease (unilateral or bilateral), a hybrid approach to reconstruction has been explored. Endophlebectomy and patch angioplasty of the common femoral vein for postthrombotic obstruction is a technique that is commonly used as a part of more extensive deep venous reconstruction surgeries for both venous occlusion and insufficiency.[12] It has been used as an adjunct to angioplasty and stenting of the iliac vein for occlusive disease. This was shown to have good short-term primary and secondary patency in a case series of 6 subjects, 83% and 100%, respectively, at a mean of 15 months follow-up,[12] and improved clinical severity and quality of life scores at 6 months.[13] However, in the experience of other investigators, longer term outcomes have been less promising with 30% 2-year secondary patency in 12 subjects. This approach is currently not recommended except as a last resort.[1]

For patients with unilateral iliac occlusions, the Palma procedure (cross-femoral venous bypass) is one of the more successful techniques for surgical deep venous reconstruction. The 5-year patency rate is almost 80%[1,8] and there is a case report of patency in 1 patient 22 years after surgery.[9] This procedure was originally described in 1960[14] and it involves using a vein graft (generally the GSV from the unaffected side) to bypass from the femoral vein distal to the obstruction to the contralateral femoral vein with end-to-side anastomoses. PTFE has been suggested as an alternative if GSV is inadequate (less than 5 mm in diameter or damaged), but PTFE has a much lower patency rate; 50% secondary patency at 1 year in 1 series.[8] Endoscopic vein harvest and creation of an adjunct arteriovenous fistula (AVF) at the inflow anastomosis have been associated with decreased primary patency rates.[1] This was a surprising finding with respect to the AVF and might well be influenced by the tendency to use this adjunctive technique in those thought prone to failure (eg, poor inflow, hypercoagulable, or prosthetic conduit use) and is based on uncontrolled retrospective evaluation only. The use of an AVF remains controversial but continues to be recommended in patients in whom the inflow to either an autologous or a prosthetic bypass is judged to be poor.

For patients with IVC obstruction, bilateral iliac disease, or iliac occlusion lacking a good vein, a variety of other open reconstructions have been used. These include the

femoroiliac, iliocaval, or femorocaval bypasses with vein or PTFE or complex reconstructions involving some combination of bypasses. Keep in mind that many of these
patients have had an attempt at an endovascular repair that was unsuccessful (generally the first interventional option) and, even in the largest series, case numbers are
small. For short iliac occlusions in patients who might otherwise have been considered
for a Palma procedure and either lacked adequate conduit or had contralateral venous
disease, short iliocaval or femoroiliac bypasses with PTFE have demonstrated good
outcomes with a secondary patency of 86% at 5 and 10 years.[1] Spiral saphenous
vein grafts were occasionally also used for such short-segment iliac or femoral reconstruction but do not have documented long-term patency[8,11] and require the sacrifice
of another lower extremity venous segment, which might be difficult to justify in these
patients. Laparotomy, with or without groin access, adds complexity and risk to the
procedure. In patients with more extensive occlusions, long femorocaval bypasses
can be performed but, of course, do require open exposure of the femoral vein and
laparotomy for caval control. PTFE is typically used for these reconstructions due to
the diameter of the vessels involved. These bypasses had lower patency rates than
the Palma procedure or the short PTFE bypasses but were comparable to endovascular recanalization and stenting for chronic IVC obstruction in some series: 57%
5-year secondary patency compared with 66% for patients amenable to the endovascular approach.[1,15] Benefit has been demonstrated for the use of an AVF in the setting
of synthetic grafts[16] and long femorocaval or iliocaval bypasses.[11] AVF can typically
be ligated after 1 to 3 months or left open if there are no associated undesired clinical
sequelae.[1] For patients with extensive or bilateral obstructions, complex reconstructions using branched grafts or jump grafts that are usually synthetic have been used.
These bypasses tend to have poor outcomes with 30% 2-year secondary patency and
may be considered as last resort options.[1]

Although patency is the most frequent primary outcome evaluated following open
surgical reconstruction for venous occlusion, the clinically relevant outcomes are
those related to the patient's symptomatology and quality of life. Symptomatic
improvement following open surgical repair of venous obstruction has been noted
to be related to the patency of the bypass and the presence of underlying venous
incompetence that can be present in 60% of patients. In a series, two-thirds of subjects with leg swelling or venous claudication had resolution of their symptoms after
surgery and all subjects with ulcerations and patent grafts healed initially. Fifty percent
of these ulcers did recur, however, but were noted in subjects who either had late occlusion of their bypasses or underlying venous valvular incompetence.[1]

DEEP VENOUS VALVULAR INCOMPETENCE

Venous insufficiency is between 3 and 4 times more common than venous obstruction in some series,[17,18] although many patients have both. Management options are
based on the severity of symptoms and the anatomic location and extent of valvular
incompetence. The mainstay of treatment remains compression therapy, leg elevation, and wound therapy when applicable. For patients with venous ulcers and
deep venous insufficiency, proper therapeutic compression is sufficient to heal
more that 90% of ulcers. However, recurrence is as high as 50% and can be more
than 80% in patients who are not compliant.[19,20] Addressing concomitant perforator
and superficial disease can improve the results of conservative care, decreasing
recurrence rates to just 15% in patients not afflicted with a postthrombotic condition
(primary incompetence).[21] In a population study, 48% of patients with deep venous
disease also had superficial venous disease, an important concomitant pathologic

complication to recognize because treatment is less invasive and of proven benefit.[5] Outcomes are worse in patients with postthrombotic deep venous insufficiency than in those with primary incompetence, with recurrence rates greater than 50%.[21] This may well be because venous occlusive disease is present in 55% of patients with chronic venous insufficiency[2] and, in appropriate patients, treating iliofemoral venous occlusive disease alone can result in ulcer healing in 60% of patients.[22] For these reasons, and likely also because of the technical challenge of addressing deep venous disease, surgical repair of deep valvular incompetence often remains the treatment of last resort.[6] Per current guidelines, open reconstruction is considered for patients who have had evaluation and appropriate intervention for any perforator or superficial venous insufficiency, or venous obstruction, and who continue to have significant disease with a CEAP score of C4b or greater despite adequate compression therapy.[6] There is controversy regarding whether surgery is appropriately relegated to the last stage in the treatment algorithm but, practically, this is so in the United States.

Having selected a patient who might benefit from surgical intervention for deep venous incompetence, options include external banding, internal and external valvuloplasty, valve or vein transposition, and autogenous valve substitution. Current guidelines suggest starting with primary valve repair or valvuloplasty if there are structurally preserved deep venous valves, though external banding may also be considered in the appropriate clinical scenario. In the absence of preserved valves, valve transposition or transplantation may be considered and autogenous valve substitute can benefit patients who have no other options.[6]

In the 1970s, it was demonstrated that surgical repair of incompetent valves was both feasible and efficacious.[23,24] Since then, numerous techniques have evolved, most of which involve the basic principle of restoring competence by reducing the redundancy of valve leaflets. Importantly, valvuloplasty does require architecturally intact valve cusps present to allow repair. During surgery, the absence of valve attachment lines may indicate that the valve has been destroyed, leaving scarred and damage cusps not amenable to this technique. This situation is most commonly observed in patients with reflux secondary to deep venous thrombosis (DVT). These patients are not generally candidates for valvuloplasty.[25,26]

Internal valvuloplasty is a form of primary valve repair that involves creating a venotomy to expose and directly visualize the valve cusps. The venotomy incisions used have taken many forms consisting of a single longitudinal,[27] single supravalvular transverse,[28] a T incision,[29] or a trapdoor incision.[30] The tradeoffs of adequacy include exposure, risk of damaging the valve, and difficulty of closure with increasing incision complexity. Once the valve cusps are visualized, excess valve laxity is reefed in by tacking the lateral edges of the valve cusps to the apices of their respective commissures, effectively gathering the redundant valve to the vein wall.[27–30] Alternatively, but less commonly applied, the excess valve can be excised and the edge of the remaining valve cusps reimplanted along the edge of the venotomy.[31] In either case, leaflet length must usually be reduced by approximately 20% to restore valve competency.[32] Although being able to repair the valve under direct visualization is an advantage of internal valvuloplasty, the decision of how much redundancy to take is clearly subjective, based on experience, and valve competence cannot be tested until after the venotomy has been closed. Additionally, flawless technique is required because taking either too much or too little valve will render the effort fruitless. Failure to evert the venotomy edges during closure can leave collagen exposed with an increased risk of DVT. After closure, vein competence can be evaluated using the strip test, which consists of milking the distally clamped vein from distal to proximal and evaluating for refilling of the infravalvular vein across the valve when retrograde pressure is applied (Valsalva, proximal compression).

As opposed to internal valvuloplasty, external valvuloplasty is a technique that has the advantage of not requiring a venotomy and being able to test for restoration of valve competency as each suture is placed. The lack of direct visualization, however, makes it potentially less precise because the sutures are placed blindly and require experience for proper placement. Some surgeons report less durable results than with internal valvuloplasty.[33] In the original external valvuloplasty, competence is restored by reducing the vein diameter with sutures placed to bring together the valve attachments line starting at the apex of the commissure and effectively reducing the commissural angle. This technique can include both anterior and posterior plications, and may not actually decrease redundancy of the valve leaflets.[26,34] Transcommissural valvuloplasty was a later variation on the technique that does involve reefing of the valve cusps directly. Starting at the apex of the commissure, full-thickness sutures are placed so as to catch the edge of the valve and draw it against the vein wall, effectively tightening the valve cusps with each additional suture. This technique has used of an angioscope for direct visualization of suture placement.[35–37] This was found to mainly confirm the experienced surgeons' ability to accomplish precise suturing rather than actually aiding in the placement of those sutures and was abandoned by some after experience was gained.[38]

Overall, primary valve repair is well-tolerated and effective. Internal valvuloplasty has a documented success rate of approximately 70% at 5 years with ulcer recurrence or ulcer nonhealing occurring in 30% of patients.[33,39–43] External valvuloplasty has somewhat less impressive outcomes with clinical success in 50% to 60% of patients and a higher rate of valvular incompetence on follow-up evaluation.[33,42–45] With either approach, clinical outcome was noted to correlate strongly with valve competence on follow-up.

A third option that has been used in patients with intact valves is external banding. This technique may be considered when vasospasm secondary to dissection results in spontaneously competent valves. An external sleeve is applied to the vein at the site of the valve and its diameter is adjusted to maintain valve competence; it is then secured in place with adventitial sutures.[46,47] Outcomes are good with valvular competence in 90% and ulcer healing in 80% at a mean of 86 months in a study. It was also noted that patients did better with banding of multiple valves.[46] This technique has also been applied in conjunction with valvuloplasty to prevent postsurgical dilation and recurrent reflux at the site.[38,48]

In patients who do not have intact valves (severely foreshortened, scarred, or destroyed), vein transposition and valve transplantation are viable options. Both techniques involve the placement of an intact and competent valve proximal to the refluxing deep venous system.

For a successful vein transposition operation, there must be a competent valve in the proximal thigh. The incompetent deep vein axial system is divided proximally and anastomosed to an adjacent vein segment distal to a competent valve. The most common application of this technique involves transposition of a refluxing femoral vein system below either a competent profunda femoris vein or GSV valve.[49,50] An alternative to this is similar to the saphenopopliteal vein bypass for obstruction and involves transposing a competent GSV onto the refluxing femoral vein with ligation of the femoral vein proximally.[51] This eliminates the size discrepancy that otherwise exits between the 2 systems. Either way, the principle remains of shunting the incompetent system into a competent one. A drawback to this technique, however, is that the increased flow may result in postprocedural venous dilation and subsequent reflux at the once competent valve, and some surgeons have suggested encircling the valve with a cuff to prevent dilation. Vein transposition is overall less commonly performed than valvuloplasty and is more frequently used in patients with postthrombotic reflux.[33] Outcomes are not as favorable as primary valve repair but these outcomes remain based on retrospective analysis. Valve competence at follow-up ranges from 40% to 75% and clinical success from 50% to 75%.[39,41,51–53]

If there are no adjacent competent and patent systems, then valve transplantation can be considered and is somewhat more versatile than the transposition procedure because valves are harvested from distant locations. Potential donor sites include the axillary vein and the brachial vein of either upper extremity.[54,55] Donor veins should be evaluated carefully for valve function. A drawback to this technique, however, is that a significant portion of upper extremity valves may be found to be incompetent at the time of surgery. In such cases, valvuloplasty of the transplanted vein would be required for a successful repair but adds another layer of complexity and potential mode of failure to an already delicate operation; prophylactic or therapeutic external sleeve banding may also be considered.[26,32,48] After the vein containing the valve segment is harvested, it is recommended that the incompetent deep venous system be divided and the proximal anastomosis be completed first. This will allow evaluation of the new valve for competence by releasing the proximal clamp (no retrograde spillage of blood should result). It will also cause distention and lengthening of the transplanted vein segment such that an appropriate length of recipient vein can be removed before accomplishing a distal anastomosis free of tension and without redundant length. To decrease the risk of suture line stenosis, interrupted or partially interrupted sutures are preferred.[32] Reported outcomes of valve transplantation series are highly variable with valve competence rates at follow-up ranging from 16% to 90% and clinical success from 33% to 82%.[41–43,53,56–59] Transplantation to the popliteal location may have better outcomes because studies that included only this location had 77% to 87% valve competence with recurrent or nonhealing ulcers noted in only 20% of cases.[60,61] In general, valve transplant has inferior outcomes to other valve repairs in the same surgeons' hands[33]

Finally, in patients for whom the previous options are not possible, creation of a substitute valve seems reasonable. Variations on creating replacement valves have included the use of synthetics, xenografts, and allografts, with some showing early promise but none demonstrating convincing clinical efficacy for any length of time and not all even making it to the clinical setting. The historical development of artificial venous valves has been reviewed elsewhere in this issue.[62] A neovalve constructed from autologous vein (wholly or in major part) remains the only valve replacement demonstrated to have clinical success for any length of time and several different techniques have been described. The method described by Plagnol and colleagues[63] involves invaginating an obliquely cut stump of GSV into the femoral vein, attaching the tip of the triangular segment to the opposite wall, and then closing the GSV ostium. This creates a valve that allows proximal flow to pass on either side of the tethered vein flap while retrograde flow flares out the cusp formed by the GSV stump and prevents retrograde flow. This was shown to have good short-term results with improvement of symptoms in all subjects and valve patency in all subjects who had had adequate GSV stump for the procedure at slightly less than 1 year median follow-up. Longer term data are not available. Another method, described by Maleti-Lugli,[64] involves the creation of 1 or more valve cusps by raising an intimal dissection flap from proximal to distal of sufficient size to cover the entire vein lumen when distended to length. This was noted to be easier in thickened postthrombotic veins due to vein wall thickness, although a degree of endophlebectomy may be required to ensure a widely patent venous lumen. Depending on the anatomic consideration, a monocuspid or bicuspid valve can be created. A later refinement of the technique involves placement of stitches to hold the valve in a partially open position and prevent readherence of the flap to the wall from which it was raised. Despite exposure of subintimal layers, there was noted to be a low incidence of DVT after this procedure and after the first month patients did not require systemic anticoagulation in the opinion of the investigators. Cumulative valve competence was 85% at a median follow-up of greater than 2 years. For the subset of subject operated on before the additional stitches were incorporated into the technique, valve patency was 68% with a longer median follow-up of 54 months. Long-term data on the former subject group is still pending.[64] Opie and colleagues[65] describe the creation of a monocusp valve using a full-thickness flap of the anterior common femoral vein wall as the invaginated valve while making the vein diameter whole with a PTFE patch. The theoretic advantage is that a full-thickness flap is not as devascularized as an intimal flap might be. This technique has had promising results in 76% clinical success and 70% valve competence at a mean follow-up of 29 months.[65,66] In all, autologous valve substitutes might be a viable alternative in patients in whom no other options are available. Some surgeons might even recommend it as preferred to valve transplant.[33]

SUMMARY

The deep venous system is more difficult to approach from a surgical perspective and, therefore, has been the last system to repair if the repair of superficial or perforator systems will result in clinical relief. With the advent of endovascular methods to treat major proximal venous obstruction, open surgical techniques have been supplanted by this less invasive, less morbid, yet successful intervention. However, some patients are faced with unrelenting venous symptoms with open wounds, costly and chronic medical treatments, and a quality of life that is unacceptable. There are viable open operative procedures that do allow some expectation of relief in the short term and, in some cases, the long term. Deep venous obstruction can be bypassed at essentially every level and valvular reflux can be repaired whether or not the valve architecture has been preserved by the underlying disease process. The more complex the repair, the more risk of failure but potentially the greatest benefit. This article highlights the potential options based on disease process, available disease-free vein or valve, and patient need.

REFERENCES

1. Garg N, Gloviczki P, Karimi KM, et al. Factors affecting outcome of open and hybrid reconstructions for nonmalignant obstruction of iliofemoral veins and inferior vena cava. J Vasc Surg 2011;53(2):383–93.
2. Neglen P, Thrasher TL, Raju S. Venous outflow obstruction: an underestimated contributor to chronic venous disease. J Vasc Surg 2003;38(5):879–85.
3. Beebe HG, Bergan JJ, Bergqvist D, et al. Classification and grading of chronic venous disease in the lower limbs–a consensus statement. Organized by Straub Foundation with the cooperation of the American Venous Forum at the 6th annual meeting, February 22-25, 1994, Maui, Hawaii. Vasa 1995;24(4): 313–8.
4. Heit JA, Rooke TW, Silverstein MD, et al. Trends in the incidence of venous stasis syndrome and venous ulcer: a 25-year population-based study. J Vasc Surg 2001;33(5):1022–7.

5. Criqui MH, Jamosmos M, Fronek A, et al. Chronic venous disease in an ethnically diverse population: the San Diego Population Study. Am J Epidemiol 2003; 158(5):448–56.
6. O'Donnell TF Jr, Passman MA, Marston WA, et al. Management of venous leg ulcers: clinical practice guidelines of the Society for Vascular Surgery (R) and the American Venous Forum. J Vasc Surg 2014;60(2 Suppl):3S–59S.
7. Delis KT, Gloviczki P, Wennberg PW, et al. Hemodynamic impairment, venous segmental disease, and clinical severity scoring in limbs with Klippel-Trenaunay syndrome. J Vasc Surg 2007;45(3):561–7.
8. Jost CJ, Gloviczki P, Cherry KJ Jr, et al. Surgical reconstruction of iliofemoral veins and the inferior vena cava for nonmalignant occlusive disease. J Vasc Surg 2001;33(2):320–7 [discussion: 327–8].
9. Mendes BC, Gloviczki P, Akhtar N. Patency and clinical success 22 years after the Palma procedure. J Vasc Surg Venous Lymphat Disord 2016;4(1):95–6.
10. Coleman DM, Rectenwald JE, Vandy FC, et al. Contemporary results after sapheno-popliteal bypass for chronic femoral vein occlusion. J Vasc Surg Venous Lymphat Disord 2013;1(1):45–51.
11. Gloviczki P, Pairolero PC, Toomey BJ, et al. Reconstruction of large veins for nonmalignant venous occlusive disease. J Vasc Surg 1992;16(5):750–61.
12. Puggioni A, Kistner RL, Eklof B, et al. Surgical disobliteration of postthrombotic deep veins–endophlebectomy–is feasible. J Vasc Surg 2004;39(5):1048–52 [discussion: 52].
13. Vogel D, Comerota AJ, Al-Jabouri M, et al. Common femoral endovenectomy with iliocaval endoluminal recanalization improves symptoms and quality of life in patients with postthrombotic iliofemoral obstruction. J Vasc Surg 2012;55(1): 129–35.
14. Palma EC, Esperon R. Vein transplants and grafts in the surgical treatment of the postphlebitic syndrome. J Cardiovasc Surg (Torino) 1960;1:94–107.
15. Raju S, Hollis K, Neglen P. Obstructive lesions of the inferior vena cava: clinical features and endovenous treatment. J Vasc Surg 2006;44(4):820–7.
16. Ijima H, Kodama M, Hori M. Temporary arteriovenous fistula for venous reconstruction using synthetic graft: a clinical and experimental investigation. J Cardiovasc Surg (Torino) 1985;26(2):131–6.
17. Ashrani AA, Silverstein MD, Lahr BD, et al. Risk factors and underlying mechanisms for venous stasis syndrome: a population-based case-control study. Vasc Med 2009;14(4):339–49.
18. Ashrani AA, Silverstein MD, Rooke TW, et al. Impact of venous thromboembolism, venous stasis syndrome, venous outflow obstruction and venous valvular incompetence on quality of life and activities of daily living: a nested case-control study. Vasc Med 2010;15(5):387–97.
19. Mayberry JC, Moneta GL, Taylor LM Jr, et al. Fifteen-year results of ambulatory compression therapy for chronic venous ulcers. Surgery 1991;109(5):575–81.
20. Erickson CA, Lanza DJ, Karp DL, et al. Healing of venous ulcers in an ambulatory care program: the roles of chronic venous insufficiency and patient compliance. J Vasc Surg 1995;22(5):629–36.
21. Kalra M, Gloviczki P, Noel AA, et al. Subfascial endoscopic perforator vein surgery in patients with post-thrombotic venous insufficiency–is it justified? Vasc Endovascular Surg 2002;36(1):41–50.
22. Raju S, Owen S Jr, Neglen P. The clinical impact of iliac venous stents in the management of chronic venous insufficiency. J Vasc Surg 2002;35(1):8–15.

23. Kistner RL. Surgical repair of the incompetent femoral vein valve. Arch Surg 1975; 110(11):1336–42.

24. Ferris EB, Kistner RL. Femoral vein reconstruction in the management of chronic venous insufficiency. A 14-year experience. Arch Surg 1982;117(12):1571–9.

25. Maleti O. Venous valvular reconstruction in post-thrombotic syndrome. A new technique. J Mal Vasc 2002;27(4):218–21.

26. Raju S, Hardy JD. Technical options in venous valve reconstruction. Am J Surg 1997;173(4):301–7.

27. Eklof BG, Kistner RL, Masuda EM. Venous bypass and valve reconstruction: long-term efficacy. Vasc Med 1998;3(2):157–64.

28. Raju S. Venous insufficiency of the lower limb and stasis ulceration. Changing concepts and management. Ann Surg 1983;197(6):688–97.

29. Sottiurai VS. Technique in direct venous valvuloplasty. J Vasc Surg 1988;8(5): 646–8.

30. Tripathi R, Ktenidis KD. Trapdoor internal valvuloplasty–a new technique for primary deep vein valvular incompetence. Eur J Vasc Endovasc Surg 2001;22(1): 86–9.

31. Verma H, Srinivas R, George RK, et al. Reduction internal valvuloplasty is a new technical improvement on plication internal valvuloplasty for primary deep vein valvular incompetence. J Vasc Surg Venous Lymphat Disord 2014;2(4):383–9.

32. Raju S, Fredericks R. Valve reconstruction procedures for nonobstructive venous insufficiency: rationale, techniques, and results in 107 procedures with two- to eight-year follow-up. J Vasc Surg 1988;7(2):301–10.

33. Maleti O, Perrin M. Reconstructive surgery for deep vein reflux in the lower limbs: techniques, results and indications. Eur J Vasc Endovasc Surg 2011;41(6): 837–48.

34. Kistner R. Surgical technique of external venous valve repair. Straub Found Proc 1990;55:15–6.

35. Gloviczki P, Merrell SW, Bower TC. Femoral vein valve repair under direct vision without venotomy: a modified technique with use of angioscopy. J Vasc Surg 1991;14(5):645–8.

36. Jing ZP, Cao GS, Zhou YI. Superficial femoral vein valvuloplasty under direct angioscopic vision. Zhonghua Wai Ke Za Zhi 1994;32(6):376–9 [in Chinese].

37. Welch HJ, McLaughlin RL, O'Donnell TF Jr. Femoral vein valvuloplasty: intraoperative angioscopic evaluation and hemodynamic improvement. J Vasc Surg 1992; 16(5):694–700.

38. Raju S, Berry MA, Neglen P. Transcommissural valvuloplasty: technique and results. J Vasc Surg 2000;32(5):969–76.

39. Masuda EM, Kistner RL. Long-term results of venous valve reconstruction: a four- to twenty-one-year follow-up. J Vasc Surg 1994;19(3):391–403.

40. Kistner RL, Eklof B, Masuda EM. Deep venous valve reconstruction. Cardiovasc Surg 1995;3(2):129–40.

41. Perrin M. Reconstructive surgery for deep venous reflux: a report on 144 cases. Cardiovasc Surg 2000;8(4):246–55.

42. Raju S, Fredericks RK, Neglen PN, et al. Durability of venous valve reconstruction techniques for "primary" and postthrombotic reflux. J Vasc Surg 1996;23(2): 357–66 [discussion: 366–7].

43. Tripathi R, Sieunarine K, Abbas M, et al. Deep venous valve reconstruction for non-healing leg ulcers: techniques and results. ANZ J Surg 2004;74(1–2):34–9.

44. Rosales A, Slagsvold CE, Kroese AJ, et al. External venous valve plasty (EVVP) in patients with primary chronic venous insufficiency (PCVI). Eur J Vasc Endovasc Surg 2006;32(5):570–6.
45. Wang SM, Hu ZJ, Li SQ, et al. Effect of external valvuloplasty of the deep vein in the treatment of chronic venous insufficiency of the lower extremity. J Vasc Surg 2006;44(6):1296–300.
46. Lane RJ, Cuzzilla ML, McMahon CG. Intermediate to long-term results of repairing incompetent multiple deep venous valves using external valvular stenting. ANZ J Surg 2003;73(5):267–74.
47. Camilli S, Guarnera G. External banding valvuloplasty of the superficial femoral vein in the treatment of primary deep valvular incompetence. Int Angiol 1994; 13(3):218–22.
48. Jamieson WG, Chinnick B. Clinical results of deep venous valvular repair for chronic venous insufficiency. Can J Surg 1997;40(4):294–9.
49. Kistner RL, Sparkuhl MD. Surgery in acute and chronic venous disease. Surgery 1979;85(1):31–43.
50. Raju S, Fountain T, Neglen P, et al. Axial transformation of the profunda femoris vein. J Vasc Surg 1998;27(4):651–9.
51. Cardon JM, Cardon A, Joyeux A, et al. Use of ipsilateral greater saphenous vein as a valved transplant in management of post-thrombotic deep venous insufficiency: long-term results. Ann Vasc Surg 1999;13(3):284–9.
52. Johnson ND, Queral LA, Flinn WR, et al. Late objective assessment of venous value surgery. Arch Surg 1981;116(11):1461–6.
53. Lehtola A, Oinonen A, Sugano N, et al. Deep venous reconstructions: long-term outcome in patients with primary or post-thrombotic deep venous incompetence. Eur J Vasc Endovasc Surg 2008;35(4):487–93.
54. Taheri SA, Lazar L, Elias S. Status of vein valve transplant after 12 months. Arch Surg 1982;117(10):1313–7.
55. Taheri SA, Lazar L, Elias S, et al. Surgical treatment of postphlebitic syndrome with vein valve transplant. Am J Surg 1982;144(2):221–4.
56. Eriksson I, Almgren B. Surgical reconstruction of incompetent deep vein valves. Ups J Med Sci 1988;93(2):139–43.
57. Dalsing MC, Raju S, Wakefield TW, et al. A multicenter, phase I evaluation of cryopreserved venous valve allografts for the treatment of chronic deep venous insufficiency. J Vasc Surg 1999;30(5):854–64.
58. Rosales A, Jorgensen JJ, Slagsvold CE, et al. Venous valve reconstruction in patients with secondary chronic venous insufficiency. Eur J Vasc Endovasc Surg 2008;36(4):466–72.
59. Taheri SA, Heffner R, Budd T, et al. Five years' experience with vein valve transplant. World J Surg 1986;10(6):935–7.
60. Bry JD, Muto PA, O'Donnell TF, et al. The clinical and hemodynamic results after axillary-to-popliteal vein valve transplantation. J Vasc Surg 1995;21(1):110–9.
61. Nash T. Long term results of vein valve transplants placed in the popliteal vein for intractable post-phlebitic venous ulcers and pre-ulcer skin changes. J Cardiovasc Surg (Torino) 1988;29(6):712–6.
62. Dalsing M. Artificial venous valves. In: Gloviczki P, editor. The handbook of venous disorders. London: Hodder Arnold; 2009. p. 483–90.
63. Plagnol P, Ciostek P, Grimaud JP, et al. Autogenous valve reconstruction technique for post-thrombotic reflux. Ann Vasc Surg 1999;13(3):339–42.
64. Lugli M, Guerzoni S, Garofalo M, et al. Neovalve construction in deep venous incompetence. J Vasc Surg 2009;49(1):156–62, 162.e1–2; [discussion: 162].

65. Opie JC, Izdebski T, Payne DN, et al. Monocusp - novel common femoral vein monocusp surgery uncorrectable chronic venous insufficiency with aplastic/dysplastic valves. Phlebology 2008;23(4):158–71.
66. Ignatyev IM, Akhmetzyanov RV. Long-term results of the monocusp valve formation in the common femoral vein in patients with avalvular deep veins of the lower extremities. Int Angiol 2017;36(2):116–21.

Thermal and Nonthermal Endovenous Ablation Options for Treatment of Superficial Venous Insufficiency

Misaki M. Kiguchi, MD[a],*, Ellen D. Dillavou, MD[b]

KEYWORDS

- Radiofrequency ablation • Laser ablation • Polidocanol foam • Cyanoacralate glue
- Mechanochemical ablation

KEY POINTS

- Thermal and nonthermal endovenous ablation options have revolutionized venous care.
- Thermal and nonthermal endovenous ablation options are safe and effective.
- Thermal and nonthermal endovenous ablation options are often minimally invasive and performed in ambulatory outpatient setting, allowing greater accessibility to millions of people.

 Video content accompanies this article at http://www.surgical.theclinics.com.

INTRODUCTION

Chronic venous insufficiency is a common medical condition that affects between 5% and 30% of the adult population.[1] It affects all age groups and is more prevalent than peripheral arterial disease.[2] Venous insufficiency is a progressive disease, with edema, pain, skin changes, hyperpigmentation, and ulcerations causing disability and becoming chronic burdens to the health care system.[3] Treatment is aimed at improving symptoms and correctly the underlying abnormality, if possible.

Saphenous removal, phlebectomy, and venous ligation were the historic surgical treatments for venous disease. However, these treatments often require general anesthesia, which prolongs recovery time beyond the actual procedure itself and puts the patient at systemic risk. Open surgical procedures can also be associated with infections, paresthesia, and recurrence.[4]

---

[a] Department of Vascular Surgery, MedStar Washington Hospital Center, 106 Irving Street, NW, Washington, DC 20010, USA; [b] Vascular Surgery Clinic, Duke Regional Hospital, 407 Crutchfield Street, Durham, NC 27704, USA
* Corresponding author.
E-mail address: Misaki.M.Kiguchi@medstar.net

Surg Clin N Am 98 (2018) 385–400
https://doi.org/10.1016/j.suc.2017.11.014
0039-6109/18/© 2017 Elsevier Inc. All rights reserved.

Recently, duplex ultrasound scanning has increased in resolution to be able to accurately diagnose venous insufficiency. This is now widely available. Advancements in percutaneous technology use ultrasound and have allowed endovenous modalities to be used for treatment of chronic venous insufficiency. These procedures have an excellent safety and efficacy profiles, compared with their more open surgical counterparts, with the added benefits of minimal anesthesia, low complication rates, and decreased recurrence rates.

PREOPERATIVE PLANNING

Preoperative planning begins with a comprehensive history and physical examination.

- History
  - Allergies
  - Comorbid conditions
  - Symptoms of chronic venous insufficiency
  - Personal and family history of deep vein thrombosis (DVT) and hypercoagulable states
  - Compression use
- Physical examination
  - Tactile and visual examination for varicosities
  - Assess distribution of varicosities to pinpoint sites of venous dysfunction
  - Assess for skin discoloration, swelling, and ulcers

The application of color duplex sonography is essential to the use of endovenous techniques to treat chronic venous insufficiency. Duplex ultrasound examination is necessary for the preoperative, intraoperative, and postoperative steps for endovenous procedures. The preoperative history and physical examination is followed by a duplex examination to assess for DVT and reflux (**Figs. 1** and **2**).

Venous ultrasound examination
- Should be performed standing or steep reverse Trendelenburg
- Will delineate anatomy
  - Anterior accessory vein
  - Small saphenous vein
  - Possible presence of a duplicated saphenous vein
  - Great saphenous vein
  - Remnant veins after phlebectomy and stripping
  - Deep veins
- For each of these veins
  - Assess reflux
  - Measure reflux time
  - Measure diameter
- Deep veins are imaged for
  - Acute and chronic thrombus
  - Scarring and webs
  - Reflux time
- Perforator veins in CEAP (clinical, etiologic, anatomic and pathophysiologic) classes 4 to 6 are evaluated for
  - Diameter
  - Reflux
  - In CEAP classes 1 to 3, the patient may have the same perforator vein evaluation as clinically indicated

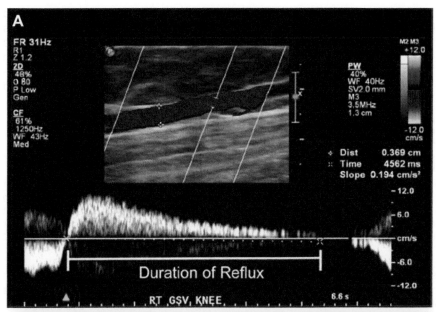

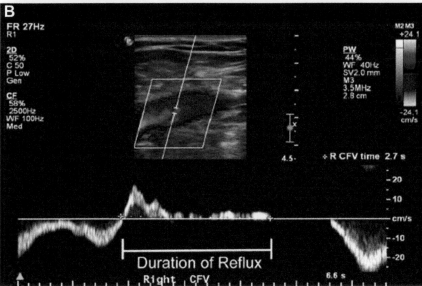

Fig. 1. (*A*) Augmentation and reflux measurement in the great saphenous vein below the knee. Reflux time of 4562 ms is well above the 500-ms threshold for significant reflux in the superficial veins. A 3.7-mm vein diameter at this location demonstrates mild dilation. (*B*) Augmentation and reflux measurement in the common femoral vein. Reflux time of 2200 ms is well above the 1000-ms threshold for significant reflux in the deep veins.

PREPARATION AND PATIENT POSITIONING FOR ABLATION
Indications

Thermal and non thermal endovenous saphenous ablation is indicated for patients with both symptoms of venous insufficiency and anatomy which demonstrates venous

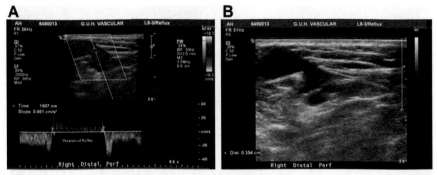

Fig. 2. (A) Augmentation and reflux measurement of a distal calf perforator. Reflux time of 1907 ms is well above the 500-ms threshold for significant reflux in the superficial veins. (B) A 3.54-mm subfascial vein diameter at this location demonstrates significant dilation. Most normal perforator veins have a subfascial diameter of less than 3 mm.[29] Reflux after augmentation of a perforator in color mode (top) and in b mode (bottom).

reflux and dilation in a distribution which corresponding to symptoms. The entirety of this topic is too broad to be adequately covered by a single chapter, but the principles of indication are described below.

Reflux of more than 500 msec in the great, small or accessory saphenous veins is considered the minimum threshold at which ablation is indicated. Many, if not most, patients with symptomatic reflux have more than 1 second of reflux time and many practitioners chose to use this as a threshold for treatment. In general, dilation of more than 5 mm is usually seen with symptomatic reflux and this size or larger is often demanded by insurance companies as a condition to finance treatment.

Symptoms consistent with axial reflux include leg swelling, heaviness, aching, tender varicosities and nighttime leg pain. Less common complaints include recurrent superficial thrombophlebitis, recurrent rash in the distribution of the reflux and itching. All of these symptoms should improve with consistent wearing of compression stockings during the day, at least 20-30 mmHg. With increasingly severe reflux there can be hemosiderin deposition, skin damage and ulceration. In general, local symptoms are commonly seen in the region of the medial malleolus for great saphenous reflux and in the lateral malleolar region for small saphenous reflux.

When assessing a patient an ultrasound is typically performed for symptoms as outlined above and/or for bulging varicosities of > 5 mm. Patients presenting with spider telangiectasias only do not suffer from symptomatic venous disease and do not need a full work up. When patients have reflux in multiple axial veins and nonfocal leg symptoms such as aching or swelling it is generally most effective to treat the most abnormal vein first. If there is not a clear source of pathology then the great saphenous is generally treated from the lowest point of reflux to the groin. This may correct or decrease reflux in other venous beds and typically results in the most symptom relief. If symptoms persist and can be attributed to other still-refluxing veins then these should be treated. Recently some insurance companies have insisted that all venous ablations be done in a single sitting. If this is the case then all refluxing veins should be treated if the practitioner feels this is safe, is clinically indicated, and the patient desires this treatment plan.

Patients are instructed to be hydrated and ambulate before the procedure to ensure maximum distention of the leg veins. The room is warmed to decrease vasospasm, with the addition of warm compresses or blankets as is needed and available.

The patient is laid supine for accessory, great saphenous, and perforator vein access. The patient is laid prone for small saphenous vein access. However, if both great and small saphenous veins are to be treated in the same sitting it is possible to prepare the entire leg and access the distal small saphenous near the ankle and perform the ablation with the leg externally rotated and bent in the supine position.

Preparation for an ablation varies by technique. Generally the entire leg is prepped for a thermal, cyanoacrylate or mechanochemical ablation, and full sterile drapes are used. For chemical ablation it is only necessary to prep a small area near the knee for cannulation. Any standard prepping agent (eg, betadine, chlorhexidine, alcohol-based solutions) is adequate.

PROCEDURAL APPROACH
Endovenous Radiofrequency Ablation

Introduced in the United States in 1999, radiofrequency ablation (RFA) is a minimally invasive technique to provide controlled thermal heat to close a refluxing vein (**Fig. 3**, Video 1). The ClosureFAST catheter (Medtronic, Minneapolis, MN) has a 3- or 7-cm bipolar electrode affixed to its distal end to treat refluxing accessory and saphenous vein (**Fig. 4**). A perforator RFA catheter has a pinpoint bipolar electrode affixed to its distal end to treat refluxing perforator veins. The electrode makes direct contact with the vein wall to deliver radiofrequency energy, causing destruction of the endothelium, contraction of the vein wall, and thrombus formation.[5]

Steps for RFA of saphenous veins
1. Prep the appropriate leg in the standard, circumferential sterile fashion.
2. An ultrasound scan is performed as the first step of the sterile procedure or before prep to map out the saphenous and assess the vein for occlusion, aneurysm, exceptionally superficial venous locations, webbing, or other anatomic details that may make the procedure difficult or less successful.

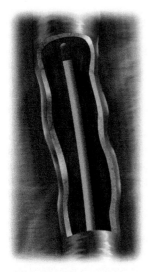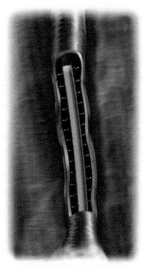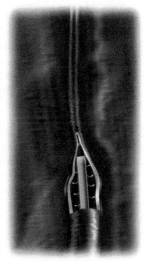

| Disposable catheter
inserted into vein | Vein heats
and collapses | Catheter withdrawn,
closing vein |

Fig. 3. Endovenous radiofrequency ablation.

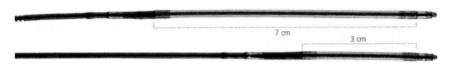

7 cm

3 cm

Fig. 4. Endovenous radiofrequency ablation catheters.

3. Access the vein percutaneously using ultrasound guidance after anesthetizing the superficial skin with lidocaine. Access is routinely initiated just below the popliteal area, or at the lowest point of reflux, on the medial calf for the greater saphenous vein. Accessing more distally on the great saphenous may be indicated for treatment of reflux along the length of the vein in patients with CEAP class 5 to 6 disease, but it increases incidence of saphenous nerve injury. Similarly, small saphenous access is typically in the mid to lower third of the calf as more distal access can result in sural nerve injury.

4. Thread the microwire through the needle and confirm its placement under ultrasound guidance.

5. Remove the needle while keeping the microwire in place.

6. Flush the introducer sheath with saline and place over the microwire into the vein.

7. Remove the inner dilator and wire. Rethread with 0.035″ introducer wire and insert a 7-F sheath. Flush the sheath.

8. Attach the catheter to the generator.

9. Flush the catheter with sterile saline and cap the Luer port.

10. Insert the catheter through the sheath and advance.

11. Optional: If the catheter does not advance easily, a 0.025-inch Glide wire (Terumo Corporation, Tokyo, Japan) may be backloaded into the catheter to guide catheter insertion. Alternatively, distal traction on the skin of the leg and stabilization of the vein with the contralateral hand frequently allows for the catheter to be passed though moderately tortuous veins.

12. Confirm the tip position with ultrasound guidance to be at least 2 cm inferior to the epigastric vein immediately distal to the saphenofemoral junction. For the small saphenous vein, the catheter tip should be positioned in the superficial portion of the small saphenous and not advanced past the point where the vein dives deep to form the saphenopopliteal junction. This point is typically at least 3 cm from the saphenopopliteal junction. The catheter and veins can be imaged in the longitudinal access, and the distance measured and recorded to ensure adequate distance.

13. Move the grommet to the end of the sheath to mark the position.

14. Administer tumescent in the perivenous tissue under ultrasound guidance, striving to create a halo of tumescence around the vein within the saphenous fascia. Tumescence should extend at least 2 cm proximal to the tip of the catheter to ensure adequate anesthesia and to form a barrier between the heat of the catheter and the deep veins.

15. Position the bed in a Trendelenburg position to facilitate vein collapse.

16. Apply compression over the length of the heating element to facilitate contact between the vein wall and heating element.

17. Press the white device button on the catheter handle to initiate treatment. Watts used during treatment cycle should decrease to less than 14 at some point during the cycle. Increasing compression can decrease the watts needed to treat the segment of vein.

18. When the treatment cycle is complete, index the catheter to the next shaft mark position. Apply compression over the entire heating element and start next treatment. Treat the segment closest to the junction twice. Consider a third cycle near the junction or a second cycle more distally if the vein is greater than 10 mm, if there are large branches or perforators exiting from the segment, or if the wattage does not decrease to less than 14. Do not treat any segment more than 3 times.
19. Repeat withdrawal, compression, and treatment.
20. Remove the sheath over the catheter once the vein is treated over the "hash" marks on the catheter.
21. Withdrawal until the last index mark is seen. Apply compression over the entire heating element and start the last treatment. Take care not to withdraw the catheter beyond the 3 hash mark area because a more superficial catheter location could possibly move the heating element too close to the puncture site and burn the skin.
22. Remove the catheter and sheath and apply compression over the access site for hemostasis.
23. Apply compression from the foot up to the thigh.
24. Review postprocedure instructions.

Technical considerations

This technique is very good for large veins (>1 cm), good for retreatment after recanalization, and may be difficult to pass through partially occluded or tortuous veins. Caution should be used in very superficial veins.

Endovenous Laser Ablation

See also http://venacure-evlt.com/varicose-veins/venacure-evlt/.

Endovenous laser ablation is similar to RFA, except that the catheter used to ablate the vein uses a fiber to deliver laser energy, rather than radiofrequency, to form the thermal energy within the vein lumen. The endothelial lining of the vessel is damaged, causing an inflammatory reaction to effectively close off the vein.[6] Different laser wavelengths have been used (ie, 910, 940, 980, 1064, 1319, 1320, and 1470 nm) to generate thermal energy. Multiple studies, however, have shown no significant difference in the efficacy in treating the refluxing vein between the wavelengths, but less pain and bruising with the higher wavelength laser treatments.[7,8]

Steps for EVLA of the saphenous veins are generally the same as for RFA. Differences related to use of the laser are described.

1. Once a microsheath is in place as per the standard protocol, advance a 0.035-inch guide wire to the saphenous deep venous junction under ultrasound guidance.
2. Remove the microsheath and select a long sheath based on the measured distance from the junction to the access site.
3. Remove the inner dilator and wire from the long sheath.
4. Advance the fiber into the sheath.
5. Connect the fiber to the generator and aim the beam toward the skin.
6. While holding the fiber in place, the sheath is withdrawn to the locking mechanism and locked in place.
7. The tip of the fiber is exposed approximately 2 cm past the end of the sheath.
8. Confirm the tip position with ultrasound guidance to be at least 2 cm inferior to the epigastric vein immediately distal to the saphenofemoral junction. For the small saphenous, the catheter tip should be positioned in the superficial portion of

the small saphenous and not advanced past the point where the vein dives deep to form the saphenopopliteal junction. This point is typically at least 3 cm from the saphenopopliteal junction. The catheter and veins can be imaged in the longitudinal access, and the distance measured and recorded to ensure adequate distance.

9. Administer tumescence as described.
10. Position the bed in a Trendelenburg position to facilitate vein collapse.
11. Once the machine is turned and set to 5 to 7 Watts from standby to ready mode, step on the foot pedal to deliver laser energy. Pull back the laser fiber and sheath together 1 cm every 3 to 5 seconds.
12. Treatment energy should be monitored as per recommendations for each laser type. The 40 J/cm (1470 nm laser) and 80 J/cm (810 nm laser) are frequently used settings
13. Stop treatment by releasing the pedal when the laser fiber is 1 to 3 cm proximal to the entry site.
14. Remove the fiber and sheath, and apply compression over the access site for hemostasis.
15. Apply compression from the foot up to the thigh.
16. Review postprocedure instructions.

Technical Considerations
This technique is good for large veins (>1 cm), good for retreatment after recanalization, and may be difficult to pass through partially occluded or tortuous veins, although it is generally better than RFA. Caution should be used in very superficial veins.

REHABILITATION AND RECOVERY
Ablation

Endovenous radiofrequency ablation and endovenous laser therapy
Postprocedural compression (20–30 mm Hg) is recommended for at least 7 days.[9,10] Patients are encouraged to ambulate as much as possible postprocedurally.

A duplex ultrasound examination should be performed within 72 hours after ablation to ensure there is no endovenous heat-induced thrombosis or DVT. Additional follow-up evaluations are at the discretion of the proceduralist, but often are at 3 months, 6 months, and 1 year after the procedure.[11,12]

Nonsteroidal antiinflammatory medication taken at regular intervals for 1 week can significantly decrease postprocedure discomfort. Narcotics are not prescribed routinely and patients generally do not have to take time off work. Athletics can safely be resumed the day after the procedure. Patients are asked to wear compression during exercise and are cautioned that they may have increased bruising and discomfort with vigorous exercise.

PROCEDURAL APPROACH
Nonthermal Ablation

Mechanochemical ablation
The use of heat energy to ablate refluxing veins has some disadvantages: the use of tumescent anesthesia and the potential for paresthesia from thermal damage to the nerves and burns of the skin. Mechanochemical ablation consists of a single-use catheter with a rotating wire at the tip that mechanically damages the endothelium of the treated vein. The treatment is initiated at least 2 cm inferior to the junction. The vein wall spasms closed by the rotating wire. As the catheter is withdrawn,

sclerosant is injected (typically 1% sodium tetradecyl sulfate) and distributes into the refluxing vein to cause further endothelial damage and result in vein closure (Video 2).

Steps for mechanochemical ablation of saphenous veins
1. The leg is prepped and vein is accessed as per the RFA ablation.
2. Place a 4-F or 5-F introducer, or a 4-F angiocath into the vein.
3. A syringe is connected to the open end of the microsheath or angiocath while preparing the catheter.
4. Flush the ClariVein (Vascular Insights, Quincy, MA) catheter with saline. Place the stopcock in the closed position on the catheter Luer lock. Have the sidearm face laterally when attached.
5. Attach the 5-mL sterile syringe containing sclerosant to the stopcock. Ensure there are no air bubbles. 1.5% sodium tetradoecyl has been more described for use in mechanicochemical ablation, however, 1% polidocanol can also be used.
6. Place the catheter into the sheath or angiocath.
7. Under ultrasound guidance, place the wire tip at least 2 cm distal inferior to the saphenofemoral junction. For small saphenous vein ablation, place the wire tip just distal to the fascial curve, within the straight segment of the small saphenous vein. If a gastrocnemius vein connects to the small saphenous vein, place the wire tip 2 cm inferior to the insertion.
8. Depress trigger briefly to test battery. An LED indicator should turn green.
9. Weld the catheter cartridge to the handle unit.
10. Pull back the cartridge wing further into the handle groove and turn slightly counterclockwise, clicking into the second stop position.
11. The tip of the fiber is exposed approximately 2 cm past the end of the sheath.
12. Four Position Speeds are available for wire rotation, with the following approximate settings: 2,000 (labeled as "L" or low), 2,500 (labeled as "M1" or medium), 3,000 (labeled as "M2" or medium-high), and 3,500 (labeled as "H" or high) rotations per minute (RPM). Determination of proper RPM setting is a clinical decision, but average speeds are generally 3000-3500 RPM. Speeds below this may be used if there is any patient discomfort, in areas of tortuosity or venous irregularity. The index finger depresses the motor trigger, while the thumb delivers sclerosant by pressing the syringe plunger after the stopcock is turned open.
13. Continue motor for 3 seconds to produce vasospasm with simultaneous pullback for 0.5 cm and initiate delivery of sclerosant after 0.5 cm pullback.
14. Continue treatment while pulling back 1.5 mm/s.
15. Treatment is stopped when 3 to 4 cm of catheter is left in the leg. A white mark on the catheter marks 6 cm distal to the catheter tip and alerts that only a short segment of catheter is remaining within the vein. Remember to pull out the access device out of the vein and skin over the catheter before the catheter tip reaches the access site to ensure treatment of distal vein segments.
16. Once the vein segment is treated, ultrasound imaging of the vein is performed to assess for vein closure.
17. If the vein is patent, immediate retreatment is accomplished by passing the sheathed catheter tip proximally again.
18. If the vein is occluded, the wire tip is resheathed by unclipping the syringe, twisting the cartridge wing clockwise, and moving the handle groove from the second lock position to the first.
19. Withdraw the catheter. Unsheath the wire and inspect.
20. Apply compression over the access site for hemostasis.[13]

Technical considerations This technique is good for veins less than 12 mm, poor for retreatment after recanalization, and may be difficult to pass and/or not able to be used in through partially occluded or tortuous veins. It is excellent for very superficial veins. There is a possibility of a valve being caught by the rotating wire. If this happens there may be resistance to the pullback and/or the patient may have pain. In this case it is usually treated by cessation of the motor, inspection with ultrasound and gentle rotation of the catheter and wire before restarting the motor.

Chemical ablation
See also https://www.btg-im.com/en-US/Varithena/Professional/About-Varithena/Learning-Center/Videos.

Varithena is a commercially prepared polidocanol microfoam used to treat incompetent great saphenous veins, accessory veins, and varicosities associated with refluxing saphenous veins. The microfoam differs from physician-compounded foam because it produces a foam that has uniform density, size, and stability.[14] The foam displaces blood and fills the lumen of the treated vein. The chemical contracts the vein by endothelial destruction and vessel thrombosis. This technique is unique in that it can treat most tortuous veins.

Steps for Varithena of the great or accessory saphenous veins
1. Prep the appropriate leg in the area of cannulation. Ultrasound examination is performed as described, with special attention to marking perforators and large branches.
2. Access the vein percutaneously using ultrasound guidance after anesthetizing the superficial skin with lidocaine. Access is routinely initiated at the most distal level of reflux.
3. Secure the intravenous catheter.
4. Elevate the leg 45°.
5. Generate the foam by connecting the syringe to the canister and activating the canister to release foam into the syringe in 5-mL increments
6. Inject the foam into the intravenous catheter while compressing the vein distally and over any perforators. Inject approximately 1 mL/s in the greater saphenous vein and 0.5 mL/s in accessory veins.
7. Monitor the dispersement of the foam into the saphenous vein during injection. Once the leading edge reaches 5 cm from the saphenofemoral junction, occlude the saphenofemoral junction with an ultrasound probe for at least 3 minutes. At this point, pressure is released from the distal aspect of the treated vein and over large branches. Pressure is continued over the perforators.
8. A maximum of 15 mL of foam is to be given in each treatment session. Patients can be brought back in as little as 24 hours to undergo repeat treatment as needed.
9. After 3 minutes, confirm with ultrasound examination that the great saphenous vein spasm has occurred.
10. Remove the intravenous catheter. Hold external compression for hemostasis.
11. Additional local injections into untreated varicosities can be performed using a 23-G butterfly needle.
12. Keep the leg elevated for 10 minutes while bandages with compression are applied.

Technical considerations This technique is good for veins less than 10 mm, excellent for retreatment after recanalization, ideal for use through partially occluded or tortuous veins. It is excellent for very superficial veins and very easy for patients to tolerate.

REHABILITATION AND RECOVERY
Chemical Ablation

Immediate foot dorsiflexion is advised to activate the calf muscle pump to clear any sclerosant from the deep veins. Postprocedural compression is recommended for at least 14 days. Patients are encouraged to ambulate as much as possible. A duplex ultrasound examination should be performed within 72 hours after ablation to ensure there is no DVT. Additional follow-up evaluations are at the discretion of the proceduralist, but often are at 3 months, 6 months, and 1 year after the procedure.

PROCEDURAL APPROACH
Cyanoacrylate Ablation

Steps for VenaSeal of the great or small saphenous veins (Video 3)
1. Prep the appropriate leg in the standard, circumferential sterile fashion.
2. Optional: a quick, sterile ultrasound scan is performed to mark the skin overlying the targeted treatment vein.
3. Access the vein percutaneously using ultrasound guidance after numbing the superficial skin with lidocaine. Access is routinely initiated at the most distal level of reflux.
4. Insert the microwire and sheath; remove the wire and dilator.
5. Advance the 0.035J-wire through the sheath into the vein and position the treatment catheter just caudal to the junction. Confirm position under ultrasound guidance.
6. Remove the microsheath over the wire and advance the 7-F introducer-dilator from the system over the J-wire to the junction.
7. Remove the wire and inner dilator.
8. Flush the sheath with sterile saline using a flushing syringe. Keep the syringe in place.
9. Position the tip of the sheath 5 cm inferior the junction under ultrasound guidance.
10. Extract the VenaSeal adhesive from its vial into a 3-mL syringe. Purge air.
11. Connect the 3-mL syringe to the 5-F catheter. Lock the 3-mL syringe attached to the catheter to the dispenser gun.
12. Prime the catheter by pulling the trigger to advance the adhesive to within 2 to 4 cm of the distal catheter tip.
13. Remove the saline-filled flushing syringe from the introducer.
14. Insert the primed catheter and gun complex into the introducer and advance until the laser mark on the catheter is at the hub of the sheath.
15. Pull the sheath caudal another 5 cm. Advance the catheter cephalad and lock the sheath to the catheter and gun complex.
16. Verify that the tip is 5 cm away from the junction.
17. Position the ultrasound probe just cephalad from the catheter tip and apply pressure to compress the junction.
18. Deliver 0.10 mL of adhesive in the vein by pulling the trigger of the gun. Hold the trigger down for 3 seconds.
19. Immediately pull back 1 cm and deliver another 0.10 mL of adhesive and hold for 3 seconds.
20. Pull back the entire system 3 cm. Hold transverse compression at the junction for a minimum of 3 minutes.
21. Locate the catheter tip position with ultrasound examination. Apply probe compression caudal to the previous injection and cephalad to the catheter tip, deliver 0.10 mL of adhesive, and hold the trigger down for 3 seconds.

22. Immediately pull back the entire system 3 cm and hold probe compression for 30 seconds.
23. Repeat steps of adhesive injection, pull back, and compression for 30 seconds, until 5 cm cephalad from access site.
24. Remove all catheters and apply manual pressure for hemostasis.

Technical considerations

This technique is good for veins less than 10 mm, can be used for retreatment after recanalization, and may be difficult in partially occluded or tortuous veins. It is excellent for very superficial veins and very easy for patients to tolerate (**Figs. 5** and **6**).

REHABILITATION AND RECOVERY
Cyanoacrylate Ablation

Postprocedural compression is optional for VenaSeal patients. Patients are encouraged to ambulate as much as possible. A duplex ultrasound examination should be performed within 72 hours after ablation to ensure there is no DVT. Additional follow-up evaluations are at the discretion of the proceduralist, but often are at 3 months, 6 months, and 1 year after the procedure (**Table 1**).

POTENTIAL COMPLICATIONS AND THEIR MANAGEMENT
Endovenous Radiofrequency Ablation

The 3-year follow-up data of the European Closure Fast Clinical Study Group reported low incidence of complications. Ecchymosis, erythema, hematoma, and phlebitis resolved within 1 week. The prevalence of paresthesias and hyperpigmentation improved significantly over the course of the 3-year follow-up.[15] Merchant and Pichot[16] reviewed the long-term outcomes of endovenous RFA to treat superficial venous insufficiency and reported a 0.9% incidence of DVT or endovenous heat-induced thrombosis, 1.2% incidence of skin burn, 2.9% incidence of clinical phlebitis, and 0.2% incidence of access site infections. Paresthesias were observed in 12.3% of all limbs treated at 1 week, but decreased to 2.6% at 5 years.

Endovenous Laser Ablation

The potential complications of EVLA are similar to RFA and include, but are not limited to, vessel perforation, DVT, pulmonary embolism, hematoma, infection, hyperpigmentation, paresthesia, and skin burns.[17,18] In a review of published clinical series, the incidence of endovenous heat-induced thrombosis and DVT was 0.3% after EVLA versus

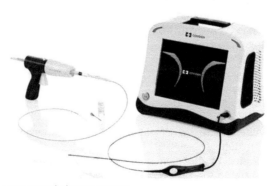

Fig. 5. Endovenous Venaseal closure system.

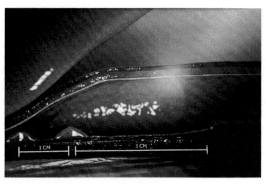

Fig. 6. Endovenous Venaseal closure system pull back.

2.1% after RFA.[19] Longer wavelength lasers are more likely to create full-thickness venous injury and cause more postprocedural discomfort than shorter wavelength lasers.[8]

Mechanochemical Ablation

The incidence of major adverse events is low with mechanochemical ablation. Studies have shown DVT, minor hematoma, indurations, and pain lasting more than 1 week as the major postprocedural complications.[13,20] Without the need for heat and tumescence anesthesia, burns and paresthesias are nonexistent.

Chemical Ablation

In addition to DVT, the most common adverse events include injection site hematoma and superficial thrombophlebitis. Severe allergic reactions to the polidocanol have been reported. Additionally, intraarterial injection or extravasation of the sclerosant can cause skin necrosis. With physician-compounded foam, there is a small but consistent reporting of neurologic complications. This incidence is increased with room air versus carbon dioxide–based foam.[21,22] There have been a few strokes

Table 1 Clinical results in the literature					
Modality	Immediate Closure (%)	Closure 12–24 mo (%)	Recanalization at 3 y (%)	Neovascularization at 3 y (%)	Significant Improvement in QoL Scores
EVLA	94[23]		6.8[24]	20[24]	+[24]
RFA	95[23]		7[24]	14.9[24]	+[24]
Mechanochemical	100[27]	94[27, a]			+[27]
Chemical–physical compounded	80[23]		26.4[24]	19.1[24]	+[24]
Chemical – commercial microfoam	86[28]				+[28]
Cyanoacrylate	99[26]	92[25, b]			+[26]
Stripping	96[23]		6.5[24]	20.2[24]	+[24]

Abbreviations: EVLA, endovenous laser ablation; QoL, quality of life; RFA, radiofrequency ablation.
[a] At 12 mo.
[b] At 24 mo.

reported that have also been thought to be due to air embolism after foam injection. Most neurologic complications reported are minor, and include visual disturbances, nausea, and coordination difficulties. These typically self-resolve in less than 30 minutes and are probably due to vasospasm rather than embolism. Patients with a right-to-left cardiac shunt and those with a history of migraine are thought to be most susceptible to embolic and vasospastic complications. In the VANISH 2 trial, there were no neurologic complications reported, raising the question of whether neurologic complications are a result of larger bubbles within foam. Without the need for heat and tumescence anesthesia, burns and paresthesias are nonexistent.

Cyanoacrylate Ablation

Potential adverse effects associated with the use of the VenaSeal system are similar to those with traditional endovenous ablation procedures. Several risks unique to the system are due to the theoretic possibility for an allergy to the adhesive, and a possible foreign body reaction to the permanent core of cyanoacrylate that remains in the vein. Approximately 8% of patients develop a phlebitic reaction after ablation, but this self-resolves and can be mitigated by nonsteroidal antiinflammatory medication. Without the need for heat and tumescence anesthesia, burns and paresthesias are nonexistent.

SUMMARY

Minimally invasive techniques for endovenous ablation of incompetent saphenous veins have proven to be safe and effective. Radiofrequency and laser ablation requires tumescent local anesthesia and have a higher risk of paresthesia or thermal complications compared with mechanochemical, cyanoacrylate ablation, or chemical ablative techniques. The nonthermal techniques have excellent early results but do not have the longitudinal history that the thermal techniques have. However, the introduction of these various endovenous techniques have provided a wide array of minimally invasive alternatives to vein stripping to those suffering from superficial venous disease.

SUPPLEMENTARY DATA

Supplementary data related to this article can be found online at https://doi.org/10.1016/j.suc.2017.11.014.

REFERENCES

1. Beebe-Dimmer JL, Pfeifer JR, Engle JS, et al. The epidemiology of chronic venous insufficiency and varicose veins. Ann Epidemiol 2005;15:175–84.
2. Gordon P, Treat-Jacobson D, Sossoman LB. Society for Vascular Nursing position statement on incorporation of vascular disease into nursing education. J Vasc Nurs 2012;30(4):135–7.
3. Heller J. Treatment of chronic venous insufficiency. Endovascular Today 2011 (October Suppl);12–5.
4. Winterborn RJ, Earnshaw JJ. Crossectomy and great saphenous vein stripping. J Cardiovasc Surg (Torino) 2006;47(1):19–33.
5. Weiss RA, Feied CF, Weiss MA. Vein diagnosis and treatment: a comprehensive approach. New York: McGraw-Hill; 2001.
6. Proebstle TM, Lehr HA, Kargl A, et al. Endovenous treatment of the greater saphenous vein with a 940nm diode laser: thrombotic occlusion after endoluminal

thermal damage by laser generated steam bubbles. J Vasc Surg 2002;35: 729–36.

7. Mauriello J, Sanchez EJ, White J, et al. Preliminary results of low energy density laser ablation treatment of incompetent truncal veins. Paper presented at the XVI World Meeting of the UIP. Monaco, August 30-September 4, 2009.

8. Kabnick LS. Outcome of different endovenous laser wavelengths for great saphenous vein ablation. J Vasc Surg 2006;43:88–93.

9. Proebstle TM. Comparison of endovenous ablation techniques. Supplement to Endovascular Today 2007;12–4. Available at: http://www.richmondveincenter.com/forms/EV_Today_Supplement_Jan07.pdf. Accessed January 8, 2018.

10. Merchant RF, Pichot O, Myers KA. Four-year follow-up on endovascular radiofrequency obliteration of great saphenous reflux. Dermatol Surg 2005;31:129–34.

11. Proebstle TM, Vago B, Alm J, et al. Treatment of the incompetent great saphenous vein by endovenous radiofrequency powered segmental thermal ablation: first clinical experience. Vasc Surg 2008;47(1):151–6.

12. Morrison N. VNUS closure of the saphenous vein. In: Bergan JJ, editor. The vein book. Boston: Elsevier; 2007.

13. Mueller RL, Raines JK. Clarivein mechanochemical ablation: background and procedural details. Vasc Endovascular Surg 2013;47(3):195–206.

14. Carugo D, Ankrett DN, Zhao X, et al. Benefits of polidocanol endovenous microfoam (Varithena®) compared with physician-compounded foams. Phlebology 2016;31(4):283–95.

15. Proebstle TM, Alm J, Göckeritz O, et al. Three-year European follow-up of endovenous radiofrequency-powered segmental thermal ablation of the great saphenous vein with or without treatment of calf varicosities. J Vasc Surg 2011;54: 146–52.

16. Merchant RF, Pichot O. Long-term outcomes of endovenous radiofrequency obliteration of saphenous reflux as a treatment for superficial venous insufficiency. J Vasc Surg 2005;42:502–9.

17. AngioDynamics, Inc: Venacure procedure kit featuring Nevertouch gold-tipped fiber instructions for use. Queensbury (NY): AngioDynamics, Inc; 2007.

18. Min RJ, Khilnani N, Zimmet SE. Endovenous laser treatment of saphenous vein reflux: long-term results. J Vasc Interv Radiol 2003;14:991–6.

19. Mozes G, Kalra M, Carmo M, et al. Extension of saphenous thrombus into the femoral vein: a potential complication of new endovenous ablation techniques. J Vasc Surg 2005;41(1):130–5.

20. Elias S. Mechanochemical Ablation (MOCA) of the Great Saphenous Vein: 2-year Results and Recommendations from the Initial Human Trial. Presented at Society for Vascular Surgery Annual meeting. National Harbor, MD, June 6–8, 2012. [abstract: SS21].

21. Guex JJ, Allaert FA, Gillet JL, et al. Immediate and midterm complications of sclerotherapy: report of a prospective multicenter registry of 12,173 sclerotherapy sessions. Dermatol Surg 2005;31:123–8.

22. Hill DA. Neurological and chest symptoms following sclerotherapy: a single centre experience. Phlebology 2014;29:619–27.

23. Rasmussen LH, Lawaetz M, Bjoern L, et al. Randomized clinical trial comparing endovenous laser ablation, radiofrequency ablation, foam sclerotherapy and surgical stripping for great saphenous varicose veins. Br J Surg 2011;98(8): 1079–87.

24. Rasmussen L, Lawaetz M, Bjoern L, et al. Randomized clinical trial comparing endovenous laser ablation and stripping of the great saphenous vein with clinical and duplex outcome after 5 years. J Vasc Surg 2013;58(2):421–6.

25. Almeida J, Javier JJ, Mackay E, et al. First human use of cyanoacrylate adhesive for treatment of saphenous vein incompetence. J Vasc Surg Venous Lymphat Disord 2013;1:174–80.

26. Morrison N, Gibson K, McEnroe S, et al. Randomized trial comparing cyanoacrylate embolization and radiofrequency ablation for incompetent great saphenous veins (VeClose). J Vasc Surg 2015;61:985–94.

27. Boersma D, van Eekeren RR, Werson DA, et al. Mechanochemical endovenous ablation of small saphenous vein insufficiency using the Clarivein device: one-year results of a prospective series. Eur J Vasc Endovascular Surg 2012;45(3): 299–303.

28. Todd KL 3rd, Wright DI, VANISH-2 Investigator Group. The VANISH-2 study: a randomized, blinded, multicenter study to evaluate the efficacy and safety of polidocanol endovenous microfoam 0.5% and 1.0% compared with placebo for the treatment of saphenofemoral junction incompetence. Phlebology 2014; 29(9):608–18.

29. Sandri JL, Barros FS, Pontes S, et al. Diameter reflux relationship in perforating veins of patients with varicose veins. J Vasc Surg 1999;30:867–74.

Phlebectomy Techniques for Varicose Veins

Daniel F. Geersen, MPAP, PA-C*, Cynthia E.K. Shortell, MD

KEYWORDS

- Ambulatory phlebectomy • Stab phlebectomy • Microphlebectomy
- Microextraction • Stab avulsion • Removal varicose veins

KEY POINTS

- Ambulatory phlebectomy is the gold standard for removal of symptomatic residual veins after truncal reflux has been treated. This can be staged or performed concomitantly.
- Phlebectomy can be performed in a clinical or operative setting with local tumescent anesthesia to augment dissection and provides adequate pain management and hemostasis.
- Complications of phlebectomy are rare and can be minimized with appropriate risk management and proper patient selection.
- Although ambulatory phlebectomy is well known and the adopted preference of most practitioners, there are other options and new emerging techniques, such as transilluminated powered phlebectomy and cyanoacrylate closure.

HISTORY

Gaius Marius, Roman statesman, general, and 7-time consul, gained an unprecedented control of the Roman Army throughout the Mediterranean. He was passionately respected by his troops, often eating with them and sharing in their labors. He marched with them through the empire, through North Africa, into the Alps, and against the Germanic tribes and the Gauls of northern and western Europe.

His recurrent rise and falls from power were renowned throughout the "modern world." Less famous is his development of severe venous disease as a result of his campaigns and refusal to undergo treatment of his contralateral leg, once completing a phlebectomy without anesthesia. He is quoted as saying that "the cure is not worth the pain."

The description of venous disease and treatment is well documented. In 400 BC, Hippocrates was the first to conceptualize phlebectomy. He described several

---

The authors have nothing to disclose.
Department of Surgery, Division of Vascular and Endovascular Surgery, Duke University Medical Center, Box: DUMC 3538, Durham, NC 27710, USA
* Corresponding author. Clinic: 10207 Cerny Street, Suite 312, Raleigh, NC 27617.
E-mail address: daniel.geersen@duke.edu

sequential punctures in the vein could be used to get rid of the "bad blood" that fed a venous ulcer. The *Ebers Papyrus* warned against treating the "Leg Serpents," describing death from presumed hemorrhage and/or infection.

Aulus Cornelius Celsus was the first surgeon to perform a phlebectomy by taking a blunt hook or cautery to destroy the veins and made large incisions with compressive bandages.[1]

Unfortunately, much of his writings were lost or destroyed, and the art of phlebectomy was lost for more than 5000 years until Robert Muller, a dermatology-trained phlebologist from Switzerland, rediscovered it. He was growing frustrated by the poor results of sclerotherapy on larger veins, and he began using small hooks from broken hemostats to remove the veins via small holes.

By 1956, Muller had refined his procedure and presented it to the French Society of Phlebology in 1967 and the International Congress of Phlebology in 1968. These presentations were not well received. He described them as "a total fiasco. Everybody agreed that it was a ridiculous method, after which I could have buried myself together with the invention."[2] It was a slow and steady group of disciples that continued the procedure and adopted it across the world and now the United States as the procedure of choice to remove these veins.[3] Today, these interventions are performed regularly on a growing population of venous disease sufferers.

AMBULATORY PHLEBECTOMY

Ambulatory phlebectomy, stab avulsion/phlebectomy, microphlebectomy, and microextraction are all interchangeable terms to describe this technique. It consists of a method by which the larger varicose veins are removed through small skin punctures and hooks specifically designed for this purpose. It is often performed in the outpatient setting using local anesthetic and tumescent anesthesia.

Tumescent anesthesia was originally developed by Klein[4] in 1987 for liposuction and was adopted by Cohn and colleagues[5] in 1995 to avoid the painful and time-consuming infiltration of local anesthetic and to reduce the risk of lidocaine overdose. This commonly contains saline, epinephrine, and lidocaine.

The authors commonly use the term stab phlebectomy and always use a tumescent anesthesia for these patients, often under general anesthesia.

The goals of therapy are to remove the residual or remaining large refluxing veins of the limb after ligation or ablation of the source of reflux. This provides an effective and economical way to provide complete treatment of the symptomatic residual veins with a good cosmetic result.

PREOPERATIVE ASSESSMENT

Upon evaluation of the patient, a complete history, including previous deep vein thrombosis (DVT), chronic edema, family history of venous insufficiency and venous thromboembolic disease, and surgical interventions, should be collected. Each patient's reflux should be identified with venous duplex, and if unilateral or deep system reflux is noted, consideration of pelvic congestion or May-Thurner should be included.

Patients with poorly controlled diabetes, hypercoagulable state, and arterial disease should be considered higher risk. Patients who are pregnant, have infection, or have severe edema should be delayed until these issues have been resolved.

Lipidermatosclerosis should be noted and quality of the skin assessed for potential wound complications. Discontinuation of anticoagulation, if possible, will reduce bruising and hematoma formation. The novel anticoagulants, such as dabigatran, rivaroxaban, and apixaban, are relatively easy to stop and restart. A period of 24 to 48 hours should be allowed between the last doses and intervention. Low-molecular-weight heparin (LMWH) bridging for warfarin should be considered in patients at high risk, previous cerebrovascular accident from atrial fibrillation, recurrent DVT, or pulmonary embolisms (PEs). The authors recommend patients completing anticoagulation for a full 3 months following a DVT or PE before engaging in a phlebectomy and withholding treatment. Anticoagulation can often be restarted 12 hours postoperativelyl.

TO STAGE OR NOT TO STAGE

There has been debate over concomitant phlebectomy with ligation or ablation, or whether a period of time following ablation of the truncal reflux should be pursued to give the patient an opportunity to avoid the invasive intervention. Monahan[6] has presented data demonstrating 13% of limbs treated by radiofrequency ablation alone had complete resolution, and on average, 34.6% of the veins that did not resolve reduced in size by 6 months. The concern with this in today's market is the need for quicker treatment resolution because insurance carriers are only allowing one treatment per lifetime per limb and limited sessions of sclerotherapy to be completed 6 months from initial ablation.[7] It is recommended to pursue concomitant treatment when the likelihood of complete resolution of the symptomatic varicosities is not likely, given the disease burden and diameter of the veins.

TREATMENT

Ambulatory phlebectomy can be performed in a variety of settings, including clinic, operating room (OR), or other ambulatory setting. It can be completed either alone or in conjunction with other procedures. Although it can be done bilaterally, if blood loss is a concern or patient tolerance of the procedure is in question, staged intervention is recommended.

The patient should have their veins marked in the preoperative area while standing using indelible ink. A nonstaining marker should be used because permanent markers have a risk of tattooing the skin postoperatively. The patient should be involved in the marking to assure all the veins of concern are addressed. Be aware of making sure the markings are not completely washed off with the skin preparation. A near-infrared imaging device or transilluminator can be used intraoperatively because these veins can shift after surgical positioning.[8] Although the authors do not use this device, there is some evidence this can speed up the intervention.[9]

Prophylactic antibiotics should be given, and the skin should be prepared by sterile technique. There have been case studies of necrotic fasciitis and need for extensive debridement and grafting from tumescent anesthetic administration and skin floral contamination.[10] Further thromboprophylaxis should be considered in all patients with a known hypercoagulable condition, or having extensive intervention with ligation, ablation, and stab phlebectomy. There is a paucity of literature on thromboprophylaxis for stab phlebectomy alone, but data for high ligation and stripping of the great saphenous veins (GSVs) show a benefit. Incidence of PE and DVT were higher in groups that did not receive prophylaxis in a study by Wang and colleagues.[11]

Although bleeding complications were higher in the group receiving LMWH, these complications were short lived. Patients should be counseled as to the risks and benefits of anticoagulation, and the authors will often administer prophylactic LMWH postoperatively or prescribe for several days after intervention prophylactic Xa inhibitors if the patient is at higher risk.

INTERVENTION

When the patient is brought to the OR, the patient's positioning should be aligned to best approach the ablation and/or cut down for ligation of the truncal refluxing veins. If not a concern, place the patient in the best positioning for the phlebectomy.

When having to perform both a GSV and a small saphenous vein (SSV) ablation, placing the patient in the supine position and then frog legging the limb to achieve exposure of the SSV can be used.

Choice of anesthesia is by practitioner and patient preference. Providing conscious sedation can be difficult because the patient may be incoherent and the limbs may be more difficult to control. It is suggested tumescent anesthesia always be used for these patients.

It was a dermatologist, J.A. Klein, who first described tumescent anesthesia as a mechanism to create a protective block of the epidermis, dermis, and subcutaneous tissues. The epinephrine causes enough prolonged vasospasm that the rate of systemic absorption of the lidocaine is reduced, permitting greater doses of lidocaine to be administered and prolonged therapeutic times with reduced risk of toxicity.

The pharmacokinetics of tumescent anesthesia results in peak plasma levels at 4 to 14 hours and lingering for up to 24 hours. With locally administered anesthetic, plasma concentrations begin to increase in 15 minutes and metabolization occurs within a few hours.[4,12]

Cohn and colleagues[5] described the use of tumescent anesthesia for phlebectomies in 1995. Infiltrating a dilute anesthesia with a long epidermal needle allows for greater administration of the vein segments and with fewer punctures. In addition, the tumescent helps isolate the vein for dissection and causes compression, leading to less hematoma and postoperative hemosiderin deposition with inflammation. Last, some investigators on the topic have postulated a reduction in infection as a result of the bactericidal properties of lidocaine.[13,14]

Administration of the tumescent can be with 60-cc syringes and long 22- to 25-gauge epidural needles or tumescent pump. The pump will facilitate larger volumes at a greater rate, and it is recommended to not keep the needle and catheter static because intraluminal volumes can be accidently administered quickly.

If the patient is undergoing an ablation or ligation before phlebectomy, it is suggested to perform the intervention in the following order:

1. Cannulate the truncal vein first, because the tumescence can cause significant vasospasm. If choosing to ligate the same vein due to larger diameters greater than 1.3 cm (to avoid windsock effect and recanalization), mobilize the catheter above the point of ligation to assist in the dissection. Pull the catheter distal to the suture before ligating.
2. If no ablation is required, ligate and cut down on the targeted vein or perforator as not to distort the surrounding tissues and obstruct ultrasound-assisted imaging.

3. Close the wound before tumescent administration to avoid loss of tumescence and increase the possibility of endovenous heat-induced thrombosis.
4. Tumesce the surrounding veins and perform ablation and stab phlebectomy. This can be performed simultaneously if 2 operators are present.

EQUIPMENT

The supplies required for the ambulatory phlebectomy in addition to those required for any cut down or ablation should include the following (**Fig. 1**):

1. Number 11 blade or 18-gauge needle
2. Phlebectomy hooks (practitioner preference)
3. Hemostats
4. 0.5-inch Steri-Strips
5. 60-cc syringe or tumescent pump
6. Fine 22-gauge spinal needle, 5 inch (micropuncture needle can be used if spinal is not available)
7. ABD bandages
8. Kerlix
9. Stretch wraps

PROCEDURE

If possible, place the patient in the Trendelenburg position. This position will assist in hemostasis. Once the tumescent is administered surrounding the previously marked varicosities, a stab incision or puncture should be made (**Figs. 2** and **3**). They should be made roughly 2 inches apart and oriented horizontally. Orient the stab sites that would favor the practitioner's dominant hand in a pulling fashion. For sites with little subcutaneous tissue, that is, patella or pretibial aspect of the leg, grasp the skin and tissue, allowing it to well, similarly to performing an injection. This should create enough space to cleanly puncture the skin and avoid hitting the osseous structures (**Fig. 4**).

To dissect the insertion site, the blunt-ended spatula found on some phlebectomy instruments or the hook itself can be inserted to dissect the tissues. Be careful not to

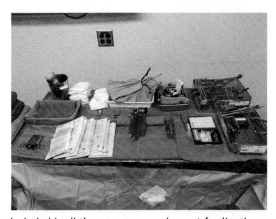

Fig. 1. Setup tray: included is all the necessary equipment for ligation and phlebectomy.

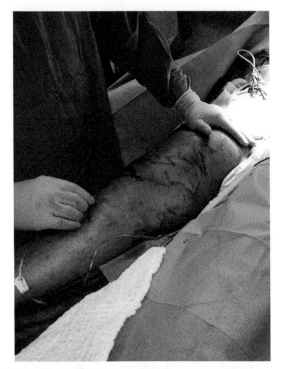

Fig. 2. Injecting tumescent anesthesia.

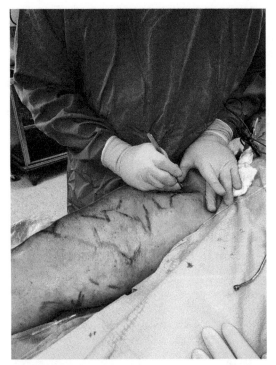

Fig. 3. Make incisions perpendicular to the vein keeping all horizontal. Place on surgeon's operative side for easy pulling.

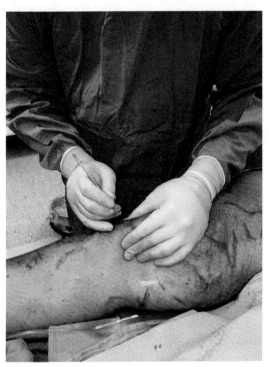

Fig. 4. Pinch the tissue over a bony prominence to avoid stabbing other structures.

disrupt the tissues surrounding the thinner subcutaneous spaces and surrounding the superficial peroneal nerve. The saphenous nerve in the calf does closely follow the medial GSV, and the sural nerve likewise follows the SSV; dissection of the calf should be more conservative than in the thigh. The hemostat should not be inserted or used to widen the stab incisions. This can cause increased distortion of the tissues and increased scarring.

Patients should be instructed before intervention that some cutaneous neuropathy may result from this intervention.

Once the hook is inserted, the practitioner should move in a sweeping motion from deep to superficial to grasp the vein. This will be performed blind. The vein, which at times is resistant to pulling up, will come up, most commonly, as a loop. The veins should be grasped with a hemostat and then pulled in a gentle back and forth motion so as to not rip the vein quickly and maximize the length removed. An alternative method is light-assisted stab phlebectomy designed to reduce recurrence from missed veins and assist in quicker identification and removal of these (**Figs. 5** and **6**).[15]

On the other hand, the hemostat can be rotated like one would rotate pasta around a fork. Two hemostats are encouraged to be used with the first anchoring the vein to keep it from reentering the skin and the other to pull (**Figs. 7** and **8**).

It is encouraged to remove as much of the vein as possible to avoid thrombophlebitis afterward. If this is not possible due to the vein shredding when removed, attempt to disrupt the vein with the hook as much as possible. As long as one

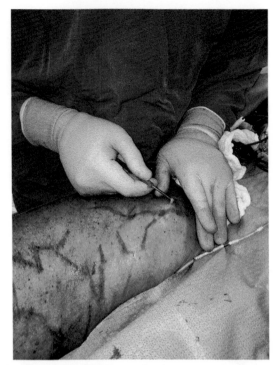

Fig. 5. Catching the vein in the phlebectomy hook.

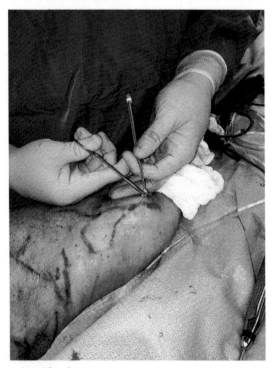

Fig. 6. Anchor the vein with a hemostat.

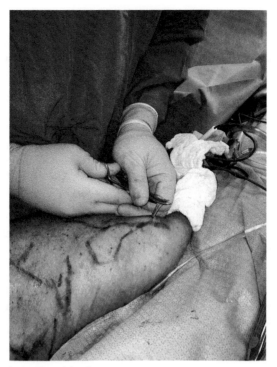

Fig. 7. Rock the vein back and forth to extract.

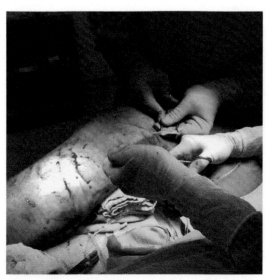

Fig. 8. A 2-surgeon team can easily be used in a larger phlebectomy case, reducing operative time.

removes or disrupts as much as possible, the patient should have an excellent result (**Fig. 9**).

The skin should then be cleaned and Steri-Strips applied. It is recommended to apply ABD dressings to absorb the higher volumes of tumescent and blood that can be seen in these cases postoperatively. Wrap the legs in Kerlix and then stretch bandages.

DISCHARGE

Postoperative hematoma formation is one of the known complications of the procedure and can be quite painful as well as result in pigmentation. Furthermore, patients and their families can be nervous about wound management and postoperative care. For these reasons, the authors are present in the post anesthesia care unit (PACU) to ambulate the patients and rewrap the leg. About 45 minutes postoperatively, the patient ambulates with the provider, and this provides assurance to the patient and their family and gives the provider an opportunity to express any hematoma before thrombosis.

The same type of dressing is reapplied in the PACU as the OR.

Provide the patient with a small amount of narcotic; typically 15 tablets of 5 mg oxycodone or similar medicine can be prescribed. Most patients do well with just acetaminophen and nonsteroidal anti-inflammatory drugs. If anticoagulation is indicated, prescribe and educate the patient on administration. After 2 days of wrapping the leg, a 20- to 30-mm Hg compression garment can be applied. This compression garment should be worn for a minimum of 2 weeks: 24 hours the first week and daily the second week.

The patient should ambulate frequently but elevate the leg at the level of the heart for the first several days. The patient should not push himself or herself, but most can return to work in 3 to 4 days. Follow-up ultrasounds should be scheduled 2 to 3 days postoperatively if ligation or ablation was performed simultaneously. If not, a 1-month follow-up can be scheduled. The Steri-Strips should

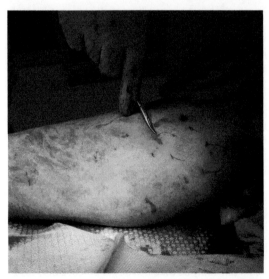

Fig. 9. Remove the residual wick to avoid poor skin healing and prevent chronic drainage.

be removed after 10 to 14 days. The patient should monitor for signs of infection and DVT or PE.

COMPLICATIONS

Complications with phlebectomy are rare. Although serious complications like DVT or PE have been documented, these are typically seen in patients who are nonambulatory postoperatively. The most common issue seen by the authors is skin allergy to the compression stocking, Steri-Strip adhesive, or skin preparation. These cases can range from mild to significant blistering and/or aseptic folliculitis. Other common complications include telangiectasial matting, hematoma formation, hemosiderin deposition, cellulitis, and neuropathy.[16,17]

Both Ramelet[16] and Olivencia[17] describe a full complement of outcomes as noted in the tabular material in later text. Ramelet published the complication rates of investigators, ranging from skin blistering being the most common and telangiectatic matting. The reports of blistering ranged from 1.3% to 20%. Sclerotherapy of this matting can be considered, although this typically results in similar formation of the blemishes. Cutaneous laser therapy may be the most appropriate treatment of this frustrating outcome.

Peripheral lymphoceles should be noted especially when forming rapidly and can be controlled with proper compression, although ambulatory drainage may be required. They are most common in the pretibial or popliteal spaces.

Certainly patients who have a predisposition to pigmentation, or matting, will have higher incidence of this and should be educated of this before intervention. Missed veins are less common but can easily be addressed with sclerotherapy afterward. Again, patients who are at risk for hypercoagulable state, that is, hormone replacement therapy, obesity, auto-inflammatory conditions like ulcerative colitis or lupus, and those who smoke or have to travel long distances home should receive prophylactic anticoagulation.[18,19]

Postoperative complications
Cutaneous
Skin blisters
Pigmentation
Scars
Contact dermatitis
Skin necrosis
Vascular
Hematoma
Phlebitis
Matting
Lymphatic pseudocyst
Deep vein thrombosis
Edema
Neurologic
Pain
Paresthesia

TRANSILLUMINATED POWERED PHLEBECTOMY

TriVex is a powered phlebectomy device and property of LeMaitre Vascular. It was developed by Greg Spitz when he used an orthopedic shaver and applied it to the removal of veins. It provides a transillumination and tumescent delivery with a powered phlebectomy system.[20] The concept is that by making 2 incisions, one on either side of the grouping of veins, rather than many incisions, this is quicker and less invasive.[21] The company claims faster intervention, better visualization, and a more complete vein removal.[22] Several studies are cited reporting 99.7% of patients claimed good outcomes and patient satisfaction. There were no recurrences at 3 months, and because of fewer incisions, this resulted in less postoperative pain and improved cosmetic results.[21,23]

Other studies showed no statistical significance in postoperative pain scores, and that in randomized trials there was no difference in cosmetic results.[24,25]

CYANOACRYLATE CLOSURE

VenaSeal is a nontumescent, nonthermal, nonsclerosant procedure that is the property of Medtronic. It uses an injector via a catheter that is placed in the superficial veins of the leg after a local anesthetic is administered. A cyanoacrylate glue is then injected into the veins and followed by ultrasound guidance using a few drops every inch or two. It currently has no procedure code and is not reimbursed by insurance. Patients pay out of pocket.[26]

Two studies, both industry funded, demonstrated that 94.3% and 88.5% of veins treated with VenaSeal glue remained closed after 2 years and 3 years, respectively.[27,28]

Although the market for this technology is for truncal reflux, the accessory veins are also treated commonly with the adhesive. Patients can still experience pain secondary to inflammation, but sites describe that it is unnecessary to use stockings, there is no neuropathy, and patients can resume regular exercise the day of the intervention.[29]

SUMMARY

Although the treatment of accessory veins with ambulatory phlebectomy is changing and new technologies are brought to bear, stab phlebectomy remains the gold standard for care of these patients. It continues to provide a very fulfilling result with excellent results and few complications.

REFERENCES

1. Carradice D. Superficial venous insufficiency from the infernal to the endothermal. Ann R Coll Surg Engl 2014;96:5–10.
2. Muller R. History of ambulatory phlebectomy. In: Ricci S, Georgiev M, Goldman MP, editors. Ambulatory phlebectomy. Boca Raton (FL): Taylor Francis Group; 2005. p. 33–60.
3. Kabnick LS. Phlebectomy. In: Gloviczki P, editor. Handbook of venous disorders. 3rd edition. London: Hodder Arnold; 2009.
4. Klein JA. The tumescent technique for lipo-suction surgery. Am J Cosmet Surg 1987;4:4.
5. Cohn MS, Seiger E, Goldman S. Ambulatory phlebectomy using the tumescent technique for local anesthesia. Dermatol Surg 1995;21(4):315–8.
6. Monahan DL. Can phlebectomy be deferred in the treatment of varicose veins? J Vasc Surg 2005;42:1145–9.

7. BlueCross BlueShield of North Carolina. Varicose Veins, Treatment for. Corporate Medical Policy. Last CAP Review 11/2016.
8. Zharov VP, Ferguson S, Eidt JF, et al. Infrared imaging of subcutaneous veins. Lasers Surg Med 2004;34:56.
9. Weiss RA, Goldman MP. Transillumination mapping prior to ambulatory phlebectomy. Dermatol Surg 1998;24:447–50.
10. Humber MG, Koch H, Haas FM, et al. Necrotizing fasciitis after ambulatory phlebectomy performed with use of tumescent anesthesia. J Vasc Surg 2004;39: 263–5.
11. Wang H, Sun Z, Jiang W, et al. Postoperative prophylaxis of venous thromboembolism (VTE) in patients undergoing high ligation and stripping of the great saphenous vein (GSV). Vasc Med 2015;20:117.
12. Klein JA. Tumescent technique for regional anesthesia permits lidocaine doses of 35 mg/kg for liposuction. J Dermatol Surg Oncol 1990;16:248–63.
13. Schmidt RM, Rosenkranz HS. Antimicrobial activity of local anesthetics: lidocaine and porcaine. J Infect Dis 1970;121:597–607.
14. Parr AM, Zoutman DE, Davidson JS. Antimicrobial activity of lidocaine against bacteria associated with nosocomial wound infection. Ann Plast Surg 1999;43: 239–45.
15. Lawrence P, Vardanian A. Light-assisted stab phlebectomy: report of a technique for removal of lower extremity varicose veins. J Vasc Surg 2007;46:1052–4.
16. Ramelet AA. Complications of ambulatory phlebectomy. Dermatol Surg 1997;23: 947–54.
17. Olivencia JA. Complications of ambulatory phlebectomy. Review of 1000 consecutive cases. Dermatol Surg 1997;23:51–4.
18. Heit JA, Silverstein MD, Mohr DN, et al. Risk factor for deep vein thrombosis and pulmonary embolism. Arch Intern Med 2000;160(6):809–15.
19. Bernstein CN, Blanchard JF, Houston DS, et al. The incidence of deep venous thrombosis and pulmonary embolism among patients with inflammatory bowel disease: a population-based cohort study. Thromb Haemost 2001;85(3):430–4.
20. Spitz GA, Braxton JM, Bergan JJ. Outpatient varicose vein surgery with transilluminated powered phlebectomy. Vasc Surg 2000;34:547–55.
21. Aremu MA, Mahendran B, Butcher W, et al. Prospective randomized controlled trial: conventional versus powered phlebectomy. J Vasc Surg 2004;39:88.
22. Available at: http://www.lemaitre.com/medical_TRIVEX_transilluminated_powered_phlebectomy.asp#. Accessed December 15, 2017.
23. Franz RW, Knapp ED. Transilluminated powered phlebectomy surgery for varicose veins: a review of 339 consecutive patients. Ann Vasc Surg 2008;23(3):303–9.
24. Luebke T, Brunkwall J. Meta-analysis of transilluminated powered phlebectomy for superficial varicosities. J Cardiovasc Surg (Torino) 2008;49:757.
25. Scavee V. Transilluminated powered phlebectomy not enough advantages? Review of the literature. Eur J Vasc Endovasc Surg 2006;31:316.
26. Available at: http://medtronicendovenous.com/patients/7-2-venaseal-closure-procedure/.
27. Morrison N, Gibson K, Vasquez M, et al. VeClose trial 12-month outcomes of cyanoacrylate closure versus radiofrequency ablation for incompetent great saphenous veins. J Vasc Surg Venous Lymphat Disord 2017;5(3):321–30.
28. Morrison N, Gibson K, McEnroe S, et al. Randomized trial comparing cyanoacrylate embolization and radio frequency ablation for incompetent great saphenous veins (VeClose). J Vasc Surg 2015;61(4):985–94.

29. Gibson K, Ferris B. Cyanoacrylate closure of incompetent great, small and accessory saphenous veins without the use of post-procedure compression: Initial outcomes of a post-market evaluation of the VenaSeal System (the Waves Study). Vascular 2017;25(2):149–56.

Liquid and Foam Sclerotherapy for Spider and Varicose Veins

Kathleen Gibson, MD*, Krissa Gunderson, BS

KEYWORDS

- Sclerotherapy • Telangiectasia • Spider veins • Varicose veins
- Foam sclerotherapy

KEY POINTS

- Sclerotherapy has diverse application in the treatment of cutaneous telangiectasia, superficial venous insufficiency, pelvic venous reflux, and venous malformations.
- It has an important role in the treatment of venous disease in all stages.
- It is an important tool for physicians treating venous disease, and familiarity with sclerotherapy indications, contraindications, and techniques is an important part of any vein practice.
- Management of patient expectations regarding symptom relief, improvement in appearance, and expectation of recurrent disease is of critical importance.

INTRODUCTION

Patients with venous insufficiency may present with symptomatic varicosities or advanced disease (skin changes, ulceration) or may just have cosmetically bothersome varicose or spider veins.[1,2] Techniques for treating superficial venous insufficiency include surgical stripping, microphlebectomy, and endothermal (laser and radiofrequency) and nonendothermal ablation. These techniques all have important places in the treatment of venous disease; however, sclerotherapy has the broadest role because it can be used in the treatment of venous disease at every stage of severity. Sclerotherapy is an effective and widely used modality to diminish the appearance of cosmetically bothersome lower-extremity telangiectasias.[3] Truncal saphenous incompetence can be treated with sclerotherapy, which offers an advantage over other saphenous ablation techniques in that incompetent tributary veins can be treated simultaneously with the same modality.[4] With advanced venous disease, nests of

Disclosure: Dr. Gibson receives research support from Medtronic, Angiodynamics, and Vascular Insights. She is a consultant for Medtronic and BTG.
Lake Washington Vascular Surgeons, 1135 116th Avenue Northeast, Suite 305, Bellevue, WA 98004, USA
* Corresponding author.
E-mail address: drgibson@lkwv.com

abnormal veins are often present in the dermal and subdermal beds of active and healed ulcers. Because of the thickening associated with the diseased overlying skin, microphlebectomy of these veins may not be possible, and foam sclerotherapy offers a straightforward treatment approach.[5] Foam sclerotherapy has also been used in the treatment of pathologic perforator veins.[6] Sclerotherapy has an important role in the treatment of vascular malformations throughout the body,[7] and in the treatment of pelvic venous reflux.[8] Given the diverse applications of liquid and foam sclerotherapy in the treatment of venous disease, it is important for physicians caring for venous patients to have familiarity with its potential benefits, limitations, contraindications, and side effects.

THE DEVELOPMENT OF SCLEROTHERAPY

Sclerotherapy induces injury to the venous intima, which is followed by eventual fibrosis of the vessel. A variety of sclerosants have been used in the past, but in the United States, the most commonly sclerosing agents used today are hypertonic saline, sodium tetradecyl sulfate (STS), and polidocanol (POL). Both liquid and foam sclerotherapy are widely used throughout the world.[9]

POL and STS are detergent sclerosants and can be turned into a foam by mixing them with a gas, usually room air, CO_2, O_2, or a CO_2/O_2 mixture. In 1944, Orbach described mixing room air with a sclerosant[10]; however, this technique did not gain popularity until its "rediscovery" some 50 years later. Both Cabrera Garrido and colleagues[11] of Spain and Monfreux[12] of France published papers in 1997 describing their techniques in the use of foam sclerosants.[11,12] Today, the most widely used technique is the "double-syringe" method described by Lorenzo Tessari of Italy in 2000.[13]

The techniques described by Cabrera Garrido, Monfreux, and Tessari were applied by clinicians to compound foam in their own clinical settings (physician compounded foam, PCF). A standardized proprietary foam sclerosant (Varithena; BTG, West Conshohocken, PA, USA) was approved by the US Food and Drug Administration (FDA) for the treatment of great and accessory saphenous vein and tributary vein incompetence in 2013.[14] Potential advantages of this commercially available proprietary foam is more consistent foam characteristics (bubble size, sclerosant strength) and assured sterility.[15]

SCLEROTHERAPY BASICS
Agents

The most frequently used sclerosants are outlined in **Table 1**. In the United States, the most commonly used agents are STS, POL, and hypertonic saline. Both STS and POL are FDA-approved sclerosants, whereas the use of hypertonic saline is considered to be an off-label use. The mechanism of action of endothelial injury varies depending on the sclerosing agent used. Hyperosmolar agents, such as hypertonic saline, cause diffusion of water from the intracellular space to the extracellular space, causing nonspecific cell destruction as well as hemolysis. The 2 commonly used detergent sclerosants, STS and POL, cause protein theft denaturation, which lyses of the cell wall, without hemolysis. Corrosive sclerosants are less commonly used and have a direct cytotoxic effect on the endothelium. Platelet aggregation is stimulated by all sclerosants, which then produces a dense network of platelets and fibrin, then eventually, vessel fibrosis.[16] If the process of fibrosis fails to occur, the sclerotherapy will not be successful. Selection of the appropriate concentration of sclerosant for the size of the treated vessel increases the chance for successful treatment.

Each sclerosant has different dosing, different advantages and disadvantages, as shown in **Table 2**. STS is a synthetic surfactant (soap); POL is a nonester local

Table 1
Sclerosing agents

Agent	Hypertonic Saline	Saline/Propylene Glycol	STS	POL	Sodium Morrhuate	Chromated Glycerine	Polyiodinated Iodine
Class	Hyperosmolar	Hyperosmolar	Detergent	Detergent	Detergent	Corrosive	Corrosive
Trade name	Not available	Sclerodex	Sotradecol	Asclera	Scleromate	Sclermo	Sclerodine
Distributer	Multiple	Omega Laboratories (Canada)	Mylan	Merz	Glenwood, LLC	Omega Laboratories (Canada)	Omega Laboratories (Canada)
FDA/US status	Off-label	Not applicable	Approved	Approved	Approved	Not applicable	Not applicable

Table 2
Advantages and disadvantages of sclerosing agents

Agent	Hypertonic saline	STS	POL
Advantages	Inexpensive Minimal allergy potential	Minimal pain Able to treat larger veins	Nearly painless Ulceration rare Allergy very rare
Disadvantages	Painful Ulceration with extravasation Can cause hyperpigmentation	Allergy less rare Contraindicated with severe asthma Can cause hyperpigmentation	Limited in size of veins to treat Can cause hyperpigmentation

anesthetic,[17] and hypertonic saline has only a local effect and then is rapidly diluted. Both STS and POL are deactivated quickly after injection because they are bound to circulating blood proteins.

With injection of judicious volumes of these 2 agents, the rapid binding/deactivation provides protection against systemic action on the deep veins, and the incidence of thrombotic complications with sclerotherapy is low.[18] Although they are more expensive, STS and POL are less painful upon injection than hypertonic saline, which increases patient acceptability.[19]

Concentration

Sclerosant concentration should be guided by the size of the vein to be treated. **Table 3** outlines suggested concentrations by vein diameter. In the United States, POL is available only in 0.5% and 1.0% concentrations; however, higher concentrations of POL are available in other parts of the world. STS is available in concentrations of up to 3% in the United States. More complex venous disease patterns, such as pelvic venous reflux and venous malformations, may warrant a stronger concentration of sclerosant; therefore, in these situations, STS may be the agent of choice.[7,8]

FOAM SCLEROSANTS
Physician Compounded Foam

The preponderance of foam sclerosants used throughout the world today is PCFs. PCFs are considered an "off-label" use of FDA-approved liquid sclerosants because the drug is fundamentally changed by mixing it with a gas. Because of the presence of gas, foams are echogenic with ultrasound, which allows them to be used in a controlled and directed fashion. PCFs are inexpensive and easy to produce, but they are not standardized and their composition can vary widely depending on which sclerosant and gas are selected and which technique is used to produce them. Injected foam pushes blood out of the vessel for a short distance and forms a "vapor lock" that arrests the flow of blood and keeps the active drug in contact with the venous endothelial for a longer period than would occur with the injection of a liquid.

Table 3
Sclerotherapy concentration by vein diameter

Vein diameter	<1 mm	1–3 mm	>3 mm
Detergent, %	STS 0.1–0.3 POL 0.3–0.5	STS 0.5–1.0 POL 1.0	STS 1.0–3.0 POL 1.0 (or foam)
Hypertonic saline, %	11.7	23.4	—

This "trapped drug" is not deactivated as quickly as a liquid drug would be because it has delayed contact with circulating plasma proteins. This prolonged contact with the vessel wall allows the use of lower concentrations and volumes of sclerosant when compared with liquid sclerosants.[4]

The Tessari technique of foam production is shown in **Fig. 1**. A sclerosant of the detergent case is forcibly mixed with air or physiologic gases (CO_2, O_2, or a mixture of both) through either a 3-way stopcock or a "female-to-female" stopcock (double syringe technique). The small aperture produces small sclerosant encapsulated gas bubbles. The ratio of gas to liquid is 1:4 or 1:3 depending on whether "wet" versus "dry" foam is preferred. The size of the circulating gas bubbles and the stability of the foam are dependent on the method of foam production, the gas chosen for use, and other factors, including atmospheric pressure and temperature.[20] Nitrogen gas is less soluble than O_2 or CO_2 because the amount of nitrogen in the gas used to create foam increases, the foam is more stable, but the bubbles are also less soluble in blood.[21]

Although liquid sclerosants are usually preferred for treating spider telangiectasias, foam sclerotherapy has been shown to be superior in terms of closure rates of varicose veins and truncal veins, such as the great saphenous vein (GSV). Closure rates of GSVs treated liquid POL were as low as 40% and 26% at 3 weeks and 6 months in a prospective randomized trial comparing liquid to foam sclerotherapy published in 2003. The foam sclerotherapy group had elimination GSV reflux in 84% and 80% of limbs at 3 weeks and 6 months.[22] Duplex closure rates of the GSV using foam sclerotherapy are highly variable in the literature, and differing patient populations and disease severities make comparisons between studies difficult. GSV closure rates after treatment with foam sclerotherapy range from 69% to 91%, depending on the agent

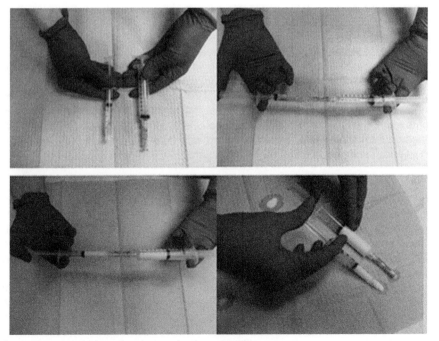

Fig. 1. Tessari technique for the production of PCF.

used, the concentration, the number of treatment sessions administered before assessing closure, and the time at which closure was assessed.[23–27] Until recently, most studies did not provide outcome assessments, such as venous clinical severity scores (VCSS) and quality-of-life (QOL) instruments. Rasmussen and colleagues'[28] often referenced trial randomized patients to surgical stripping, endothermal laser ablation (EVLT), radiofrequency ablation (RFA), or ultrasound-guided foam sclerotherapy (UGFS). All groups had similar improvements in QOL scores, but recanalization and the need for additional treatments were most common in the group treated with UGFS.[28] van der Velden and colleagues[29] performed a randomized trial comparing EVLT and conventional surgery with UGFS. The GSV was obliterated in 85%, 77%, and 23% in the surgical, EVLT, and UGFS groups, respectively. At 5 years, QOL scores in the UGFS groups were inferior compared with the other groups.

One concern for the use of PCF is a rare but serious adverse event or events, particularly neurologic injuries (strokes and transient ischemic attacks [TIAs]), that have been reported. As previously noted, when air is used to produce PCF, the compound is high in nitrogen, an insoluble gas. Most cases of reported neurologic injury occurred with the use of air-based foam. With further investigation, some patients were found to have structural cardiac defects such as a patent foramen ovale or atrial septal aneurysm.[30–33] There are some data demonstrating fewer visual disturbances and other side effects when physiologic gases are used.[34] These data, as well as the reported cases of neurologic injury with air-based foams, have led some to recommend the use of physiologic gases (CO_2 or CO_2/O_2) to produce PCF.[35] O_2 and CO_2, the "physiologic gases," have minimal nitrogen content and are rapidly absorbed in the circulation. There is little downside to using physiologic gases other than the cost of the gas itself.

Right-to-left shunts are quite common in the general population and theoretically place patients at higher risk of cerebral embolization with foam sclerotherapy. It is estimated that roughly 25% individuals have a right-to-left shunt; however, they are more common in patients with varicose veins. A study of 221 patients with varicose vein showed that 58.5% of the individuals had a right-to-left shunt with bubble testing.[36] The overall rarity of neurologic events with foam sclerotherapy, and the high prevalence of such shunts in patients with varicose veins, makes screening for shunts before foam sclerotherapy impractical and unnecessary. Caution should be used, however, in performing foam sclerotherapy in patients with a known right-to-left defect and is contraindicated if the patient has a history of previous events that led to the detection of the defect. Good standard practice in the performance of foam sclerotherapy is to use foam with no grossly visible bubbles and to limit injection volumes.

Proprietary Endovenous Microfoam

A desire to standardize and market a consistent endovenous microfoam for clinical use led to the development of Varithena. This product gained FDA approval for treatment of incompetence of the GSV, accessory saphenous veins (ASV), and their tributaries after several clinical trials proving safety and efficacy. Although it tempting to extrapolate the results of PEM trials to PCF, caution should be used in doing so because the techniques for producing PCF are not standardized. In vitro testing in a bench-top vein model has been performed, and proprietary endovenous microfoam (PEM) gas bubbles are smaller overall, with a narrower distribution of sizes when compared with PCF bubbles, and the stability of PEM foam is superior to PCF. Stable foam is easier to work with, and decreased circulating bubble size may decrease the chance of neurologic complications.[21]

To date, there have been no published reports of stroke or TIA in patients treated with PEM. During the development of PEM, the FDA expressed concern for the possibility of neurologic injury with treatment because of demonstration of bubbles in the left heart on echocardiography in some patients treated with PEM. This concern led to a phase 2 clinical trial to assess the neurologic safety of the use of PEM for the treatment of GSV incompetence. To qualify for the trial, patients with symptomatic GSV incompetence had to have a right-to-left shunt as demonstrated with a transcranial Doppler bubble test. Sixty-one patients had a demonstrated shunt and underwent diffusion-weighted MRI testing (very sensitive to the presence of edema formation) at baseline, and at 24 hours and 1-month after treatment. There were no changes in MRI findings, visual fields, or neurologic examinations after PEM treatment in any of the study patients.[37] Following the encouraging safety results from this trial, phase 3 testing of PEM with 2 pivotal trails was completed. After presentation of the pivotal trials, the FDA approved Varithena for use in November of 2013.[38]

The 2 pivotal single-blind randomized trials, VANISH-1 (275 patients)[39] and VANISH-2 (230 patients),[39] used patient-reported outcomes (PRO) as the primary study endpoint, along with change in appearance of the leg as assessed by both an independent physician reviewer and the patients themselves. The primary and secondary outcome measures were assessed at 8 weeks. GSV or ASV duplex closure was assessed, and studies compared PEM to placebo. The VANISH-1 study randomized patients to 3 differing doses of POL (0.5%, 1.0%, and 2.0), whereas VANISH-2 randomized patients to 0.5% or 1.0% POL. VANISH-2 patients could have 2 treatment sessions, separated by 1 week. Highly statistically significant improvements (P<.0001 for both endpoints) in PRO scores and appearance compared with placebo were achieved in both trials. At 8 weeks, the duplex closure rate was 80.4% in the VANISH-1 trial (with 1% POL)[39] and 86.2% for the VANISH-2 trial.[40] The VANISH-2 group was followed out to 1 year, and symptom improvement was sustained.[41] Adverse events were monitored in these trials, and other than headache, there were no neurologic events. The most common adverse events were superficial thrombophlebitis in 5.4% of patients and deep vein thrombosis (DVT) in 4.7% of patients. Most DVTs were asymptomatic and discovered as part of the study follow-up protocol with mandated detailed duplex examinations. None of the patients developed postthrombotic changes, and there were no pulmonary emboli.

PEM has several advantages over traditional heat ablation techniques in that it allows treatment of truncal incompetence and side tributaries with a single-treatment modality. It does not require a tumescent anesthesia and can treat tortuous veins through which an ablation device could not travel. In addition, because there is no risk of thermal injury, it can be used to treat veins near the dermis. In the authors' practice, PEM is often their "go-to" treatment for recurrent varicose veins and neovascularization. Disadvantages include dosing limitations, a somewhat lower duplex closure rate (although there are no head-to-head studies published comparing this modality to endothermal ablation), and a higher rate of thrombotic events (DVT and superficial thrombophlebitis), when compared with historic endothermal ablation data. A final disadvantage to PEM is cost, especially when compared with PCF.

Barriers still exist in terms of widespread adoption to PEM in that some insurers consider it to be "investigational." A dedicated current procedural technology code for billing for PEM is anticipated to be available soon, and such a code should help make carrier coverage and reimbursement more predictable.

PATIENT WORKUP AND TREATMENT
Diagnostic Workup

As with any patient evaluation, a good history and physical examination are the first step to successful treatment. A history should begin with addressing why the patient is seeking treatment, and what their goals for treatment are—whether for symptom relief or to improve the appearance of their legs. Patients without advanced venous disease and without symptoms do not require treatment (except for cosmesis) and may just be seeking reassurance that their spider and/or varicose veins are not a life- or limb-threatening health concern.

Patients should be asked about previous treatments and response to those treatments, including any adverse events they may have encountered. The risks and benefits of the procedure should be outlined and balanced next to the patient's treatment goals. Expected results should be realistically addressed as should potential recurrence of spider and varicose veins. The pretreatment consultation is a key factor to avoiding unrealistic expectations on the part of the patient, and the patient should understand that multiple sclerotherapy sessions may be required for them to achieve their goals.

A review of medical history and medications should be done to alert the provider to any contraindications the patient may have for treatment. Sclerotherapy should not be performed in a patient with active infection or acute deep or superficial thrombosis. Minocycline, often prescribed for adult acne, can cause permanent hyperpigmentation in the areas of treated veins and should be stopped several weeks before a sclerotherapy session and not resumed for about a month afterward.[42] Sclerotherapy should not be performed in pregnant women or women who are breast-feeding unless the benefit clearly outweighs the risk, which is seldom if ever the case for venous treatment. Allergic reactions are not common, but may occur.[43,44] STS is contraindicated in patients with asthma. All clinical sites where sclerotherapy is performed should have a readily available and up-to-date emergency kit in the event of an anaphylactic reaction to a sclerosant. Sclerotherapy has been reported to cause visual disturbances or migraine headache,[45] and patients with a history of migraine (especially migraine with aura) are cautioned that therapy could possibly trigger symptoms. In the authors' practice, they advise patients with a history of migraine with aura to bring any medications that they would usually take in the event of a migraine with them to their sclerotherapy session.

Sclerosant Volumes/Concentration

Both STS and POL have a maximum volume per session of 10 cc, regardless of concentration (STS in the United States is available as 1% and 3% concentrations, and POL is available as 0.5% and 1% concentrations). Multiple injections of small volumes of sclerosant are preferred to fewer injections of large volume. The lowest concentration (effective dose) of sclerosant to achieve the desired effect should be used. **Table 3** lists suggested sclerosant concentration by vein diameter. Side effects, such as matting, ulceration, and venous thrombosis, can occur when high volumes, high concentrations, or forceful injections are used.

Telangiectasias

Although spider telangiectasias rarely cause significant health issues, treatment of this most minor of venous disorders often has the steepest learning curve. With proper technique and patient preparation, sclerotherapy of spider veins is safe and effective. Target veins can be quite small, sometimes a millimeter or less, so stability of the injecting hand is very important because any extraneous movement may dislodge the needle from the vein. The sclerotherapist should position himself or herself in a favorable ergonomic position in relation to the target vein. It is a 2-handed technique, with the nondominant hand stabilizing and stretching the skin, and the dominant hand bracing the elbow, wrist, and hypothenar eminence of the dominant hand against a solid surface to ensure stability. This positioning is shown in **Fig. 2**. In the authors' practice, spider veins are treated using small needles (30 or 32 gauge) and a small-volume (3-cc) syringe. The angle of injection is shallow, with the bevel up. Bending the needle to allow a more acute angle of entry can be helpful. The liquid should be injected with very low pressure to prevent extravasation into the surrounding tissues. Typically, patients will have pain with extravasation, and a wheal will appear. Commercially available tools to aid in visualization of telangiectasias include the Syris system, Veinlite, and Venoscope (transillumination aids) and the Veinviewer (near infrared light).

Instructions for after-sclerotherapy care are not standardized evidence based. There is a paucity of data regarding exercise, bathing, and sun exposure following sclerotherapy. Most practitioners recommend compression after sclerotherapy, but the type, strength, and duration of compression use is highly variable. A randomized trial of 100 patients compared results in women treated with 3 weeks of 23 to 32 mm Hg compression stockings versus no stockings following sclerotherapy of telangiectasias and reticular veins. The study found no difference in adverse events between the 2 groups, but did find a significant difference ($P = .026$) in favor of compression in terms of improvement in appearance as rated by blinded observers.[46]

Varicose Veins

PCF treatment of varicose veins is facilitated by UGFS; however, it can be performed with confirmation of needle placement with blood return. Advantages to the use of ultrasound are confirmation of intravenous needle placement, demonstration of spasm in the treated vein, and the ability to follow the PCF as it travels through the vein. The authors typically mark the veins with an indelible pen with the patient in the standing position and use a 23- or 25-gauge butterfly needle when treating varicose veins. Multiple injections with small volumes are recommended, to avoid inadvertent boluses of foam into the deep system. Ultrasound images of a varicose vein treated with PCF showing needle placement and vasospasm are shown in **Fig. 3**. The authors' practice places patients in a 20- to 30-mm Hg stocking with or without underlying pressure

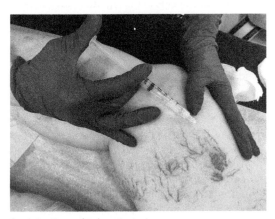

Fig. 2. Positioning for injection of telangiectasias.

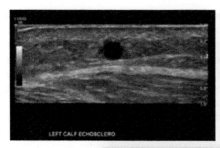
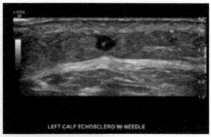
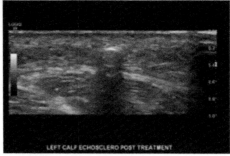

Fig. 3. Ultrasound-guided foam sclerotherapy.

pads for 2 weeks after treatment. Patients walk for 10 minutes after the procedure and are encouraged to walk/be physically active hourly during the first 2 weeks after treatment.

UGFS can be a helpful treatment in advanced venous disease in patients with lipodermatosclerosis or ulceration as an adjunct to truncal ablation and compression therapy.[47] Society for Vascular Surgery/American Venous Forum (SVS/AVF) guidelines recommend treatment of pathologic perforator veins (those >3.5 mm in diameter with >500 ms of reflux near an open or healed ulceration) to aid in ulcer healing and prevent recurrence in patients with CEAP clinical class 5 or 6 disease.[48] UGFS can be used to treat nests of subdermal varices as well as pathologic perforator veins. One study showed a 75% improvement in patients' VCSS and venous disability scores with treatment of pathologic perforator veins with UGFS.[6]

Nonsaphenous source varicose veins in the leg often have a pelvic source.[49] UGFS can be used to treat pelvic source varicose veins in the perineum and leg. PCF has been used extensively for both treatment of pelvic venous insufficiency on its own and as an adjunct to coil embolization of the gonadal veins.[50] A final essential use of sclerosants is the treatment of vascular malformations.[51] Vascular malformations may require multiple sclerotherapy sessions, and recurrence is not uncommon.

Saphenous Incompetence

As described previously in this article, PCF can be used to treat saphenous incompetence, but no standardization of technique exists. In contrast, the technique for GSV or ASV ablation with PEM is standardized and outlined in its instructions for use.[52] Access into the truncal vein is performed in a standard fashion with ultrasound guidance using either a micropuncture set or an angiocatheter. For the GSV, the tip of the catheter is usually in the mid thigh. After blood return is confirmed and the catheter is flushed, the limb is elevated to 45°. After preparation of the PEM, compression is held caudal to the access site and the injection is performed with a silicone-free syringe. During injection, a second individual visualizes the saphenofemoral junction (SFJ) in longitudinal view. The PEM will arrive as a bright white column, and when visualized 2 to 3 cm from the SFJ, the junction will be compressed with the ultrasound probe to hold the PEM in place and prevent premature entry into the deep veins. The distal compression is then released. The SFJ is compressed until the GSV or ASV is visualized with ultrasound and found to be in complete spasm along the treatment length, with no areas of patency. Pressure is continued for about 3 to 5 minutes, and a typical GSV can be treated with 4 to 7 cc of PEM. Up to 15 cc of PEM can be used in one session and can include injections into tributaries.

Following treatment of the truncal vein in the thigh, it can be treated more caudally by either pulling the access catheter back slightly, compressing above the tip of the catheter and injecting retrograde through the catheter, or accessing the vein in another location. Side branches are then accessed using a butterfly or other needle, and injecting small volumes of PEM (1–2 cc per injection) while compressing any large perforator veins associated with the side branches being treated. Following completion of treatment, the leg is wrapped with a short-stretch bandage, a compression pad, and a compression stocking. Patients are instructed to walk or be active for 5 to 10 minutes out of every waking hour for the first 2 weeks after the procedure. More than one treatment session may be required for optimal results in patients with extensive branch varicosities.

ADVERSE REACTIONS

Strokes, the most dreaded sclerotherapy complication, are fortunately rare. Migraines and visual disturbances, however, are more commonly reported and can occur with the use of either liquid or foam sclerotherapy. It is estimated that the prevalence of transient visual disturbance with sclerotherapy ranges from 0.09% to 2% in a recent review of the literature.[53] There are several proposed mechanisms for visual disturbance and migraine with sclerotherapy, including gas and particle microemboli, or the release of endothelin from the treated veins. Rat models show that circulating endothelin, a potent vasoconstrictor and bronchoconstrictor, is increased with foam sclerotherapy.[54] The endothelin hypothesis is especially intriguing because it helps explain why visual disturbances may occur with liquid sclerotherapy.

DVT can occur following sclerotherapy, with either liquids, PCF, or PEM. The prevalence of reported DVT and pulmonary embolism after sclerotherapy was 0.8% and 0.2%, respectively, in a review of nearly one million subjects undergoing venous procedures. These rates were lower than reported rates for endothermal ablation (RFA and EVLT) and surgery.[55] A common adverse event after sclerotherapy is superficial phlebitis. Superficial phlebitis can be uncomfortable for the patient but is rarely dangerous. Early drainage of trapped coagula using an 18-gauge needle or a number 11 blade may provide quick relief of discomfort and decrease the extent of hyperpigmentation following sclerotherapy.

Cutaneous necrosis can cause disfiguring scars. It can occur with any sclerosant, but is more common with hypertonic saline when compared with STS or POL.[56] Mechanisms of cutaneous necrosis include extravasation of contrast, and inadvertent injection into a small arteriole or arteriovenous fistula. Most ulcerations, fortunately, are small and will heal with appropriate wound care; however, large areas of necrosis may require advanced wound techniques to achieve healing.

Both hyperpigmentation and telangiectatic matting are cosmetically adverse events that can decrease patient satisfaction. Matting has the appearance of fine red or purple veins that occur over areas of treatment and can occur after sclerotherapy in 10%

to 30% of patients. Hyperpigmentation is common following sclerotherapy and will generally gradually lighten and improve over time. Spontaneous resolution will typically occur in 70% of patients by 6 months and 99% of patients by 1 year.[57] Conservative therapy with observation should be the first approach to the patient with hyperpigmentation after sclerotherapy. As with hyperpigmentation, patients should be reassured that resolution with time is typical.

In general, sclerotherapy is safe and well tolerated, and it is likely that the most common "adverse event" following treatment is failure to meet the patient's expectations in terms of cosmesis. One of the most important considerations in terms of patient satisfaction is educating patients in regards to realistic outcomes. Patients should be counseled that immediate improvement in appearance is not likely, and that improvement is usually gradual and incremental. Multiple treatment sessions, especially for telangiectasias, may be necessary for the patient to achieve their desired results. Preprocedural counseling should be thorough and include showing patients photographic examples of both ideal and nonideal outcomes.

Fortunately, serious complications from sclerotherapy are rare, and the more common adverse events will almost always improve over time. The most common "adverse event" with sclerotherapy is a failure of the treatment to live up to the patient's expectations. It is important that patients have a thorough understanding of the gradual and incremental improvements that are the norm with sclerotherapy. Multiple sclerotherapy sessions may be required to achieve a good result. Photographic examples of ideal as well as nonideal sclerotherapy outcomes can be helpful in educating patients in regards to realistic expectations.

SUMMARY

Sclerotherapy has diverse application in the treatment of cutaneous telangiectasias, superficial venous insufficiency, pelvic venous reflux, and venous malformations. It has an important role in the treatment of venous disease in all stages. It is an important tool for physicians treating venous disease, and familiarity with sclerotherapy indications, contraindications, and techniques is an important part of any vein practice.

REFERENCES

1. Rabe E, Guex JJ, Puskas A, et al, Coordinators VCP. Epidemiology of chronic venous disorders in geographically diverse populations: results from the Vein Consult Program. Int Angiol 2012;31:105–15.
2. Porter JM, Moneta GL. Reporting standards in venous disease: an update. International Consensus Committee on Chronic Venous Disease. J Vasc Surg 1995; 21(4):635–45.
3. Parlar B, Blazek C, Cazzaniga S, et al. Treatment of lower extremity telangiectasias in women by foam sclerotherapy vs. Nd:YAG laser: a prospective, comparative, randomized, open-label trial. J Eur Acad Dermatol Venereol 2015;29(3): 549–54.
4. Gibson K, Ferris B, Pepper D. Foam sclerotherapy for the treatment of superficial venous insufficiency. Surg Clin North Am 2007;87(5):1285–95.
5. Campos W, Torres I, da Silva E, et al. A prospective randomized study comparing polidocanol foam sclerotherapy with surgical treatment of patients with primary chronic venous insufficiency and ulcer. Ann Vasc Surg 2015;29(6):1128–35.
6. Masuda EM, Kessler DM, Lurie F, et al. The effect of ultrasound-guided sclerotherapy of incompetent perforator veins on venous clinical severity and disability scores. J Vasc Surg 2006;43(3):551–6.

7. Park HS, Do YS, Park KB, et al. Clinical outcome and predictors of treatment response in foam sodium tetradecyl sulfate sclerotherapy of venous malformations. Eur Radiol 2016;26(5):1301–10.

8. Pieri S, Agresti P, Morucci M, et al. Percutaneous treatment of pelvic congestion syndrome. Radiol Med 2003;105(1–2):76–82.

9. Rathbun S, Norris A, Morrison N, et al. Performance of the endovenous foam sclerotherapy in the USA. Phlebology 2012;27(2):59–66.

10. Orbach EJ. Sclerotherapy of varicose veins: utilization of an intravenous air block. Am J Surg 1944;66:362–6.

11. Cabrera Garrido JR, Cabrera Garcia-Olmedo JR, Garcia-Olmedo Dominguez MA. Elargissement des limites de la schlerotherapie: nouveaux produirs sclerosants. Phlebolgie 1997;50:181–8.

12. Monfreux A. Traitement sclerosant des troncs saphenies et leurs collaterals de gros caliber par le methode MUS. Phlebologie 1997;50:355–60.

13. Tessari L. Nouvelle technique d'obtention de la sclero-mousse. Phlebologie 2000; 53:129.

14. Varithena (prescribing information). Provensis LTD, a BTG International Group Company; 2013. Available at: https://www.btgplc.com/media/1266/varithena-media-fact-sheet-us-var-2013-0835-3.pdf.

15. Carugo D, Ankrett DN, O'Byrne V, et al. The role of clinically-relevant parameters on the cohesiveness of sclerosing foams in a biomimetic vein model. J Mater Sci Mater Med 2015;26(11):258.

16. Worthington-Kirsch R. Injection sclerotherapy. Semin Intervent Radiol 2005;22(3): 209–17.

17. Feied CF. Sclerosing solutions. In: Fronek H, editor. The fundamentals of phlebology, venous disease for clinicians. 2nd edition. American College of Phlebology; 2007. p. 23.

18. Parsi K, Exner T, Connor DE, et al. Lytic effects of detergent sclerosants on erytrocytes, platelets, endothelial cells and microparticles are attenuated by albumin and other plasma components in vitro. Eur J Vasc Endovasc Surg 2008;36(2): 216–32.

19. Peterson JD, Goldman MP, Weiss RA, et al. Treatment of reticular and telangectatic leg veins: double-blind prospective randomized comparative trial of polidocanol and hypertonic saline. Dermatol Surg 2012;38(8):1322–30.

20. Patel SB, Ostler AE, Dos Santos SJ, et al. Effects of environmental and compositional manipulation on the longevity of Tessari-made foam for sclerotherapy. J Vasc Surg Venous Lymphat Disord 2015;3(3):312–8.

21. Carugo D, Ankrett DN, Zhao X, et al. Benefits of Polidocanol endovenous microfoam (Varithena®) compared with physician-compounded foams. Phlebology 2016;31(4):283–95.

22. Hamel-Desnos C, Desnos P, Wollmann JC, et al. Evaluation of the efficacy of polidocanol in the form of foam compared with liquid form in sclerotherapy of the greater saphenous vein: initial results. Dermatol Surg 2003;29(12):1170–5.

23. Bergan J, Pascarella L, Mekenas L. Venous disorders: treatment with sclerosant foam. J Cardiovasc Surg 2006;47(1):9–18.

24. Darke SG, Baker SJ. Ultrasound-guided foam sclerotherapy for the treatment of varicose veins. Br J Surg 2006;68(2):182–3.

25. Darvall KA, Bae GR, Adam DJ, et al. Duplex ultrasound outcomes following ultrasound-guided foam sclerotherapy of symptomatic recurrent great saphenous varicose veins. Eur J Vasc Endovasc Surg 2011;42(1):107–14.

26. Blaise S, Bosson JL, Diamond JL. Ultrasound-guided sclerotherapy of the great saphenous vein with 1% vs. 3% polidocanol foam: a multicentre double-blind randomised trial with 3-year follow-up. Eur J Vasc Endovasc Surg 2010;39(6): 779–86.

27. Gonzalez-Zeh R, Armisen R, Barahona S. Endovenous laser and echo-guided foam ablation in great saphenous vein reflux: one-year follow-up results. J Vasc Surg 2008;48(4):940–6.

28. Rasmussen L, Lawaetz M, Serup J, et al. Randomized clinical trial comparing endovenous laser ablation, radiofrequency ablation, foam sclerotherapy, and surgical stripping for great saphenous varicose veins with 3-year follow-up. J Vasc Surg Venous Lymphat Disord 2013;1(4):349–56.

29. van der Velden SK, Biemans AA, De Maeseneer M, et al. Five-year results of a randomized clinical trial of conventional surgery, endovenous laser ablation and ultrasound-guided foam sclerotherapy in patients with great saphenous varicose veins. Br J Surg 2015;102(10):1184–94.

30. Bush RG, Derrick M, Manjoney D. Major neurological events following foam sclerotherapy. Phlebology 2008;23(4):189–92.

31. Forlee MV, Grouden M, Moore DJ, et al. Stroke after varicose vein foam injection sclerotherapy. J Vasc Surg 2006;43(1):162–4.

32. Hahn M, Schultz T, Jünger M. Late stroke after foam sclerotherapy. Vasa 2010; 39(1):108–10.

33. Leslie-Mazwi TM, Avery LL, Sims JR. Intra-arterial air thrombogenesis after cerebral air embolism complicating lower extremity sclerotherapy. Neurocrit Care 2009;11(2):247–50.

34. Morrison N, Neuhardt DL, Rogers CR. Comparisons of side effects using air and carbon dioxide foam for endovenous chemical ablation. J Vasc Surg 2008;47(4): 830–6.

35. Wong M. Should foam made with physiologic gases be the standard in sclerotherapy? Phlebology 2015;30(9):580–6.

36. Wright D, Gibson K, Barclay J, et al. High prevalence of right-to-left shunt in patients with symptomatic great saphenous vein incompetence and varicose veins. J Vasc Surg 2010;51(1):104–7.

37. Regan JD, Gibson KD, Rush JE, et al. Clinical significance of cerebrovascular gas emboli during polidocanol endovenous ultra-low nitrogen microfoam ablation and correlation with magnetic resonance imaging in patients with right-to-left shunt. J Vasc Surg 2011;53(1):131–7.

38. FDA access data in: Available at: http://www.accessdata.fda.gov/drugsatfda_docs/nda/2013/205098Orig1s000SumR.pdf. Accessed November 28, 2017.

39. King JT, O'Byrne M, Vasquez M, et al, the VANISH-1 Investigator Group. Treatment of truncal incompetence and varicose veins with single administration of a new polidocanol endovenous microfoam preparation improves symptoms and appearance. Eur J Vasc Endovasc Surg 2015;50(6):784–93.

40. Todd KL III, Wright DI, the VANISH-2 Investigator Group. The VANISH-2 study: a randomized, blinded, multicenter study to evaluate the efficacy and safety of polidocanol endovenous microfoam 0.5% and 1.0% compared with placebo for the treatment of saphenofemoral junction incompetence. Phlebology 2014;29(9): 608–18.

41. Todd KL, Wright D, Orfe E. The durability of polidocanol endovenous microfoam treatment effect on varicose vein symptoms and appearance in patients with saphenofemoral junction incompetence: one-year results from the VANISH-2 study. J Vasc Surg Venous Lymphat Disord 2014;2(1):112.

42. Green D. Persistent post-sclerotherapy pigmentation due to minocycline. Three cases and a review of post sclerotherapy pigmentation. J Cosmet Dermatol 2002;1(4):173–82.
43. Feied CF, Jackson JJ, Bren TS, et al. Allergic reactions to polidocanol for vein sclerosis. Two case reports. J Dermatol Surg Oncol 1994;20(7):466–8.
44. Bzoza Z, Kasperska-Zajac A, Rogala E, et al. Anaphylactoid reaction after the use of sodium tetradecyl sulfate: a case report. Angiology 2007;58(5):644–6.
45. Sarvananthan T, Shepherd AC, Willenberg T, et al. Neurological complication of sclerotherapy for varicose veins. J Vasc Surg 2012;55(1):243–51.
46. Kern P, Ramelet AA, Wutschert R, et al. Compression after sclerotherapy for tel-angiectasias and reticular leg veins: a randomized controlled study. J Vasc Surg 2007;45(6):1212–6.
47. Kulkarni SR, Slim FJ, Emerson LG, et al. Effect of foam sclerotherapy on healing and long-term recurrence in chronic venous leg ulcers. Phlebology 2013;28(3): 140–6.
48. Gloviczki P, Comerta A, Dalsing M, et al. The care of patients with varicose veins and associated chronic venous diseases: guidelines of the Society for Vascular Surgery and the American Venous Forum. J Vasc Surg 2011;53(5 Suppl):2S–48S.
49. Whiteley AM, Taylor DC, Dos Santos SJ, et al. Pelvic venous reflux is a major contributory cause of recurrent varicose veins in more than a quarter of women. J Vasc Surg Venous Lymphat Disord 2014;2(4):411–5.
50. Daniels JP, Champaneria R, Shah L, et al. Effectiveness of embolization or sclero-therapy of pelvic veins for reducing chronic pelvic pain: a systematic review. J Vasc Interv Radiol 2016;27(10):1478–86.
51. Qui Y, Chen H, Lin X, et al. Outcomes and complications of sclerotherapy for venous malformations. Vasc Endovascular Surg 2013;47(6):454–61.
52. Varithena® instructions for use: Available at: http://varithena.com/Portals/VarithenaHCP/assets/Varithena_Instructions_for_Use.pdf.
53. Willenburg T, Smith PC, Shepherd A, et al. Visual disturbance following sclero-therapy for varicose veins, reticular veins and telangiectasias: a systematic liter-ature review. Phlebology 2013;28(3):123–31.
54. Frullini A, Felice F, Burchielli S, et al. High production of endothelin after foam sclerotherapy: a new pathogenetic hypothesis for neurological and visual distur-bances after sclerotherapy. Phlebology 2011;26(5):203–8.
55. O'Donnell TF, Eaddy M, Raju A, et al. Assessment of thrombotic adverse events and treatment patterns associated with varicose vein treatment. J Vasc Surg Venous Lymphat Disord 2015;3(1):27–35.
56. Goldman MP, Sadick NS, Weiss RA. Cutaneous necrosis, telangiectatic matting, and hyperpigmentation following sclerotherapy: etiology, prevention, and treat-ment. Dermatol Surg 1995;21(1):19–29.
57. Davis LT, Duffy DM. Determination of incidence and risk factors for postsclero-therapy telangiectatic matting of the lower extremity: a retrospective analysis. J Dermatol Surg Oncol 1990;16(4):327–30.

Moving?

Make sure your subscription moves with you!

To notify us of your new address, find your **Clinics Account Number** (located on your mailing label above your name), and contact customer service at:

Email: journalscustomerservice-usa@elsevier.com

800-654-2452 (subscribers in the U.S. & Canada)
314-447-8871 (subscribers outside of the U.S. & Canada)

Fax number: 314-447-8029

Elsevier Health Sciences Division
Subscription Customer Service
3251 Riverport Lane
Maryland Heights, MO 63043

*To ensure uninterrupted delivery of your subscription, please notify us at least 4 weeks in advance of move.

Printed and bound by CPI Group (UK) Ltd, Croydon, CR0 4YY

03/10/2024

01040398-0008